made INCREDIBLY

Children & Young People's Nursing

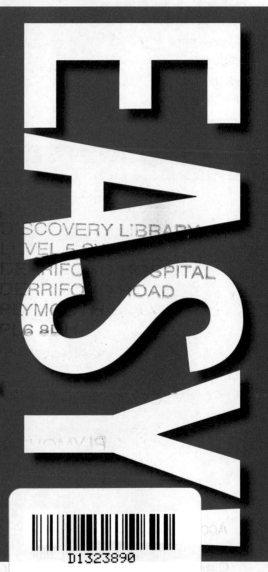

Adapted for the UK by

Patric Devitt, RSCN, RGN, BA (hons), MSC

Senior Lecturer, in Children and Young
  People's Nursing
School of Nursing and Midwifery
University of Salford

and

John Thain, BSc, MSc, PGCEd, RGN, RSCN

Senior Lecturer in Children's Nursing
School of Health and Wellbeing
University of Wolverhampton

First UK Edition

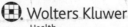

D1323890

Wolters Kluwer | Lippincott Williams & Wilkins
Health

Philadelphia · Baltimore · New York · London
Buenos Aires · Hong Kong · Sydney · Tokyo

Staff

Acquisitions Editor
Rachel Hendrick

Academic Marketing Executive
Alison Major

Production Editor
Kevin Johnson

Proofreader
Helena Engstrand

Illustrator
Bot Roda

Text and Cover Design
Designers Collective

For information, write to Lippincott Williams & Wilkins, 250 Waterloo Road, London SE1 8RD

British Library Cataloging-in-Publication Data. A catalogue record for this book is available from the British Library
ISBN-13: 978-1-901831-09-2
ISBN-10: 1-901831-09-4

Contents

Acknowledgements

Reviewers of the UK edition

Cheryl Clarke, RNC, BSc, MSc, PGCE High Ed.
Lecturer Practitioner for Advanced Practice Acute and Critical Care, Critical Care, Alder Hey Children's Hospital, Faculty of Health and Applied Social Science, Liverpool John Moores University

Wendy Dubbin, MSc, PG Dip (Teaching and Learning), BSc (Hons), RSCH, RGN
Course Director/Lecturer Children's Nursing, School of Nursing and Midwifery, University of East Anglia

Liz Gormley-Fleming, MA, PG Dip HE, RNT BSc (Hons), RGN, RSCN
Senior Lecturer, Nursing, Midwifery & Social Work, University of Hertfordshire

Fiona Horrox, RSCN RGN BSc (HONS) MSc, PGCHEPR, ENB 415, 998
Senior Lecturer Children's Nursing/Lead Clinical Skills & Simulation, Department of Children's nursing, Faculty of Health & Social Care, London South Bank University

Teresa Hughes RGN, RN Child, BSc(Hons), PGCE(A) MSc Psych
Child Health Tutor, Division of Health and Social Care, University of Surrey

Honor Nicholl, PhD, MEd, BSc, RCN
Lecturer/Head of Discipline Children's Nursing, School of Nursing and Midwifery, University of Dublin, Trinity College

Maxine Pryce-Miller, MA Ed, PGDip, PGCE, BSc (Hons), RSCN Rgn
Senior Lecturer-Child Health, School of Health & Well Being, University of Wolverhampton

Foreword

Certain words have the power to wreak havoc in the nurse's mind: research, evidence-based practice, theoretical underpinnings … all the concepts that form the foundation of nursing care for children, young people and their families. However, making such concepts usable in daily nursing practice can be quite challenging.

That's where Children's and Young People's Nursing Made Incredibly Easy! comes in. Research has shown that we absorb core knowledge when the material is meaningful, easily understood, and fun to learn. The editors of this book have found a way to put the important information in an easy-to-read format, with humorous artwork, checklists, and illustrations to aid the reader.

While some nurses choose to work in children's nursing, others have to assume these responsibilities on an occasional basis. Children's and Young People's Nursing Made Incredibly Easy! provides a unique, concise point of reference that answers your critical questions even if you only have time for a quick review.

You'll find more than 100 of the most commonly encountered childhood problems presented in an organised format. Chapters include concepts in pediatric nursing care; infancy; early childhood; middle childhood and adolescence; communicable and infectious diseases; and neurologic, cardiovascular, respiratory, urinary, musculoskeletal, GI, endocrine and metabolic, hematologic and immunologic, and dermatologic problems.

This informative reference assists the nurse in dealing with situations unique to children's nursing care - psychosocial structures of families, common milestones in development, childhood hospitalisations and terminal illnesses, and dosage calculations and techniques for administering medications to children.

Children's and Young People's Nursing Made Incredibly Easy! is loaded with useful features. Colour illustrations of the pathophysiology of paediatric disorders help you visualise how patients are affected. Memory joggers offer simple tricks to help you remember key information.

In addition, icons draw your attention to important issues:

Advice from the experts – presents tips for children's nurses from the professionals

It's all relative – offers teaching topics for children and their families to promote wellness

 Growing pains – provides age and stage descriptions, expectations, and dangers

 Cultured pearls – identifies unique aspects of care by cultural group.

This book is a valuable resource for students, for those returning to the health care field, and for novice and experienced nurses. The research, evidence, and theory are so well integrated, you won't even know how much you've learned until you test your knowledge with the Quick quiz at the end of each chapter. Then you'll realise just how much material applies to your practice – and how much you and your patients of all ages will benefit!

Patric Devitt, RSCN, RGN, BA (hons), MSC
Senior Lecturer, in Children and Young
   People's Nursing
School of Nursing and Midwifery
University of Salford

and

John Thain, BSc, MSc, PGCEd, RGN, RSCN
Senior Lecturer in Children's Nursing
School of Health and Wellbeing
University of Wolverhampton

Contributors and consultants to the US edition

Peggy D. Baikie, RNC, MS, PNP, NNP
Clinical Coordinator, Lake School Based
    Clinic
St. Anthony's Hospitals
Denver
Adjunct Professor
Metropolitan State College of Denver

J. Mari Beth Barr, RN, BC, MSN, PhD
Associate Professor of Nursing
Missouri Southern State University
Joplin

Vera C. Brancato, RN, BC, MSN, EdD
Associate Professor of Nursing
Kutztown (PA) University

Gloria Clocklin, RN, EdD, PNP, FNP
Professor of Nursing
Northern Michigan University
Marquette

Marsha L. Conroy, RN, BA, MSN, APN
Nursing Educator
Cuyahoga Community College
Cleveland
Kent (OH) State University

Sherrill Anne Conroy, RN, BN, MEd, DPhil
Assistant Professor, Faculty of Nursing
University of Alberta
Edmonton, Canada

Vera V. Cull, RN, DSN
Assistant Professor, Coordinator of Child
    Heath Course
University of Alabama at Birmingham
School of Nursing

Doreen S. DeAngelis, RN, MSN
Associate Professor
Community College of Allegheny County,
    South Campus
West Mifflin, PA

Cheryl L. DeGraw, RN, MSN, CRNP
Instructor
Florence-Darlington Technical College
Florence, SC

Michelle Johnson, RN, MSN
Assistant Professor
Northern Michigan University
Marquette

Vicki Clarkson Keller, RN, MSN, PhD(c)
Assistant Professor
Ball State University School of Nursing
Muncie, IN

Geeta Maharaj, APRN, MSN, CPNP
Assistant Professor (Clinical)
University of Utah College of Nursing
Salt Lake City

Kristie Nix, RN, EdD
Associate Professor and Faculty-in-
    Residence
The University of Tulsa (OK)

Georgia McCoy O'Neal, RN, MSN
Instructor in Nursing
Jefferson State Community College
Birmingham, AL

Sondra L. Raubacher, RNC, MSN, CPNP, APNP
PNP Coordinator
Faculty Women Neonates & Children
    Program
Wayne State University
Detroit

Linda F. Samson, RN, BC, PhD, CNAA, BC
Dean, College of Health Professions
University Professor of Nursing
Governors State University
University Park, IL

Shelia Savell, RN, MSN
Clinical Instructor
University of Arkansas for Medical
    Sciences
College of Nursing
Little Rock

Martha M.Z. Shemin, RN, BSN, MS
Nursing Instructor & Facilitator, Parent/
    Child Health Nursing Course
Holy Name Hospital School of Nursing
Teaneck, NJ

Ralph Vogel, RN, PhD, CPNP
Clinical Assistant Professor
Pediatric Specialty Coordinator
University of Arkansas for Medical
    Sciences
College of Nursing
Little Rock

Julee Waldrop, RN, MS, FNP, PNP
Clinical Assistant Professor
School of Nursing
University of North Carolina
Chapel Hill

Karen Wilkinson, RN, MN, ARNP
Pediatric Nurse Practitioner, Pain
    Management Program
Children's Hospital and Regional Medical
    Center

① Introduction to nursing children

Just the facts

In this chapter, you'll learn about:

♦ the role of the children's and young people's nurse

♦ the philosophy of family-centred care

♦ types of family structures

♦ sociocultural influences that affect children's health.

Role of the children's and young people's nurse

In this chapter, we will discuss children's and young people's nursing and nurses, but for ease the term 'CYP nurse' will be used throughout. Children's and young people's nursing involves providing care for infants, children and young people on a continuum from health to illness through recovery and, when needed, rehabilitation. Care and interventions now take place in various settings from hospitals to prisons and so CYP nurses have to respond to a range of differing needs in differing environments.

However, providing care doesn't stop with the child; CYP nurses should ensure that parents and other family members, where appropriate, are included in planning and delivering the child's care. This approach is known as family-centred care.

In providing care, nurses will work very closely with colleagues in health as well as in social care, education and voluntary sector. This is particularly so when working together to safeguard children.

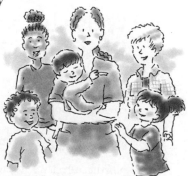

Children's nursing includes babies and teens and everyone in between!

Being in the know

When providing care and interventions for children and families, all CYP nurses must fulfil their professional responsibilities, so the following are crucial sources of information/policy for practising effectively and within one's sphere of competence:

Nursing and Midwifery Council

This is the regulatory body under which all nurses practise and is specifically concerned with protecting the public. It sets standards and provides guidelines which inform professional practice which all nurses are expected to follow particularly The code: standards of conduct, performance and ethics for nurses and midwives (NMC, 2008). Student nurses are also required to adhere to professional conduct requirements identified in the 'Guidance on professional conduct for nursing and midwifery students' (NMC, 2009), although they are supervised by a registered practitioner.

Department of Health and Department for Education

The governmental bodies regulate health care and latterly policies for children and young people in England and Wales. These are jointly responsible for developing guidelines and policies on a range of issues affecting children and, in particular, health and safeguarding.

Scottish government (Riaghaltas na h-Alba)

Scotland has a devolved government which sets out it's own policies and guidelines for the well-being and health of children and young people in the country. Scottish law also differs and this will impact on the way children and families are supported and cared for.

Welsh assembly government (Llywodraeth Cynulliad Cymru)

Wales has a devolved government which sets out it's own policies and guidelines for the well-being and health of children and young people in the country although the UK government still has overall powers in some areas.

Northern Ireland government

Northern Ireland also has a devolved government which sets out it's own policies and guidelines for the well-being and health of children and young people in the country although the UK government still has overall powers in some areas.

NHS National Institute for Health and Clinical Excellence

NIHCE is concerned with providing guidance on a range of health, medical and other interventions whilst also promoting good health and preventing and treating ill health.

Scottish Intercollegiate Guidelines Network

The network publishes evidenced-based guidelines specifically for NHS Scotland but these are equally applicable in other parts of the UK.

Royal College of Nursing

This is a professional organisation and union which represents nurses and provides valuable resources, guidance and advice on a wide range of issues which affect nurses and nursing care. It works closely with many other organisations and, in particular, the Royal College of Paediatrics and Child Health to produce joint nursing and medical guidance.

British National Formulary for Children

This is a publication which brings together information and provides guidelines on medicines used in childhood. This document should be referred to when checking any medications, dosages or for other information when giving medication to children.

Contact a Family

This is a charitable organisation which provides information, advice and support to families with a disabled child. The Contact a Family Directory provides information on many condition and disease-specific support organisations, so it is often a starting point to finding out more.

All of the above are part of the nurse's armoury and so you should refer to them regularly to identify contemporary guidance, evidence and policy which determine your practice. Don't forget that parents and children also have access to them!

Standards of care

It has been recognised since the Platt report (MoH, 1959) that children are not mini adults and as such need to be cared for in an age and developmentally appropriate way. The report had many implications for nursing children, e.g. a move towards sick children being looked after at home and the relaxed visiting arrangements on children's wards. One of the major things was the recognition that those providing nursing care for children must be specifically educated to undertake this role. This has been reinforced by national reports, enquiries and the Nursing and Midwifery Council. Now the UK is one of the very few countries that educate CYP nurses as a primary qualification. It is these people who can ensure the continued high standard of care for children whether sick or well at hospital or in the community.

Policy framework

The care of children takes place within an increasingly complex framework, especially as the different governments within the UK pass their own legislation. You must get to know the policy that governs where you work. The National Service Framework (NSF) for Children, Families and Maternity Services (DH, 2004) provides the framework for care in the health service in England and Wales and provides a set of standards for delivering high-quality care. Wales has it's own version published in 2005 and in Scotland the action framework 'Delivering a Healthy Future' is similarly facilitating the development of services.

The NSF is a component of Every Child Matters which contains core concepts relevant to every children's nurse (See *What Every Child Matters actually means*) and establishes a set of outcomes that all children should achieve. These outcomes can be used in various situations in order that professionals and organisations can work together to enable children's health and development. At the time of writing, a new government is in place and the continuation of such policies is being debated, so nurses should keep abreast of health-related news.

Family-centred care

Essential to caring for children is the principle that nurses, parents and the child negotiate care and how it is provided. In family-centred care, the family's input should be the major driving force behind the development of the child's care plan. Family-centred care recognises that parents or those in a parenting capacity are usually the constant in a child's life and are generally considered experts in the care of their child. As such, interventions are geared towards respecting, supporting and encouraging the family's ability to provide care to their child throughout illness, recovery or for specified needs.

All of these activities will be based on the family and the child's ability to participate; however, the nurse must be aware of inadvertently placing too

What Every Child Matters actually means

Outcomes	Aims	Support
Be healthy	• Physically healthy • Mentally and emotionally healthy • Sexually healthy • Healthy life styles • Choose not to take illegal drugs	Parents, carers and families promote healthy choices
Stay safe	• Safe from maltreatment, neglect, violence and sexual exploitation • Safe from accidental injury and death • Safe from bullying and discrimination • Safe from crime and anti-social behaviour • Have security, stability and are cared for	Parents, carers and families provide safe homes and stability
Enjoy and achieve	• Ready for school • Attend and enjoy school • Achieve stretching national educational standards at primary school • Achieve personal and social development and enjoy recreation • Achieve stretching national educational standards at secondary school	Parents, carers and families support learning
Make a positive contribution	• Engage in decision making and support the community and environment • Engage in law-abiding and positive behaviour in and out of school • Develop positive relationships and choose not to bully or discriminate • Develop self-confidence and successfully deal with significant life changes and challenges • Develop enterprising behaviour	Parents, carers and families promote positive behaviour
Achieve economic well-being	• Engage in further education, employment or training on leaving school • Ready for employment • Live in decent homes and sustainable communities • Access to transport and material goods • Live in households free from low income	Parents, carers and families are supported to be economically active

HM Government. *Every Child Matters: Change for Children*. London: Department for Education and Skills, 2004.

Benefits of family-centred care

Family-centred care benefits the child and the family as well as the health care professional.

Benefits to families

- Less stress and heightened feelings of confidence and competence in caring for their children
- Less dependence on professional caregivers
- Empowerment to develop new skills and expertise in the care of their children
- Child is more settled as it continues family relationships

Benefits to health care professionals

- Greater job satisfaction
- Empowerment to develop new skills and expertise in children's nursing

---

much responsibility on them. The ability of the child or the young person to participate will vary and so nurses will need to use various skills to facilitate his or her involvement. Over time, it is expected that young people will be more responsible and knowledgeable about their needs and nurses will work with them in partnership to manage their needs and to assist them with the transition to adult services.

It is important when practising family-centred care to recognise that families are diverse and in some the child or the young person might be a carer or even a parent. Practising family-centred care means being observant and responsive to the real needs of the family!

Power to the people

Empowering and enabling are two important concepts in family-centred care. Empowering is allowing parents/carers to maintain, or helping them to develop, a sense of control over their child's care. Enabling refers to the practices that help family members to acquire the new skills necessary to meet the needs of their child.

These two concepts foster the teamwork between the family and the health care professionals that serves to benefit the child, both physically and emotionally. (See *Benefits of family-centred care*.)

A closer look at the family

Family is defined as the structure, or the relationship between individuals, that provides the financial and emotional support needed for social functioning. Individuals don't have to have blood relationships in order to be a family. Many different family structures exist in our society which is now multicultural and so each type of family may provide a unique set of challenges to the nurses who care for their children.

Nuclear family

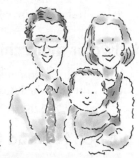

A nuclear family (also known as a 'traditional family') consists of a husband, a wife and their child or children (biological or adopted). The nuclear family was the most common type of family in previous years, but it's becoming less common with the rise in divorce rates, single parenthood and alternative lifestyles.

The nuclear family serves as a support system for its members who share roles and responsibilities as well as financial obligations. One disadvantage of some nuclear families is the absence of additional support that may be needed in times of crisis.

Extended family

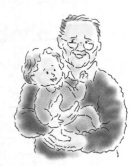

An extended family (also called a 'multigenerational family') includes at least one parent, a child or children and any combination of grandparents, aunts, uncles or cousins. In this type of family, the family group provides the support although this should not be assumed. This type of family is becoming less common as geographical mobility increases.

Single-parent family

A Single-parent family is composed of one parent living at home with a child or children. Because of such factors as the rise in divorce rates, the single-parent family is becoming more common. In a single-parent family, the parent and the child are each other's source of support. This can create close bonds but can also lead to strain for the single parent in terms of the parental role he or she plays. If a child becomes ill, childcare difficulties may arise. There may also be financial constraints related to limited income. Issues may also arise concerning an absent parent's rights to be informed or consulted about a child's care.

Being a single parent can be rewarding – and exhausting!

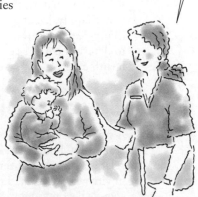

... and ready for a nap

The single parent can become exhausted from being responsible for all of the tasks involved in raising children and particularly if they have extra medical or nursing needs. Single parenting can also lead to low self-esteem, as the parent tries, and sometimes fails, to provide everything for the child that some two-parent families are able to provide.

Blended family

A blended family consists of a father with a child or children from a previous relationship and a mother with a child or children from a previous relationship, who marry and live together.

Add two or more children, mix well …

A blended family provides emotional support and allows for shared roles within the household. It also provides the opportunity for the family members to learn how to work together and discover new ways of accomplishing tasks.

… but don't spread too thin

Financial responsibilities can be shared but can also produce strain if support must be provided to the previous spouse or children of either adult, or both.

Cohabitation family

A cohabitation family is one in which a man, a woman and a child or children live together as a nuclear family while the man and the woman remain unmarried. In the past, this type of relationship tended to be viewed as temporary but, with increased societal acceptance, more relationships of this type are lasting for longer periods.

This type of family provides emotional and financial support to its members. However, the risk exists that one individual may feel threatened by the partner's real or perceived lack of commitment.

Foster family

A foster family is designed to care for a child whose biological or adoptive family can't do so. Ideally, foster care is provided on a temporary basis until the biological or adoptive family can resume its role.

Unfortunately, the foster child may be shuffled from foster family to foster family, lacking the stability that comes from being with the same family (biological, adoptive or foster) for an extended period. It can also be difficult to determine who's responsible for making decisions about the foster child's health care.

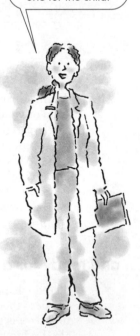

Foster care is based on the idea that the foster home will be a temporary one for the child.

Gay or lesbian family

A gay or lesbian family consists of same-sex adults and a child or children. Children in this type of family come from previous heterosexual relationships, have been adopted or are the product of surrogate mothers or in vitro fertilisation. The number of gay and lesbian families is increasing as society becomes more accepting of same-sex relationships.

Transient or the no family...

Some children and young people are homeless, living off the streets and may be exposed to a range of risks and dangers. They come into contact with services on and off and often their families are fellow homeless people.

The don't know family

The UK has seen an increase in the number of children, who may have no identifiable family, such as those who are seeking asylum and victims of human trafficking and sex trade. Their only support may have been the people around them and so they have no specific family.

In all these family structures, concerns may arise about identifying who is the legally responsible individual for issues such as consent and ongoing care. In addition, the nurse will need to consider the needs of those children who are in the care of the local authority be that through fostering, children's services or in secure accommodation.

Sociocultural influences on children's health

Sociocultural influences on children's health include:
- ethnicity
- socioeconomic factors
- religion
- school
- peers
- the family's health-related beliefs and practices.

Ethnicity

Ethnicity refers to belonging to or believing in a group with customs, languages and characteristics that differ from those in other sections of society. The UK is an ethnically diverse country. The children's nurse must be aware that different ethnic groups tend to view health, illness and health care differently although this mustn't be assumed!

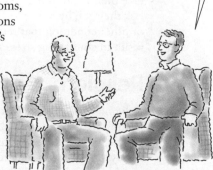

My family doesn't make decisions without me. In my ethnic group, what the man says, goes.

Father knows best

In some ethnic groups, the adult male is the decision maker. When a child is brought in for treatment, no decisions can be made until he arrives.

Grin and bear it

Other ethnic groups believe that pain shouldn't be shown. Children from these ethnic groups may be up and walking or conversing, or may appear stoic, despite being in pain. This can make it difficult for the nurse to assess, or even detect, pain.

Watch what you eat

Diet is another area in which ethnic influence can be strong. For instance, meat products may need to be prepared in line with religious beliefs. The CYP nurse should undertake a thorough dietary/nutritional assessment relating to the family's beliefs in order to respond to their specific cultural needs. (See *Putting cultural care into practice*.) Bear in mind that dietary requirements may vary not only with cultural but also with religious and social practices such as vegetarianism.

Socioeconomic factors

Socioeconomic influences on children's health can result from income levels which may be low or may be about how much is spent or is not spent on appropriate things, e.g. when parents misuse alcohol. Poverty is the lack of money or resources necessary for survival. Whilst health care is free within the UK, the level of family income and where a child lives both within the country and within a region have a major impact upon a child's expected health.

Calling in sick

Another area of concern arises when both parents work, as is common in today's economy. One or both parents may not be able to afford to take time off from work to take their child to the General Practitioner's surgery or hospital, or they may risk their job by doing so. This is particularly so when the child has a chronic or other condition that requires frequent hospital stays or visits and this can result in continuing stress for the family.

Religion

Religious beliefs can affect when, where and even if an individual will seek health care. Because religious beliefs guide health care practices for many people, the CYP nurse must be aware of what beliefs the individual, and family, holds and should help ensure that these needs are met in a way that provides the child with the care needed.

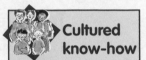

Cultured know-how

Putting culturally sensitive care into practice

Awareness and knowledge are the first steps towards incorporating culturally sensitive care into your daily nursing practice. To facilitate your care, develop your own cultural reference folder that could include

- brief descriptions of pertinent cultures
- views on health, illness, diet and other matters
- lists of interpreters, ethnic community services and other sources for quick reference

School

School typically provides the child with his or her first exposure to the concept of right and wrong, or moral values. School commonly helps children learn rules and regulations and introduces them to the concept of an authority figure.

School is a powerful influence on children's lives and can be very positive in terms of developing confidence, awareness and a good support mechanism. On the other hand, children can be exposed to negative experiences such as bullying, intimidation and racism.

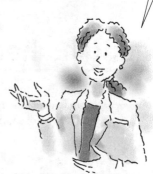

When both parents work because of socioeconomic reasons, they find it hard to take time off for their child's illness.

Peer influences

Peer relationships are the relationships a child has with other individuals in the same age group. A child's ability to be part of a peer group is influenced by his or her having the same beliefs or attitudes as the others in their group.

A child may try to change his or her beliefs or behaviours to feel a part of the group or the norm. He or she may partake in behaviours that risk his or her health to conform to the group. For example, a child's experimentation with smoking, drinking alcohol or using drugs can be heavily influenced by the behaviours of his or her peers.

Health-related beliefs and practices

Health-related beliefs and practices of the family have a strong influence on how often they will seek health care for their child. If family members hesitate to seek health care for themselves, they may not seek health care for their child until they become seriously ill, although this may be viewed with some concern as it is expected that parents act responsibly.

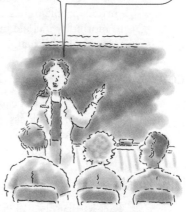

A bad experience at school can lead to more than detention. It can make children fear hospitals, too.

Once bitten

Sometimes, a family's health-related beliefs and practices are based on previous experiences with health care services and professionals. Negative experiences can make family members reluctant to seek health care for themselves and for their child.

These experiences may include:
- real or perceived poor quality of care
- real or perceived insensitivity of health care professionals
- physical or emotional pain or trauma
- death of a family member in hospital.

The CYP nurse can help to make a family's health-related beliefs more positive by
- asking family members about their health care experiences and acknowledging their concerns
- stressing the ways the current situation differs from past situations
- encouraging family members to participate actively in their child's health care and praising them for the care they're already providing.

Changing health patterns

Advances in medicine, technology and health care more broadly as well as better nutrition and environmental health have led to major changes in the lives of children, morbidity and mortality rates.

Childhood morbidity

Morbidity is defined as the number of people in a population who are faced with a specific health problem at a particular point of time.

Morbidity rates for many illnesses that previously caused severe problems for children, such as poliomyelitis and measles, have been dramatically reduced through immunisations. However, success in preventing children dying from specific conditions has meant that they may have to live with chronic problems, e.g. cystic fibrosis. Other conditions studied in relation to morbidity include injuries, acute illness, human immunodeficiency virus infection and sexually transmitted diseases.

Acute isn't cute

The most common causes of acute ill health in childhood include:
- respiratory illness
- injuries
- infections other than respiratory.

Risky business

Factors that place children at risk for increased morbidity include:
- chronic illness
- obesity
- homelessness or poor living conditions
- prematurity
- low birth weight
- poverty
- adoption from a foreign country.

Childhood mortality

Mortality refers to the number of deaths from a specific cause in a given year. Accidents are the leading cause of death in all age groups of children (older than age 1) in the UK. The most recent figures show a death rate of 15 deaths per 100,000 children (ONS, 2010). Infant mortality rates are the number of infant deaths during the first year of life per 1,000 live births. Whilst infant mortality rates have decreased dramatically in the UK, the nation still lags behind other developed countries that have even lower infant mortality rates. The most recent figures show that there were 4.85 deaths per 1,000 children, with more than two-thirds occurring in the first 28 days of life (ONS, 2010). The majority of these are directly linked to a lack of development as a result of premature birth or congenital defects.

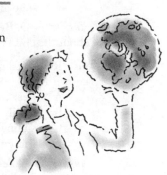

Quick quiz

1. The phrase infant mortality rates refers to the:
   A. number of children faced with any given health problem.
   B. number of infant deaths in any given year.
   C. nutritional health of a population of infants.
   D. socioeconomic status of a population of infants.

Answer: B. Infant mortality rates refer to the number of infant deaths per 1,000 live births in any given year.

2. A child is admitted for surgery. On your admission assessment, the mother tells you that her family is composed of herself, the patient (her daughter), her new husband and her stepson. What type of family is this?
   A. Nuclear family
   B. Cohabitation family
   C. Blended family
   D. Foster family

Answer: C. A family composed of a mother with children from a previous relationship who marries a father with children from a previous relationship is called a blended family.

3. A 5-year-old child is in the hospital following an appendicectomy. He is recovering well and doesn't appear to be in pain; however, analgesia is given initially as children do not always verbalise their discomfort. The mother states that he is fine and doesn't need painkillers! Which action is the nurse's best response?
   A. Explain to the mother that such analgesia is needed after surgery and it has been prescribed.
   B. Respect the mother's wishes and do not give the analgesia.

C.   State that you will ask a medical practitioner to discuss this with her.
D.   Review with the mother how the child feels pain and how she can help and work together.

Answer: D. By allowing the mother to participate in making decisions about the child's care, the nurse is fostering family-centred care.

4.   Relationships that a child has with others in their age group are known as:
A.   peer relationships.
B.   family relationships.
C.   sibling relationships.
D.   caregiver relationships.

Answer: A. Peers are those of a person's own age group. Peers can heavily influence the behaviour of a children as they attempt to conform to the norms of the group.

Scoring

☆☆☆   If you answered all four items correctly, congratulations! Your introduction to CYP nursing is empowering.

☆☆   If you answered three items correctly, good work! Tell your peers that you have are beginning to understand children and young people's nursing.

☆   If you answered fewer than three items correctly, don't get morbid! You have 14 more chapters to create a positive CYP nursing experience.

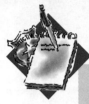

Issues in children and young people's nursing care

2

Just the facts

In this chapter, you'll learn:

♦ factors influencing growth and development

♦ methods of preparing and administering medications to children

♦ how to assess and manage pain in the child

♦ needs of the hospitalised and the child with special needs

Principles of growth and development

Growth and development occur throughout the lifespan. Growth implies an increase in size, such as height and weight. Development refers to the acquisition of skills and abilities that takes place throughout life. (See *Patterns of development*, page 16.)

Growth and development are essential parts of the nursing assessment of children. Problems that may initially seem insignificant might actually have severe consequences in later life if not dealt with early.

Stages of development

There are five stages of development during childhood:

Infancy is the period from birth to 1 year of age.

The toddler stage is the period from 1 to 3 years of age.

The preschool stage lasts from 3 to 5 years of age.

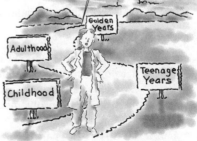

Whether you're 5 or 50, growth and development continue to occur.

Patterns of development

This chart shows the patterns of development and their progression and gives examples of each.

Pattern	Path of progression	Examples
Cephalocaudal	From head to toe	Head control precedes the ability to walk.
Proximodistal	From the trunk to the tips of the extremities	The neonate can move his/her arms and legs but can't pick up objects with his/her fingers.
General to specific	From simple tasks to more complex tasks (mastering simple tasks before advancing to those that are more complex)	The child progresses from crawling to walking to skipping.

 School age refers to children 5 to 11 years of age.

 Adolescence is the period from 12 to 19 years of age.

Factors that influence growth and development

From birth onwards, children normally accomplish a series of developmental tasks during the stages of growth. As a child matures, he/she develops a readiness to master new, age-appropriate tasks.

Task master

A child's ability to master these tasks is affected by environmental, social, cultural and relational factors. Without the appropriate stimuli or environment, these tasks might not be accomplished, and development may be arrested or may occur in a maladaptive manner.

Family

The family environment in which a child is raised greatly influences his/her development. For example, a child who has been abused or neglected may experience attachment disorders, as well as emotional, psychological and physical health problems that continue into adulthood.

Health status

A child's physiological state can significantly affect his/her development. Children with chronic health conditions may experience developmental delays in acquiring skills relating to cognition, communication, adaptation and social and motor functioning. The extent to which a health condition affects a child's development depends on a range of factors including the type, effects on anatomy and physiology and whether it is life-limiting.

Socioeconomic status
A family's socioeconomic status can have a significant impact on a child's growth and development as well as his/her achievement of the Every Child Matters (ECM) outcomes.

No time, no money

Parents who are dependent on social benefits, work long hours or have varying shift patterns can find it difficult to provide basic necessities and may have little time or money to allow their children to participate in a wide range of activities. This can disadvantage some children and have an impact on their development and well-being, although this is not always the case. Parents who focus on work and acquisition of materials may neglect the needs of their children and thus influence their growth and development.

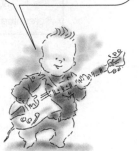

I'm singing the blues. My parents can't afford lessons. Who knows how far my talent would have taken me!

I could have been a winner

A lack of time and funds can also limit a child's ability to pursue special interests such as art, music and sports.

Cultural background
A family's cultural beliefs and circumstances also affect a child's growth and development. Culture influences the way children are socialised, learn values and experience the world. The child's developing beliefs, customs, mode of communication and dressing and actions are influenced by and vary according to culture.

Normal to me, taboo to you

Practices vary from culture to culture; what's acceptable in one culture may be taboo in another. It's extremely important for nurses to become knowledgeable about and respectful of cultural beliefs that differ from their own. This knowledge enables nurses to develop strategies for effective interventions. (See *Cultural influences on developmental assessment*, page 18.)

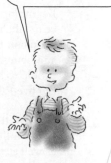

Ya know, I think I need to take it easy and get some more sleep so I can reach my highest potential.

Basic necessities
A child must have such basic necessities as sleep, rest and proper nutrition to reach his/her highest potential.

Cultured know how

Cultural influences on developmental assessment

Tools for measuring development might not take into account cultural influences. For example, Southeast Asian children may be considered delayed in the area of personal–social development on the Denver II test because of a lack of familiarity with games such as pat-a-cake, a game well-known to other cultures.

No single tool can take into account all the factors that contribute to the child's development. Variables that will impact on the assessment of a child's development must be considered when performing developmental screenings.

Children need more sleep than do adults, and nurses should keep in mind that sleep deprivation can impact performance on growth and development assessments. Chronic sleep deprivation can result in negative physiologic consequences.

Brain food

Appropriate feeding, including breastfeeding, weaning and nutrition, is crucial for the health, development and well-being of all children and so nutritional guidelines should be followed when supporting and advising parents, as well as for the child as they develop. The Department of Health follows the WHO/UNICEF UK Baby Friendly Initiative as the standard for encouraging breastfeeding as the best start for children.

Teach your children well

Beginning in infancy and continuing throughout the early years of childhood, the nurse, parents and other significant people in the child's life can teach habits of healthy eating and living. These healthy habits may prevent serious health problems as the child grows and allow him/her to achieve the five ECM outcomes.

Other influences

Other influences on growth and development include genetics and heredity as well as the inborn personality or temperament of the child.

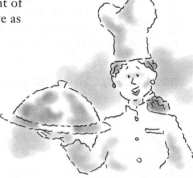

Teach parents and children good nutritional habits. Bon appetite!

Theories of development

According to most theories of personality and cognitive development, certain tasks must be mastered before a child can advance to other more advanced tasks. This process is similar to the patterns of biological development (cephalocaudal, proximodistal, general to specific). (See *Theories of development*.)

Psychosocial development

A developmental framework for the entire lifespan was first proposed by Erik Erikson in 1959. Erikson's psychosocial theory has been further refined but essentially remains the same today.

Erikson believed that the psychosocial development of an individual is a function of ego (the conscious part of the personality and the part that most immediately controls thought and behaviour) as well as social and biologic processes. At given times in the life cycle, the interaction between these processes cause psychosocial crises by placing a demand on the individual. In order for the person to grow, he/she must resolve these crises and master the task at hand.

Growing pains

Theories of development

The child development theories discussed in this chart shouldn't be compared directly because they measure different aspects of development. Erik Erikson's psychosocial-based theory is the most commonly accepted model for child development, although it can't be empirically tested.

Age group	Psychosocial theory	Cognitive theory	Psychosexual theory	Moral development theory
Infancy (birth to age 1)	Trust versus mistrust	Sensorimotor (birth to age 2)	Oral	Not applicable
Toddlerhood (ages 1 to 3)	Autonomy versus shame and doubt	Sensorimotor to preoperational	Anal	Preconventional
Preschool age (ages 3 to 5)	Initiative versus guilt	Preoperational (ages 2 to 7)	Phallic	Preconventional
School age (ages 5 to 12)	Industry versus inferiority	Concrete operational (ages 7 to 11)	Latency	Conventional
Adolescence (ages 12 to 19)	Identity versus role confusion	Formal operational thought (ages 11 to 15)	Genitalia	Postconventional

He trusts me, he trusts me not

These tasks occur in eight different stages, five of which pertain to childhood. Each stage is characterised by a specific positive identity issue, such as trust in the infancy stage, and a contrasting negative attribute that may emerge from that issue, such as mistrust in the infancy stage. The prominence of either positive or negative attributes determines mastery of the crisis.

Weighing the pros …

If the positive attribute emerges, the individual has a better chance of experiencing unimpaired development.

… and the cons

If the negative attribute predominates, the individual may have problems with later attitudes and personal strength. Some negative attributes are, however, necessary to completely master the task at hand. As the person deals with each task, they assume both increased vulnerability and increased potential, which develops new strength and pushes them on to the next level.

Hopeful today, caring tomorrow

Optimal development depends on the proper resolution of each task in the appropriate sequence. For example, the trust developed in infancy leads to a sense of hope, which forms a foundation for the emerging trait of fidelity in adolescence, and an ability to care in adulthood.

Stages of psychosocial theory

The five childhood stages of psychosocial theory are the following:

trust versus mistrust (birth to 1 year). The child develops trust as the primary caregiver meets their needs.

autonomy versus shame and doubt (1 to 3 years). The child learns to control their body functions and becomes increasingly independent, preferring to do things themselves.

initiative versus guilt (3 to 5 years). The child learns about the world through play and develops a conscience.

industry versus inferiority (5 to 12 years). The child enjoys working on projects and with others, and tends to follow rules; competition with others is keen, and forming social relationships takes on greater importance.

identity versus role confusion (12 to 19 years). Changes in the child's body are taking place rapidly, and the young person is preoccupied with how they look and how others view them; while trying to meet the expectations of their peers, they're also trying to establish their own identity.

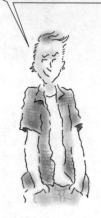

Hey, it isn't my fault if my attitude stinks. Blame it on my predominant negative attribute. (Can I get grounded for that?)

Cognitive development

According to Jean Piaget, cognitive or intellectual acts occur when an individual is adapting to and organising the perceived environment around him/her. Piaget thought a child moves through four stages of cognitive development. As the child moves through each stage, he/she builds on structures gained from the previous stages, moving from relatively simple to very complex operations.

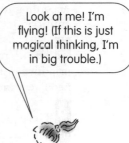

Who am I? What's my role? Will my skin ever clear up? I made it through Erikson's other four stages, but I could have done without number five!

Some people never grow up!

Piaget noted that all individuals have the capability to achieve the most advanced levels of functioning, although not all will reach the final stages of development!

No problem too big

It's through experience with the environment that development is pushed ahead. The child incorporates new ideas, skills and knowledge into familiar patterns of thought and action.

When faced with a problem that's new or too complex to fit into his/her existing pattern of thought, the child accommodates (draws on past experiences that are closest to his/her current problem to solve it).

Sensorimotor stage
The sensorimotor stage spans birth to 2 years. During this stage, the child progresses from reflex activity, through simple repetitive behaviours, to imitative behaviours. Concepts to be mastered include:
- object permanence – the understanding that objects and events continue to exist, even when they can't be seen, heard, or touched directly
- causality – the relationship between cause and effect
- spatial relationships – the recognition of different shapes and the relationships between them (e.g. placing a round object in a round hole).

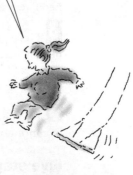

Look at me! I'm flying! (If this is just magical thinking, I'm in big trouble.)

Preoperational stage
The preoperational stage starts at 2 years and ends at around 7 years. This stage is marked by egocentricity (the child can't comprehend a point of view different from their own). It's a time of magical thinking and increased ability to use symbols and language. Concepts to be mastered include:
- representational language and symbols
- transductive reasoning – generalisation to the extent that items that share characteristics are labelled the same.

Concrete operational stage

During the concrete operational stage (7 to 11 years), children's thought processes become more logical and coherent. They can use inductive reasoning (using facts gathered from one or more specific experiences to draw a general conclusion about a situation) to solve problems but still can't think abstractly. The child is less self-centred during this stage. Concepts to be mastered include sorting, ordering and classifying facts to use in problem-solving.

Formal operational thought stage

The formal operational thought stage, from 11 to 15 years, is characterised by adaptability and flexibility. The young person can think abstractly, form logical conclusions from their observations and establish and test hypotheses. Concepts to be mastered include abstract ideas and concepts, possibilities, inductive reasoning and complex deductive reasoning.

Psychosexual development

Development of human sexuality is influenced by physical, emotional and cultural aspects in the society in which we live. Sexuality is part of the total person, which develops over time. It's expressed through many avenues, including a person's attitudes, feelings, beliefs and self-image.

Sexual feelings

Sigmund Freud theorised that sexual feelings are present in some form from the newborn period through adulthood. He felt that human nature has two sides: rational intellect and irrational desires.

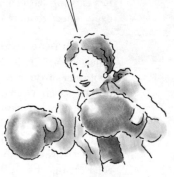

Between the id, ego and superego, there's always a battle going on. Are you up for the challenge?

Id, ego and superego

According to the psychosexual theory, personality is composed of three entities:

The id, the largest portion of the mind, is the centre of our primitive instincts and requires immediate gratification (e.g. the neonate wants feeding now!).

The ego develops in infancy and is the conscious, rational part of the personality; it's less inward-seeking than the ego, and recognises the larger picture. (The ego acts as a censor to the id; if there's conflict between the id and the ego, mental health problems may develop.)

The superego represents the person's conscience and ideals; therefore, it's in continuous battle with the id.

Five stages of development

Freud proposed five stages of development; these stages centre around the early years of the person's life and the parent–child relationship. At each stage, sexual energy, what Freud called instinctual libido, is focused on a different area of the body.

Each stage also centres around a conflict that must be resolved before the child can progress to the next stage. If the conflict isn't resolved, the child becomes fixated in that stage and development is halted.

I can't get no ... satisfaction

Satisfaction must be achieved before a person can move on to the next stage. If not fully satisfied, it's possible that they may never fully complete the stage.

How the individual responds to others depends on which stage they are in. This was an important theory in the field of psychology, although it's relatively limited in its scope.

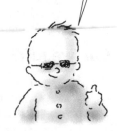

So many stages, so little time. Thanks to Dr. Freud, I have my work cut out for me.

Oral stage
In the oral stage (birth to 1 year), the child seeks pleasure through sucking, biting and other oral activities. Oral stimulation reduces tension and provides sensual satisfaction.

Anal stage
The anal and urethral areas are of great interest in the anal stage (1 to 3 years). The child goes through toilet training and learns control.

Phallic stage
During the phallic stage (3 to 6 years), the child is interested in their genitalia and various sensations and discovers the difference between boys and girls. The child may love the opposite-sex parent and consider the parent of the same sex a rival. This is known as the Oedipal (boys) or Electra (girls) complex.

Latency period
In the latency period (6 to 12 years), the child expands on traits developed in earlier stages and concentrates on playing and learning. The child doesn't focus on a particular area of the body during this stage.

The Oedipal or Electra complex eventually disappears, and the child forms close relationships with other children of the same age and gender. Energy is directed towards physical and intellectual interests.

Genitalia stage
The production of sex hormones becomes intense during the genitalia stage (12 years and older), and the reproductive system reaches maturation. During this stage, the young person develops the capacity for love and maturity.

Moral development

Lawrence Kohlberg's ideas of moral reasoning (the basis for ethical behaviour) are based on the work of Piaget and the American philosopher John Dewey.

Born free ... of morals, that is!

Kohlberg's theory is based on the premise that, at birth, all beings are devoid of morals, ethics and honesty. Then, through different stages, the family, and then the larger society, instil values, morality and a sense of right and wrong. As the child's intelligence and ability to interact with others mature, their patterns of moral behaviour mature as well.

Kohlberg, along with Piaget, believed that most moral development occurs through social interaction; he felt that development could be promoted through formal education.

Can we talk?

According to Kohlberg, it's important to present a person with moral dilemmas for discussion, which helps him see the reasonableness of the next higher stage and progress towards it. Kohlberg based this discussion approach on the insight that a person develops as a result of cognitive conflicts in his/her current stage.

Three levels of moral development

Kohlberg proposed three levels of moral development through which the person must pass. As the child comprehends and understands a stage, he/she can then progress to the next stage.

Preconventional level of morality

At the preconventional level (2 to 7 years), the child attempts to follow rules set by those in authority. He/she tries to adjust his/her behaviour according to good and bad and to right and wrong.

Conventional level of morality

At the conventional level (7 to 12 years), the child seeks conformity and loyalty. He/she attempts to justify, support and maintain the social order, and he/she follows fixed rules.

Postconventional autonomous level of morality

At the postconventional level (12 years and older), the adolescent strives to construct a personal and functional value system independent of authority figures and his/her peers.

Social development

A more recent theory, which is gaining acceptance, is that formulated by Len Vygotsky and puts forward the view that culture and society are important for promoting cognitive development. It is based around three themes.

Social interaction

Social interaction plays a major role in the process of cognitive development as he/she believed social learning precedes development. Children use tools including reading, speech and writing developed from their culture to interact with and mediate their environments.

More knowledgeable other (MKO)

The MKO is anyone who has a better understanding or a higher-level ability than the child with respect to a particular task or process.

Zone of proximal development (ZPD)

The ZPD refers to the space between the activities a child can perform with help and his/her ability to perform independently. Learning and development occurs as the child is facilitated to develop independence in achieving the task or process.

Watch that development

Being familiar with theories of growth and development may help you to focus your nursing skills of communication, observation and interaction to best meet the differing needs of children and young people – but don't forget that adults are also developing as well!

Caring for the hospitalised child

Hospitalisation can be a major stressor for any individual, especially for a child. The child is in an unfamiliar surrounding, with unfamiliar people. His/her routine is disrupted, and he/she is not able to do things that he/she normally do.

Added to these stressors may be the fear, pain and discomfort associated with his/her illness or injury and, in many cases, the diagnostic and therapeutic interventions used. What's more, even a minor illness may be perceived by the family as life-threatening. This perception can trigger fears that may overwhelm the family's coping skills and lead to crisis.

No matter what the developmental stage of the child, interventions should be geared towards helping him/her and family cope with this very stressful time.

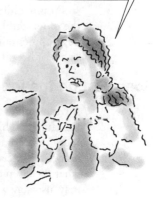

Everyone has stress – even kids. We all have to find a way to deal with it.

No place like home

Separation of the child from their parents, siblings and usual support systems further adds to the emotional stress and discomfort a child feels when hospitalised. Parents (and siblings) should be allowed to spend as much time as possible with the hospitalised child. The opportunity for a parent to stay with or close to the child should be provided. However, it should also be recognised that parents may also have responsibilities that prevent them from staying.

Minimising the trauma of hospitalisation

Preparing a child for hospitalisation and any interventions can help him/her cope more effectively and make it easier to trust health care professionals responsible for his/her care.

The importance of play

One of the most important aspects of a child's life is play. Play can become even more important to a child who's hospitalised. It can serve several functions:

- Play is an excellent stress reducer and tension reliever. It allows the child freedom of expression to act out his/her fears, concerns and anxieties.
- Play provides a source of diversional activity, alleviating separation anxiety.

- Play provides children with a sense of safety and security because, while they're engaging in play, they know that no painful procedures will occur.
- Developmentally appropriate play fosters the child's normal growth and development, especially for children who are repeatedly hospitalised for chronic conditions.
- Play puts the child in the driver's seat, allowing him/her to make choices and giving a sense of control.

Always be prepared

When possible, it's better to prepare the child for admission to the hospital. The timing of the preparation and the amount of teaching given depends on his/her age, developmental stage, personality and the length of the procedure or treatment.

Young children may need only a few hours of preparation, whereas the older child may benefit from several days of preparation. The use of developmentally appropriate activities may also help the child cope with the stress of hospitalisation. (See *The importance of play*.)

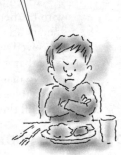

I'm trying to follow my parents' rules, but this preconventional stuff isn't easy.

Specialist on the job

Most hospitals have a play specialist, who can arrange a preadmission visit for the child and his/her parents allowing them to the children's unit and helping them to become familiar with the sights, sounds and smells of the hospital. The play specialist, an expert in child development, then explains, step-by-step, what the child can expect – especially relating to any planned procedures – and may also stay with the child during procedures.

Keep it in the family

To reduce the fear that accompanies hospitalisation, the nurse can help the child and family cope by:
- explaining procedures in a language and ways appropriate to understanding
- answering questions openly and honestly
- minimising separation from the parents
- structuring the environment to allow the child to retain as much control as possible.

Family-centred care permits the family to remain as involved as possible and helps give the child and his/her family a sense of control in a difficult and unfamiliar situation. It may also help alleviate separation anxiety and reassure the child that all care is intended to help them. The child needs reassurance that the illness isn't his/her fault and that fear is a normal response. All children should be encouraged to express their feelings, and the play specialist is a good resource person to help facilitate this.

Caring for the child with special needs

All children go through times in their lives when parents, family and others need to adapt to certain outside influences. How the child copes with these influences, either positive or negative, is determined by their strengths, personality, developmental stage and support systems.

Chronic illness and disability

When a child has a chronic illness or is disabled, family members experience additional stress that has lasting implications for the child, his/her parents and his/her siblings.

Flexibility required

Chronic or terminal illnesses, disabilities or acute conditions that impact daily living require the family and the child to adapt their normal process of living and being; they also require health care professionals to adapt their usual way of providing care.

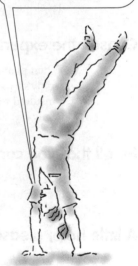

Always stay flexible when providing care to children with special needs.

On the rise

About 12 in every 10,000 children in the UK have a condition that falls into these categories. This percentage is increasing because of improved technology, health care and treatments that increase survival rates.

Barriers to optimal care level

Children with special needs often require continuous and complex care. Management of care is usually provided by specialists who may or may not take into account alterations in development or the child's response to the illness. Occasionally, this may mean that the child doesn't receive preventive health services. Other barriers to optimal health care for this group of children include family finances, navigating through the health care system and knowledge barriers. For these reasons, it's especially important for the nurse to ensure that the child is up to date on immunisations and routine health care on top of any specialist intervention.

Impact on the family

The diagnosis of a chronic condition may cause extreme distress in the family. Parents grieve over the loss of their 'healthy' child, feel guilty and may perceive him/her as vulnerable. This view may hinder the child in meeting the tasks required to grow and develop as normally as possible. Helping the family to understand the condition and its impact on normal growth and development will help the child achieve his/her highest level of ability.

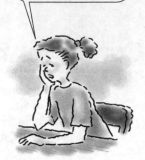

When you have a sick brother or sister, it's easy to get lost in the shuffle.

Hey, what about me?

Having a sibling with a chronic condition may elicit feelings of stress, helplessness, guilt or depression. Siblings should be included in the family assessment of coping and should be provided with appropriate support. Older siblings often participate in providing care to a child with chronic health care needs at home as much as the parents do. They must be included when providing care and teaching to the child.

Nursing strategies

Care and nursing interventions should be adapted to the child's level of development.

Consult the experts

When planning interventions, the nurse should take into consideration the family's expertise in providing care for their child; the parents should be consulted for advice about their child's routine, care preferences and special needs.

Be all that you can be

The child should receive interventions aimed at helping him/her to achieve his/her maximum potential.

A little help, please

It's important to remember that a child with a disability or chronic illness faces many challenges. Encouraging the use of such resources as support groups may help the child and family interact with others who are experiencing, or who have managed, the same issues.

Understanding that the child's condition realigns the hopes and expectations of the family and the assigned roles within that family, the nurse can help provide interventions to help the child and family cope. To this end, the nurse can show respect and caring by:
- supporting family coping strategies
- providing education in a forthright, honest manner
- helping the family access specific services
- promoting preventive health measures.

Caring for the terminally ill child

The dying child elicits many different emotions in the child, family and nurse. A perception exists in society that children aren't supposed to die. For the nurse, this can be a painful and awkward situation.

Dealing with a terminal illness

An understanding of how the child and his/her family have managed health and illness in the past may provide the nurse with clues about how the family may cope with having a dying child.

Impact on the family

The death of a child is viewed by most people as the worst possible thing that can happen to a parent. Family members of a terminally ill child must deal with a range of emotions while still trying to deal with everyday needs, such as those related to jobs, the household and the needs of their other children.

To stay or to go – that is the question

These stressors can bring families closer together, but they can also tear families apart. It can lead to separation or divorce after the death of a child, at a time when they need each other's support more than ever.

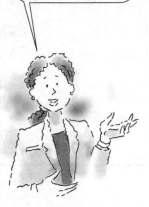

It's difficult to imagine how parents must feel when their child is terminally ill.

It's a roller coaster ride

Parents may experience a range of emotions, from fear and anger (sometimes directed at health care professionals) to guilt and disabling grief even before their child dies. Siblings may feel unloved or forgotten, as their parents focus their attention on the dying child. They may then feel guilty about having those feelings.

Nursing strategies

The child who's dying has the same emotional and developmental needs as any other child of the same age – as well as other needs related to his/her prognosis. The nurse should develop care plans based on family input to meet these needs at the child's developmental level. Adaptations in care must be made and must be based on the child's physiologic and psychological status.

Tell me no lies

Communication should be honest. Understanding the developmental level of the child in relation to his/her concept of death will help foster appropriate communication techniques. (See *Concepts of death in childhood*, page 30.)

Growing pains

Concepts of death in childhood

A child's concept of death depends on his/her developmental stage.

Developmental stage	Concept of death	Nursing considerations
Infancy	• None	• Be aware that the older infant will experience separation anxiety. • Help the family cope with death so they can be available to the infant.
Early childhood	• Knows the words 'dead' and 'death' • Reactions are influenced by the attitudes of parents	• Help the family members (including siblings) cope with their feelings. • Allow the child to express his/her own feelings in an open and honest manner.
Middle childhood	• Understands universality and irreversibility of death • May have a fear of parents dying	• Use play to facilitate the child's understanding of death. • Allow siblings to express his/her feelings.
Late childhood	• Begins to incorporate family and cultural beliefs about death • Explores views of an afterlife • Faces the reality of own mortality	• Provide opportunities for the child to verbalise fears. • Help the child discuss concerns with his/her family.
Adolescence	• Adult perception of death, but still focused on the 'here and now'	• Use opportunities to open discussion about death. • Allow expression of feelings of guilt, confusion and anxiety. • Support and maintain self-esteem.

A positive and helpful approach should be maintained, and the family should be included in all aspects of care. All procedures and therapies should be explained before carrying them out.

Maximum control

Pain control is an essential component in the management of a terminally ill child. The nurse should serve as the child's advocate to ensure that the child receives the most effective pain management possible. Where appropriate children and families should be referred to the children's palliative care team as well for possible for hospice or respite care.

Helping families cope

The nurse can help the family cope during this very difficult time by:
• encouraging all family members to express their feelings, even though they might be difficult to hear

- allowing families to spend as much time as possible with the dying child (including overnight stays)
- allowing and encouraging parents to continue to take an active role in their child's care.

We can cope! Not always!

The nurse can also help the family cope by:
- reminding parents that they don't always have to be strong and that asking for help is a sign of strength, not weakness
- helping parents to talk with their child about dying if he/she's ready to do so
- providing parents and siblings with information about support groups and professionals who can help them with their grief
- contacting other health care professionals (social workers, play therapists, art and music therapists) and volunteers who may be able to help the child, their siblings and their parents in coping with practical daily needs (such as transportation, sibling care and special arrangements)
- reassuring parents that you understand how difficult this must be, but avoiding such phrases as 'I know how you feel'
- remaining as accessible and available as possible and facilitating contact and communication with other individuals on the child's health care team.

   Nurses have the unique opportunity to impact on the child in every stage of his/her life. Using the principles of caring for the whole person will help the child and his/her family deal with the most difficult stage, that of the dying child.

An art therapist can help a child cope.

Pain and children

Pain is a subjective experience; for infants and children, it's possibly the most bewildering and frightening occurrence in their young lives. Until 3 years of age or so, children can't grasp abstract concepts, such as time, cause and effect and quantification. Consequently, it's impossible for them to understand why pain occurs, or that relief is just around the corner. They only know that something hurts right now.

My kingdom for a word

What makes the experience particularly distressing is that infants and young children lack the language skills needed to tell someone that they're in pain, where it hurts and how much, or to ask for help.

   In this respect, infants and children are uniquely dependent on the ability of their parents and health care professionals to recognise the physiological

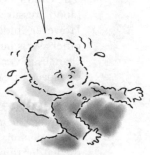

Hey, give me a break! I have no idea that I'll feel all better in 10 minutes. I live in the here and now, baby! Whaah!

and behavioural signs of pain and to react by relieving their discomfort. Similarly, children should reasonably expect these same professionals to anticipate and prevent or minimise painful experiences whenever possible.

Assessing pain

A growing number of health professionals who work with children talk about pain as a fifth vital sign, one that should be assessed early and often to ensure prompt, effective relief.

Assessing pain in infants and young children requires the cooperation of the parents and the use of age-specific assessment tools. If the child can communicate verbally, they can also aid the process.

Health history and physical examination

A nursing assessment involves a health history that includes a description of any pain and palliative measures. During assessment you must then ask parents about the child's health history and background experience of pain. This is in addition to the physical assessment the nurse will undertake and when the skills of communication and observation are crucial in recognising pain and discomfort.

Wanna play 20 questions?

To help you better understand the child's pain, ask the parents these questions:
- What kinds of pain has your child had in the past?
- How does your child usually respond to pain?
- How do you know that your child is in pain?
- What words does your child use to say that they are in pain?
- What do you do when they are hurting?
- What does your child do when he or she is hurting?
- What works best to relieve your child's pain?
- Is there anything special you'd like me to know about your child and pain?

No wonder they call 'em vital

The child's vital signs can be pain indicators. Elevated pulse, blood pressure or respirations can be signs of pain and stress. However, findings here must be viewed in conjunction with other assessment data because nonpainful stimuli can elicit changes in vital signs as well. For example, just touching an infant can speed or calm his/her pulse rate.

Assessment tools

A number of validated assessment tools have been designed for a child or young person. Many of these tools seek to quantify the child's pain, one of the harder things to accomplish during assessment and observation. Using an

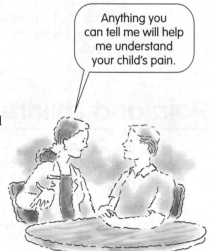

Anything you can tell me will help me understand your child's pain.

assessment tool will help, but quantifying pain in the infant or preverbal child will still be difficult.

Where's that toolbox?

Pain assessment tools are described as being unidimensional (assessing one indicator) or multidimensional (assessing multiple indicators). Composite measures of pain include physiological, behavioural, sensory and cognitive indicators. These tools tend to be especially useful when assessing children younger than 3 years or older children with cognitive deficits.

Painful measures

Because of the complexity of assessing pain in children, there's no single pain measurement tool that works well for all. As such, there are different tools that may be 'self-report', which is where the child scores his/her own pain and discomfort, or behavioural whereby the level of pain is assessed in relation to the child's behaviour. There aren't any specific physiologically based assessment tools but physiological readings (pulse, blood pressure and so on) form part of the assessment of pain.

There are several pain measurement tools that can be utilised depending on the child's age, status and condition as well as events, such as surgery, which may take place. The 'Recognition and assessment of acute pain in children' published by the Royal College of Nursing (2009) provides information on a range of tools that can be utilised with children and young people.

Pulling faces

In nonverbal children, the assessment of pain relies on observation and assessment of their behaviour as well as being informed, where possible, by the history from parents. In some situations the child's status, such as being premature, limits the information available to assess pain and so specific tools may help. Three tools that have proved to be quite effective are:

- CRIES Neonatal Postoperative Pain Measurement Scale
- Neonatal Infant Pain Scale
- Premature Infant Pain Profile (See *Measuring pain in infants*, page 34.)

Speaking of pain

For the child capable of speaking, typically age 3 years, the task is somewhat easier. Several simple and effective pain-measuring scales can help the child identify a level of pain. These include a:

- faces pain-measuring scale
- visual analogue scale
- chip pain-measuring tool
  (See *Measuring pain in young children*, page 35.)

Measuring pain in infants

Assessing pain in infants can be challenging for health care providers. This chart describes three assessment tools that can help you meet this challenge.

Assessment tool	Factors measured
CRIES Neonatal Postoperative Pain Measurement Scale	• Crying (C) • Oxygen saturation (R – requires oxygen to maintain saturation above 95%) • Heart rate and blood pressure (I – increased) • Expression (E) • Sleeplessness (S)
Neonatal Infant Pain Scale	• Facial expression • Crying • Breathing patterns • State of arousal • Movement of arms and legs
Premature Infant Pain Profile	• Gestational age • Heart rate • Oxygen saturation • Behavioural state • Brow bulge • Eye squeeze • Nasolabial furrow

Behavioural responses to pain

Behaviour is the language infants and children rely on to convey information about their pain. Areas of behaviour that change because of pain include body positioning, facial expression, patterns of eating and sleeping, attention level and vocalisation.

Look at that face!

In an infant, facial expression is the most common and consistent behavioural response to all stimuli, painful or pleasurable, and may be the single best indicator of pain for the provider and the parent. Studies indicate that facial expression is a more reliable pain indicator than crying, heart rate or body position and movement.

Facial expressions that tend to indicate that the infant is in pain include:
• mouth stretched open
• eyes tightly shut
• brows and forehead knitted (as they are in a grimace)
• cheeks raised high enough to form a wrinkle on the nose.

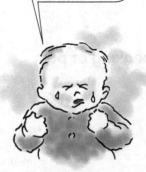

Can you tell I'm in pain? Until I can say it, this is the best way I can let you know.

Measuring pain in young children

For children who are old enough to speak and understand sufficiently, three useful tools can help them communicate information for measuring their pain. Here's how to use each one:

Faces scale

The child 3 years and older can use the faces scale to rate pain. When using this tool, make sure that they can see and point to each face and then describe the amount of pain each face is experiencing. If able, the child can read the text under the picture; otherwise, you or his/her parent can read it to him/her.

Avoid saying anything that might prompt the child to choose a certain face. Then, ask the child to choose the face that shows how he/she's feeling right now. Record the response on your pain assessment form.

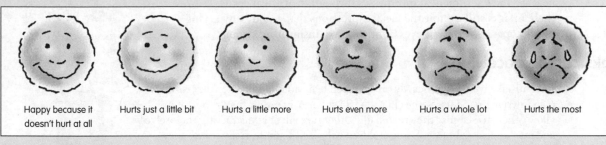

| Happy because it doesn't hurt at all | Hurts just a little bit | Hurts a little more | Hurts even more | Hurts a whole lot | Hurts the most |

Visual analogue scale

A visual analogue pain scale is simply a straight line with the phrase 'no pain' at one end and the phrase 'the most pain possible' at the other. Children who understand the concept of a continuum can mark the spot on the line that corresponds to the level of pain they feel.

No pain   The most pain possible

Older signs

In young children, facial expression is joined by other behaviours to convey pain. In these patients, look for such signs as:
- narrowing of the eyes
- grimace or fearful appearance
- frequent and longer-lasting bouts of crying, with a tone that's higher and louder than normal
- less receptiveness to comforting by parents or other caregivers
- holding or protecting the painful area.

Hush-a-bye, why do you cry?

Enlist the parents' help in interpreting the child's crying. Pain may be the cause, but hunger, anger, fear or a wet nappy can also elicit crying. Typically, parents can distinguish among the different cries of their child and help narrow down the possible causes. Some young children, however, are incessant criers and no specific cause can be identified, but this causes parents ongoing stress and sleepless nights! Crying associated with pain is distinguished by frequency, duration, pitch and intensity. Cries of pain are usually short, sharp, higher in pitch, tense, harsh, nonmelodious and loud.

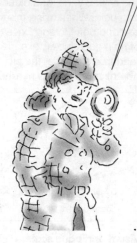

It takes a little detective work to solve a crying mystery. Thank goodness the parents can offer some clues!

Silent cry

On the other hand, some infants don't cry in response to pain, even pain associated with an invasive procedure. Also, some treatments make crying impossible. Intubated infants, for example, can't produce an audible cry because the endotracheal tube passes through their vocal cords. However, these infants still exhibit the facial expressions that accompany crying – mouth opened wide and eyes tightly closed, insinuating crying.

Looks can be deceiving

It's a mistake to rely too heavily on observed behaviour alone when assessing pain in young patients. Some children will suffer pain rather than report it or allow others to see that they're in pain. Others are adept at distracting themselves and may appear pain free. Some children will sleep soundly, not because they have no pain, but because they're physically and emotionally exhausted.

Translation needed

A child who has mastered the rudiments of language can provide some useful information. However, keep in mind that his/her language skills are very basic and that he/she may not understand the words you use; you may call it pain, but he/she may think of it as a hurt or boo-boo. Find the words that work best by talking with the parents as well as the child.

Check the mirror

Remember that children who are just learning to talk have a great deal more skill in reading the facial expressions and body language of their parents and caregivers. After all, they've been reading this language since birth.

Be sure that your expression and body posture are conveying a message consistent with your words. If you or the child's parents appear concerned, he/she may feel that there's something to fear, and this may colour his/her description of the pain he/she's feeling.

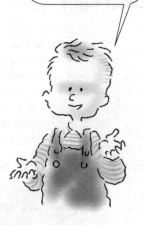

I have a boo-boo on my doo-dah and it's foo-foo! Do you need a translation? Ask my Mum!

Managing pain

Infants and young children may experience acute pain, cancer pain or chronic pain associated with an underlying disorder. Pain management is most effective when it prevents, limits or avoids noxious stimuli and involves administering analgesics. Children and parents often report that effective pain management is not provided, so focusing on this is crucial and particularly as Standard 6 of the National Service Framework for Children, Young People and Maternity Services (DH 2007) states that children 'have a right to appropriate prevention, assessment and control of their pain'.

Regardless of the underlying cause, pain management for children seeks to:
- identify and relieve existing pain
- anticipate and prevent or minimise pain related to hospitalisation, procedures and treatments
- optimise pharmacologic and nonpharmacological interventions to reduce stress, increase comfort and enhance healing.

All professionals should refer to relevant evidence and guidelines when managing pain, such as the British National Formulary for Children (http://bnfc.org) and for nurses the NMC Standards for Medicine Management (http://www.nmc-uk.org). When caring for children with specific pain issues then the ACT (Association for Children's Palliative Care) guidelines on Basic Symptom Control in Paediatric Palliative Care (2011) are invaluable.

Pharmacological intervention

Pharmacological therapy is the mainstay of pain management for an infant or a child. Selection of the medications, dosages and administration routes depends on the specific needs of the child, his/her status and any interventions such as surgery.

On the outside

If the pain or discomfort is, or going to be, related to an intervention then the use of a local anaesthetic should also be considered, unless the situation is so urgent as to preclude their use. Ametop or EMLA, local anaesthetics, can be applied to the skin prior to the insertion of needles for venepuncture or administration of medication.

Take a deep breath

Entenox (nitrous oxide) is a useful analgesic that is inhaled and can provide some temporary relief from pain and discomfort but it does need cooperation from the child and his/her parents.

A spoonful of sugar makes the medicine go down ...

Oral sucrose is now used in neonates prior to painful procedures such as heel pricks. This has been demonstrated to dampen the pain associated with such procedures.

Opioid analgesics

Opioid analgesics are highly effective pain relievers and constitute the core of most pharmacological interventions to manage acute pain (especially postoperative pain) in infants and children.

Choose your weapon ...

Morphine and fentanyl are the two opioids used most commonly in children. While they're thought to be equivalent, morphine may provide better sedation and a lower risk of chest wall rigidity than fentanyl.

... and pick a route

Opioid analgesics are available in oral, sublingual, rectal, nasal, subcutaneous (SC), transdermal, intravenous (IV) and epidural forms, which makes it relatively easy to find an acceptable route. Finding a route also means avoiding pain and discomfort so important to consider how best to give the medication. Your unit should have protocols for managing children's pain so check these out.

> OK, guys, this is it. Get ready to wipe out some pain.

Hip hooray for PCA!

Patient-controlled analgesia (PCA) can be useful in managing pain, provided the parents are involved and they (and, if appropriate, the child) are trained in the administration and proper use of this equipment. PCA allows for the maintenance of a therapeutic level of the prescribed analgesic at all times. It has proven effective in children ages 5 years and older.

Parent-controlled analgesia is an effective way to allow the use of IV PCA for children younger than 5 years and for those with a developmental delay.

Nonopioid analgesics

Nonopioid analgesics, which include paracetamol and nonsteroidal anti-inflammatory drugs (NSAIDs), are prescribed to manage mild to moderate pain. In instances of severe pain, nonopioid analgesics can be used in conjunction with opioid analgesics to reduce the required dosage of the opioid drug.

Infants and children metabolise nonopioid analgesics in the same manner and at the same rate as adults; consequently, the selection criteria, effects and possible adverse effects are the same as they are for adults.

Paracetamol anyone?

Paracetamol is the drug of choice for treating mild pain. It has the added benefit of helping reduce fever and is safe, even for neonates. Paracetamol has few adverse effects or contraindications. However, long-term use can increase the risk of liver damage, and it's possible to reach a point at which additional doses no longer provide an analgesic affect. On the plus side, it is available in suppository, liquid, soluble and tablet form, making it easy to administer and appropriate for most situations.

Who said NSAIDs?

NSAIDs relieve mild to moderate pain and also act as anti-inflammatory agents. The most commonly prescribed NSAID is ibuprofen (Brufen), and it is approved for use in children. Its possible adverse effects include inhibition of platelet aggregation, exacerbation of asthma symptoms and gastrointestinal (GI) irritation.

Adjuvant therapy

A range of medications are prescribed as adjuvant therapy usually when treating cancer pain in infants and children. Positive results from such therapy have made adjuvant therapy more acceptable as a component of pain management in other chronic conditions as well, such as neuropathies, headache and recurrent abdominal pain.

Types of drugs used for adjuvant therapy, and their therapeutic effects, include:

• antianxiety medications, such as lorazepam, diazepam and midazolam, which are used to enhance the effect of opioids
• anticonvulsants, such as phenytoin or carbamazepine, which are used to treat neuropathies caused by certain diseases or trauma
• corticosteroids, which help alleviate severe inflammation and bone pain
• neuroleptic drugs, which are antipsychotic, tranquilising, sedative and analgesic and help relieve pain associated with cancer, certain neuralgias, phantom limb and muscular discomfort
• topical or local anaesthetics, which are given before procedures, such as IV insertion, to reduce procedural pain.

Nonpharmacologic interventions

For the infant and young child, nonpharmacologic interventions pick up where drug therapies stop (or haven't started) – by reducing stress and anxiety and increasing comfort and security. Typically, these measures are just as critical to the child's well-being as pain relief.

Nonpharmacologic interventions cause no adverse effects, require no special equipment and can be used at any time. These interventions have another benefit: they can give the parents an opportunity to shine in the care of their child. It is important that these approaches are used 'as well as' and not as an opt-out to giving analgesia!

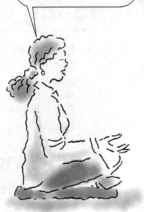

There's nothing like a little relaxation to relieve stress in children—and in nurses too!

Cognitive–behavioural therapies

Cognitive–behavioural interventions for the infant include positioning, containment or swaddling, distraction, touching and gentle massage.

Wrap 'em up

Placing an infant in a midline or supine position has a calming effect, as does wrapping him/her snugly in a soft blanket. Providing distraction – for example, with a bedside mobile or a safe, colourful toy or stuffed animal – helps the infant focus on something enjoyable rather than their pain. Maintain their safety when using the 'wrap em up' approach!

You're getting sleepy – very sleepy

For a toddler, distraction, hypnosis, guided imagery, gentle massage, snuggling with Mom and Dad and curling up in bed listening to a story are all methods of moving the child's focus away from their pain towards more serene, safe and comforting thoughts.

Physical therapy

Thermotherapy is the most common form of physical therapy used with infants. Applying warm and cold to painful areas can make them feel better. Heat promotes circulation, and cold helps reduce swelling and provides a limited amount of numbing.

Complementary therapies

Complementary therapies, such as music or aromatherapy, are gaining acceptance because of the influence music and aromas can have on emotions and state of mind. Similarly acupuncture can be helpful but as it involves needles children may not like it.

Charms to soothe

For the infant or child, soothing music has a calming effect and can help them drift off to sleep at nap time. More lively music can stimulate memories or encourage singing, which distract the child for a time. Smells that remind them of home can be comforting as well. An alternative is the Snoezelen Sensory room, which is equipped with a range of equipment that can help the child, the parents and staff to relax …

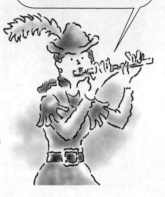

A little music goes a long way toward soothing or distracting a child in pain. (And they probably won't even notice if you're off-key!)

Preparing children's medications

Medications are used throughout the lifespan to treat health problems (including pain), combat disease and promote health. Many health care professionals have expressed concerns about medication use in infants and children. These concerns are gradually beginning to fade, primarily because our understanding of medications, pharmacokinetics and pharmacodynamics in infants and young children has significantly improved in recent years.

Pharmacokinetics and pharmacodynamics

The pharmacokinetic (how a drug acts and how it moves through the body) and pharmacodynamic (study of drug mechanisms that produce biochemical or physiologic changes in the body) properties of medications include:

- absorption
- distribution
- protein-binding capacity
- metabolism
- elimination.

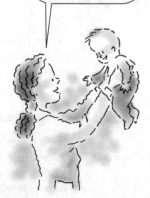

Children aren't little adults. Their bodies absorb, distribute and metabolise medication differently.

Medication metabolism in young children

It's important to understand how the unique physiology of young children affects pharmacokinetics and pharmacodynamics. Infants and young children are still developing physiologically, which affects the way their bodies absorb, distribute and metabolise drugs. The metabolism of an infant or young child differs significantly from that of an older person.

Acid, protein and water … oh my!

A better understanding of how medications are used and metabolised in children will lead to safer medication administration in children:
• Because gastric acidity doesn't stabilise until approximately 3 years of age, the absorption and concentration of drugs that require an acid environment to be fully assimilated may be affected.
• Protein binding, which aids in the distribution of drugs in the body, is lower in infants and children than in older patients.
• Compared with adults, infants have proportionately more water weight and extracellular water, less fat and less muscle tissue. In infants, hepatic (liver) metabolism is slower and renal clearance is delayed. These factors can increase the potential for drug toxicity.

Dosage calculations

To calculate and verify the safety of children's drug dosages, use either the dosage per kilogram of body weight method or the body surface area (BSA) method. Other methods, such as those based on age, are less accurate and typically aren't used unless in an emergency.

Whichever method you use, remember that, as a nurse, you're professionally and legally responsible for checking the safety of a prescribed dose before administration.

Dosage per kilogram of body weight

Information about specific drug dosages for children are provided with the medication, by the pharmacy and in guidelines such as the BNF for Children (2010). Dosages are usually stated in milligrams per kilogram of body weight. This measurement is the most accurate and common way to calculate paediatric dosages.

Children's drug dosages are usually expressed as mg/kg/day or mg/kg/dose. Based on this information, you can determine the dose by multiplying the child's weight in kilograms by the required number of milligrams of drug per kilogram.

Shifting weight

Children's weights should be measured and recorded in kilograms. If you must convert from pounds to kilograms before calculating the dosage per kilogram of body weight, remember that 1 kg equals 2.2 lb. Parents usually think in pounds and ounces so get converting …

Real-world problems

The following example shows how to calculate a mg/kg/dose for one-time or as-needed (p.r.n.) medications, and how to calculate mg/kg/day

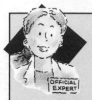

Advice from the experts

What's in a nomogram?

Body surface area (BSA) is critical when calculating dosages for children or for drugs that are extremely potent and need to be given in precise amounts. The nomogram shown here lets you plot the child's height and weight to determine the BSA. Here's how it works:

- Locate the child's height in the left column of the nomogram and his/her weight in the right column.
- Use a ruler to draw a straight line connecting the two points. (The point where the line intersects the surface area column indicates the patient's BSA in square metres.)
- For an average-size child, use the simplified nomogram in the box. Just find the child's weight in kilograms on the left side of the scale, and then read the corresponding BSA on the right side.

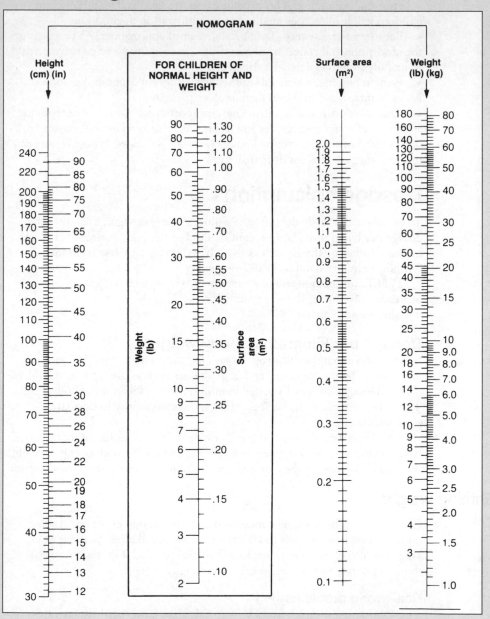

for doses given around the clock to maintain a continuous drug effect.

Penicillin problem

Penicillin oral suspension is prescribed at 56 mg/kg/day in four divided doses for a child who weighs 25 kg. The suspension that's available is penicillin 125 mg/5 ml. What volume should you administer for each dose?

First, determine the total daily dosage.

Weight multiplied by dose per kilogram

$$25 \times 56 = 1,400 \text{ mg}$$

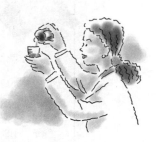

- The child's daily dosage is 1,400 mg. Now, divide the daily dosage by four doses to determine the dose to administer every 6 hours:

$$1,400 \div 4 = 350$$

The child should receive 350 mg every 6 hours.
- then work out the amount of the medicine to be given

$$\frac{\text{What you want} \times \text{what it is in}}{\text{What you got}} = \text{amount to be given}$$

$$\frac{350 \times 5}{125} = 14 \text{ ml should be administered.}$$

You should practice drug calculations until you are confident and competent. The Nursing and Midwifery Council make it clear that you should be able to perform them without relying on a calculator.

> I guess my math teacher was right. You really do have to solve for X in the real world.

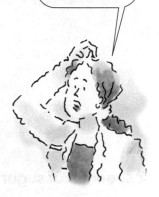

Administering children's medications

The methods used to prepare drugs and administer them to children differ from the methods used for adults, depending on which route is used. There are specific administration guidelines and precautions for each route. (See *Giving medications to children*, page 44.) Also, nurses must adhere to the NMC Standards for Medicine Management (NMC, 2007) and refer to the Children's BNF when administering any type of medication. Importantly, the standards emphasise the need to fully assess the child or young person in relation to his/her medication needs and select, with him/her, the most suitable method of administration.

Wet, Soap, Wash, Rinse, Dry

Before and after all procedures hand hygiene is crucial to stop crossinfection.

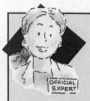

Advice from the experts

Giving medication to children

When giving oral and parenteral medications to children, safety is essential. Keep these points in mind:

- Check the child's mouth to make sure that he/she has swallowed the oral medication.
- Carefully mix oral drugs that come in suspension form.
- Give intramuscular (IM) injections in the vastus lateralis muscle of infants who haven't started walking.
- Don't inject more than 1 ml into IM or subcutaneous (SC) sites.
- Rotate injection sites.

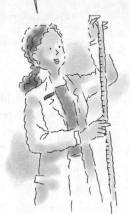

I have the height. Now I need the weight and the BSA. Will this be on the final exam?

Oral route

Infants and young children are usually given oral medication in liquid form. When a liquid preparation isn't available some tablets can be crushed and mixed with a small amount of liquid following advice from a pharmacist. However, it's important not to:
- mix crushed tablets in essential fluids, such as infant formula, because this could lead to feeding refusal
- crush enteric-coated drugs or timed-release capsules or tablets as crushing destroys the coating that causes drugs to release at the right time or prevent stomach irritation.

A spoonful of sugar

These suggestions will help to make administering medication easier for the child and the nurse:
- Allow the child as much choice as possible (for instance, which to take first or which to drink to have).
- If the medication is prepared as a suspension or as an insoluble drug in a liquid base, mix it thoroughly before you measure and administer it to ensure that none of the drug remains settled out of the solution.
- If the child can drink from a cup, measure and give liquid medications using this.
- If the child is very young or can't drink from a cup, use a syringe.
- For the infant, slowly instil liquid medication by syringe along the side of his/her tongue. Hold the infant with his/her head elevated to prevent aspiration.

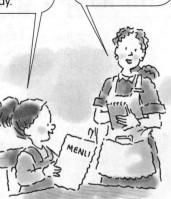

Ah, yes. I think the apple juice will go quite nicely with my paracetamol today.

Allowing choices gives the child a sense of control.

Nasal route

Administering a nasal medication to a child may not be as difficult as it sounds. Parents can also be instructed in giving nose drops and giving medication with a nasal inhaler.

Drop in the bucket?

To administer nose drops:
• Warm the medication to room temperature and warn the child that they may taste the medication.
• Draw up the proper amount of medication into the dropper.
• Have the child gently blow his/her nose if able, or clean away secretions with a tissue.
• Tilt the child's head back. (In small children, this can be accomplished by having the child lie on his/her back with a small pillow placed between the shoulders and tilting his/her head back over the top of the pillow.)
• Push up gently on the child's nose.
• Instruct the child to breathe through his/her mouth while the medication is being placed in the nose. (For infants, be sure to instil the drops in one nostril at a time because infants are obligate nose breathers.)
• Without touching the dropper to the nose, aim the dropper towards the back of the nostril and place the correct number of drops in each side of the nose.
• Keep the head tilted back for at least 1 minute (count to 60), and then allow the child to spit out any medication that has run down the back of his/her throat.

The nose knows

To give medication with a nasal inhaler:
• Place the tip of the inhaler inside the child's nostril.
• Have the child inhale; then administer the medication.
• Have the child hold his/her breath for a few seconds and then exhale through his/her mouth.
• Don't allow the child to blow his/her nose for at least 3 minutes.

Up your nose with a … sprayer

To administer a nasal spray:
• Plug one nostril and place the tip of the sprayer a short distance into the opposite nostril.
• Have the child hold his/her breath; then administer the medication.
• Tell the child to hold his/her breath for a few more seconds and then exhale through his/her mouth.
• Make sure that the child keeps his/her head tilted back for at least 1 minute, and don't allow him/her to blow his/her nose.

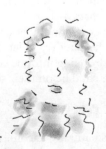

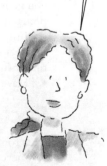

Always prepare the child and the parent for blurred vision before instilling eye ointment. Knowing what to expect makes interventions less frightening.

Optic route

The administration of eyedrops or eye ointment can be difficult for the child because of his/her natural instinct to blink. Tell the child and parents that eye ointment may cause blurred vision for a short time.

The eyes have it

To administer eyedrops or ointments:
• Clean the eye of all secretions and residual medication.
• Tilt the child's head back and have the child look at the ceiling or hold up a picture for him/her to look at.
• Using your thumb and index finger, gently pull back the lower lid to expose the conjunctival sac.
• Without touching the dropper or bottle to the eye, administer the drops into the conjunctival sac, not directly into the eye. When administering an eye ointment, apply the ointment from the inner canthus to the outer canthus of the eye.
• Have the child close his/her eyes for a few minutes; then wipe away excess ointment.
• If a second type of eyedrop or an eye ointment is required, wait 5 minutes before administering the second medication.

Eardrops

Because younger children are more prone to developing ear infections than older children, eardrops may be used. Medications that are cold may cause dizziness and nausea when placed into the ear; therefore, always warm the medication to body temperature by placing it between your hands for several minutes.

In one ear ...

To administer eardrops:
• Place the child on their side, with the affected ear facing up.
• Clean away secretions or residual medication.
• Straighten the ear canal. (In children younger than 3 years, hold the ear and gently pull down and back. In children older than 3 years, gently pull the pinna up and back.)
• Instil the correct number of drops into the ear without touching the dropper on the ear. (Try to let the drops run down the side of the canal rather than dropping into the centre of the canal.)
• Have the child lie on their side for at least 1 minute.

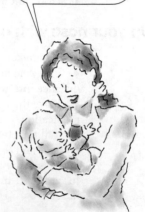

Take special care of how you hold a baby's ear when administering eardrops.

Rectal route

This route is naturally uncomfortable and embarrassing for the older child, so where possible is avoided. However, medication given rectally is absorbed fairly quickly and is useful when a child cannot be given something orally.

Rectal suppositories may be needed for a child who has been vomiting or who can't receive his/her medications orally. The rectal suppository should be firm. If it isn't, run it under cold water before unwrapping it.

How it's supposed to go

To administer a suppository:
- Remove the suppository from its wrapper.
- Assist the child to lie on his/her left side with the right knee flexed and close to his/her chest.
- Dip the suppository into water or a water-soluble lubricant such as K-Y jelly.
- Wearing gloves, gently separate the buttocks to expose the anus.
- Gently insert the smooth, rounded end of the suppository into the anal orifice.
- Push the suppository into the rectum (approximately 2.5 cm) until there's no resistance. (Use your smallest finger in a child younger than 3 years.)
- Remove your finger, ensuring that the suppository remains in place.
- Hold the child's buttocks together for 5 minutes to prevent expulsion of the medication.
- Keep the child on his/her side for approximately 20 minutes.

Nasogastric, orogastric or gastrostomy route

Administration of nasogastric (NG), orogastric (OG) and gastrostomy medications or feedings follows the same principles, and the Children's and young people's (CYP) nurse should be aware of the National Institute for Health and Clinical Excellence (NIHCE) and local guidance on undertaking these procedures. Tube placement is checked by withdrawing fluid from the tube and testing it using pH paper. It should be pH 5 or less. This is the only safe bedside test for NG tube placement. The medication or formula should be warmed to room temperature to decrease the likelihood of discomfort.

Past the lips, past the gums ...

To administer NG, OG or gastrostomy medications or feedings:
- Aspirate and measure stomach contents to determine the amount of residual stomach contents, and then return the contents to the stomach to prevent an electrolyte imbalance.
- Pinch or clamp the tubing closed to prevent air from entering the stomach.
- Remove the plunger from the barrel of the syringe and attach the barrel to the gastric tube.
- Fill the tube with the medication or formula.
- Allow the medication or formula to infuse slowly, holding the tube no more than approximately 15 cm above the stomach.
- Flush with water to clean the tubing and prevent obstruction.
- Clamp the end of the tubing when finished.

Needle and syringe selection

This chart will help you select the most appropriate needle and syringe size to use when administering medications by the intramuscular (IM) or subcutaneous (SC) route to children. Children usually require the smallest gauge possible.

Route	Needle size	Syringe size
SC	• 25G to 29G • 3¼" to 5¼"	1 ml to 3 ml
IM	• 23G to 25G • 5¼" to 1"	1 ml to 5 ml

Intramuscular and subcutaneous routes

Intramuscular (IM) and SC routes are used when medications are better absorbed outside of the gastric system; however, where possible alternative methods are used to avoid discomfort and reduce the potential for needle phobias developing. Children commonly fear needles and need lots of support when receiving parenteral medications. Unless an emergency situation a topical skin anaesthetic (such as Ametop or EMLA cream) should be applied to numb the skin. The nurse must facilitate the child to cope by explaining how he/she can help, applying ice on the injection site if necessary or teaching distraction techniques. The play therapist can be invaluable here!

Allowing the parents to hold and comfort the child may make the job easier for you, and less traumatic for the child but don't assume this as they may be just as anxious!

Always maintain the safety of the child and be prepared for him/her to jump or move around whilst you are giving the injection!

SC P's and Q's (See *Needle and syringe selection*.)

To administer an SC injection

• Select the site for administration; the typical areas used are the abdomen, the lateral and posterior aspects of the upper arm or thigh, the scapular area of the back and the upper ventrodorsal gluteal areas. (For frequent SC administration, plan rotation sites before the injections are given.)
• Clean the area with a swab.
• Grasp SC tissue between the thumb and forefinger.

- Insert the needle at a 45-degree angle. (If using a prepackaged syringe with a short needle, a 90-degree angle may be used.)
- Aspirate for blood; if none is seen, slowly inject the medication, limiting the volume to 0.5 ml.
- Withdraw the needle.

To administer an IM injection

- Select the muscle for injection. (Don't inject into the gluteus muscle until the child learns to walk, at which point the muscle will be fully developed.) (See *IM injection sites in children*, page 50.)
- Spread the skin taut between your thumb and forefinger. (In smaller children, grasp the muscle to increase muscle mass and prevent striking the bone.)
- Insert the needle at a 90-degree angle, using a quick, darting action to reduce puncture pain.
- Aspirate for blood; if none is seen, inject the medication slowly.
- Withdraw the needle quickly.

Intraosseous route

At times, venous access in a child may be a challenge. For the critically ill child in cardiac arrest or shock, the administration of fluids and medications may be lifesaving. For the child in whom venous access can't be quickly established, intraosseous infusion may be necessary. (This occurs most commonly in children younger than 5 years.) Fluids and medications that are infused into the medullary space of the long bones quickly enter the venous circulation. (See *Performing intraosseous administration*, page 51.)

The most common site for intraosseous infusion is the medial surface of the proximal tibia. Other sites include the distal tibia and the distal femur.

When the needle has been placed into the bone, fluid resuscitation should be instituted by injecting fluid under pressure via a syringe. Standard IV pumps and tubing may be used to deliver the fluids. It's important to remember that extravasation is common around the site, especially with prolonged placement and pressure infusion.

IV therapy

IV therapy is commonly used to give both fluids and medications to an ill child. Extreme caution and care must be taken in giving the prescribed amounts of fluids and medications. The rate of flow should be checked frequently, and a pump system should be used. Because extravasation of fluid or phlebitis may develop quickly, the site must be checked frequently.

Access granted

The venous system may be accessed either peripherally or centrally. After the access device is in place, the site must be kept secure and protected to provide the necessary fluids and medications.

IM injection sites in children

When selecting the best site for a child's IM injection, consider the child's age, weight and muscle development; the amount of subcutaneous fat over the injection site; the type of drug you're administering and the drug's absorption rate. Also, there should be consideration whether an alternative route such as IV can be used to reduce discomfort.

Vastus lateralis and rectus femoris

For a child younger than 3 years, you'll typically use the vastus lateralis or rectus femoris muscle for an IM injection. Constituting the largest muscle mass in this age group, the vastus lateralis and rectus femoris have fewer major blood vessels and nerves.

Ventrogluteal and dorsogluteal

For a child who can walk and is older than 3 years, use the ventrogluteal and dorsogluteal muscles. Like the vastus lateralis, the ventrogluteal site is relatively free of major blood vessels and nerves. Before you select either site, make sure that the child has been walking for at least 1 year to ensure sufficient muscle development.

Deltoid

For a child older than 18 months who needs rapid medication results, consider using the deltoid muscle. Because blood flows faster in the deltoid muscle than in other muscles, drug absorption should be faster.

Be careful if you use this site because the deltoid doesn't develop fully until adolescence. In a younger child, it's small and close to the radial nerve, which could be injured during needle insertion.

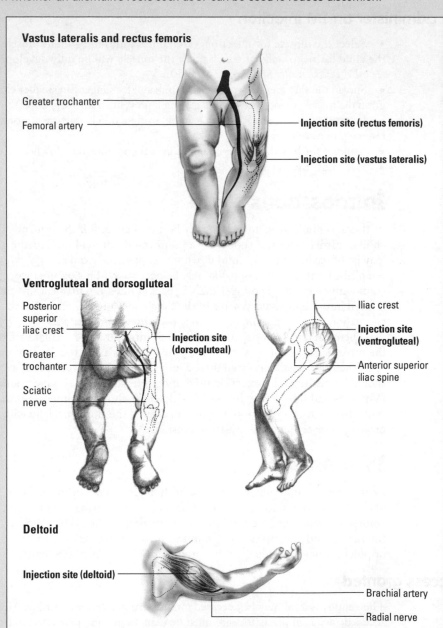

Vastus lateralis and rectus femoris

Greater trochanter

Femoral artery

Injection site (rectus femoris)

Injection site (vastus lateralis)

Ventrogluteal and dorsogluteal

Posterior superior iliac crest

Greater trochanter

Sciatic nerve

Injection site (dorsogluteal)

Iliac crest

Injection site (ventrogluteal)

Anterior superior iliac spine

Deltoid

Injection site (deltoid)

Brachial artery

Radial nerve

Performing intraosseous administration

In an emergency, intraosseous drug admin-istration may be used for a critically ill child from 5 to 6 years old. Insert a bone marrow needle (or spinal needle with stylette, trephine or standard 16G to 18G hypodermic needle) into the anteromedial surface of the proximal tibia 3¼89 to 11¼49 (1 to 3 cm) below the tibial tuberosity. To avoid the epiphyseal plate, the needle is directed at a perpendicular or slightly inferior angle.

After penetrating the bony cortex and inserting the needle into the marrow cavity, there'll be no resistance, you'll be able to aspirate bone marrow, the needle will remain upright without support and the infusion will flow freely without subcutaneous infiltration. If bone or marrow obstructs the needle, replace the needle by passing a second one through the cannula.

When the needle is properly inserted, stabilise and secure it with gauze dressing and tape. Discontinue when a secure IV line is established.

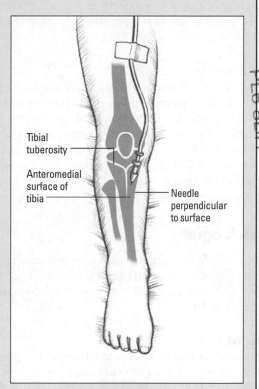

Tibial tuberosity

Anteromedial surface of tibia

Needle perpendicular to surface

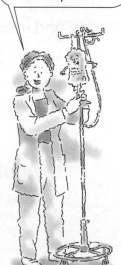

A mobile child is a happy child. Most children can become experts at getting around with an IV stand. It just takes a little teaching and some supervision.

On a short leash

The nurse must consider the sensitivity of the child's skin and limit the use of tape. The nurse should also consider the child's developmental needs, such as the desire to explore, and take steps to ensure his/her safety whilst giving as much freedom as possible after the IV is in place.

Venous access devices

Commonly used peripheral IV sites include the hands and arms; however, in some children, these might not be the most readily accessible sites.

By foot or by scalp ... we shall prevail

The feet (greater saphenous vein) or even a scalp vein in the neonate may be used. Always use the smallest needle size possible. For children, this is typically a 24G or 25G needle.

Have no fear no tourniquet here

Smaller children may be fearful of a tourniquet. In this instance, venous distention may be obtained simply by applying pressure to the area proximal to the vein.

Long-term IV therapy

Long-term IV therapy is best accomplished with a vascular access device. Such devices include infusion ports, catheters and cannulas. The type that's most appropriate in a particular situation depends on the type and length of treatment as well as the diagnosis. Children with cancer who require chemotherapy, blood transfusions, fluids and nutrition are usually given an implantable device such as a Hickman line or port. This type of device allows for frequent access to the venous system with venepuncture and multiple IV lines.

Check, check and check again

Such devices as central venous catheters also provide access for drawing blood. These catheters may remain in place for months. The nurse must check the site frequently for signs and symptoms of infection, patency, proper functioning and placement.

Infusion pumps

Infusion pumps should always be used with children. The pump doesn't depend on gravity for flow; instead, it maintains a preselected volume delivery by adding pressure to the system when necessary. If the pressure required to deliver the fluid exceeds a maximum pressure limit, an alarm sounds.

Infiltrate and irritate

Unfortunately, the use of pumps carries the danger of infiltration or vein irritation caused by the medication or solution administered under pressure. When the pump has delivered the exact volume prescribed, an alarm sounds. Many hospital policies dictate the time lapse allowed for checking the pump, the IV site and the volume of solution infused, usually this is recorded hourly.

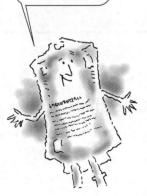

Go ahead – calculate me. It's just a matter of choosing among weight, metabolism and BSA.

Calculating children's fluid needs

Children's fluid needs are proportionally greater than those of adults, so children are more vulnerable to changes in fluid and electrolyte balance. Because their extracellular fluid has a higher percentage of water, children's fluid exchange rates are two to three times greater than those of adults, leaving them more susceptible to dehydration.

Calculation trio

Determining and meeting the fluid needs of children are important nursing responsibilities. You can calculate the number of millilitres of fluid a child needs based on:
- weight in kilograms
- metabolism (calories required)
- BSA in square metres.

Although results may vary slightly, all three methods are appropriate. Keep in mind that fluid replacement can also be affected by clinical conditions that cause fluid retention or loss. Children with these conditions should receive fluids based on their individual needs.

Fluid needs based on weight

You may use three different formulas to calculate a child's fluid needs based on his/her weight.

Fluid formula for tiny tots …

A child who weighs less than 10 kg requires 100 ml of fluid per kilogram of body weight per day.

Here's the formula:

$$\text{weight in kg} \times 100 \text{ ml/kg/day} = \text{fluid needs in ml/day}$$

… middleweights …

A child weighing 10 to 20 kg requires 1,000 ml of fluid per day for the first 10 kg plus 50 ml for every kilogram above 10. To determine this child's fluid needs, follow these steps:
- Subtract 10 kg from the child's total weight, and then multiply the result by 50 ml/kg/day to find the child's additional fluid needs. Here's the formula:

$$(\text{total kg} - 10 \text{ kg}) \times 50 \text{ ml/kg/day} = \text{additional fluid need in ml/day}$$

- Add the additional daily fluid need to the 1,000 ml/day required for the first 10 kg. The total is the child's daily fluid requirement:

$$1,000 \text{ ml/day} + \text{additional fluid need} = \text{fluid needs in ml/day.}$$

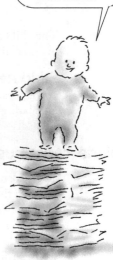

You won't need a mountain of papers to figure out my fluid needs.

… and bigger kids too

A child weighing more than 20 kg requires 1,500 ml of fluid for the first 20 kg plus 20 ml for each additional kilogram. To determine this child's fluid needs, follow these steps:
- Subtract 20 kg from the child's total weight, and then multiply the result by 20 ml/kg to find the child's additional fluid needs. Here's the formula:

$$(\text{total kg} - 20 \text{ kg}) \times 20 \text{ ml/kg/day} = \text{additional fluid need in ml/day}$$

• Because the child needs 1,500 ml of fluid per day for the first 20 kg, add the additional fluid need to 1,500 ml. The total is the child's daily fluid requirement:

1,500 ml/day + additional fluid need = fluid needs in ml/day.

Real-world problem
This problem will give you some real-world experience with calculating fluid needs based on weight.

Maintenance mystery

How much fluid should you give a 20 kg child over 24 hours to meet his/her maintenance needs?
• Subtract 10 kg from the child's weight, and multiply the result by 50 ml/kg/day to find the child's additional fluid need:

$$X = (20 \text{ kg} - 10 \text{ kg}) \times 50 \text{ ml/kg/day}$$
$$X = 10 \text{ kg} \times 50 \text{ ml/kg/day}$$
$$X = 500 \text{ ml/day additional fluid need}$$

• Next, add the additional fluid need to the 1,000 ml/day required for the first 10 kg (because the child weighs between 10 and 20 kg).

$$X = 1,000 \text{ ml/day} + 500 \text{ ml/day}$$
$$X = 1500 \text{ ml/day}$$

The child should receive 1,500 ml of fluid in 24 hours to meet his/her fluid maintenance needs.

Fluid needs based on calories
You can calculate fluid needs based on calories because water is needed for metabolism. A child should receive 120 ml of fluid for every 100 kilocalories (kcal; also called calories) of metabolism.

Calorie-conscious calculation

To calculate fluid requirements based on calorie requirements, follow these steps:
• Find the child's calorie requirements. You can take this from a table of recommended dietary allowances for children, or you can have a dietician calculate it.
• Divide the calorie requirements by 100 kcal because fluid requirements are determined for every 100 calories.
• Multiply the results by 120 ml (the amount of fluid required for every 100 kcal). Here's the formula:

$$\text{fluid requirements in ml/day} = \frac{\text{calorie requirements}}{100 \text{ kcal}} \times 120 \text{ ml}$$

Real-world problem

This problem will help sharpen your skills for calculating fluid needs based on calories. Use the information above to solve it.

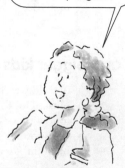

What a nice change. I'm counting calories, and it has nothing at all to do with my thighs!

Daily dilemma

Your child uses 900 cal/day. What are his/her daily fluid requirements?
• Set up the formula inserting the appropriate numbers and substituting X for the unknown amount of fluid:

$$X = \frac{900 \text{ kcal}}{100 \text{ kcal}} \times 120 \text{ ml}$$

$$X = 9 \times 120 \text{ ml}$$

$$X = 1{,}080 \text{ ml}$$

The child needs 1,080 ml of fluid per day.

Fluid needs based on BSA

Another method for determining maintenance fluid requirements is based on the child's BSA.

To calculate the daily fluid needs of a child who isn't dehydrated, multiply the BSA by 1,500, as shown in this formula:

$$\text{fluid maintenance needs in ml/day} = \text{BSA in } m^2 \times 1{,}500 \text{ ml/day/}m^2$$

Real-world problem

This problem gives you a taste of the process used to calculate fluid needs based on BSA. Use the formula above to solve it.

The child is 110 cm tall and weighs 20 kg. If his/her BSA is 0.78 m^2, how much fluid does he/she need each day?
• Set up the equation, inserting the appropriate numbers and substituting X for the unknown amount of fluid. Then solve for X:

$$X = 0.78 \text{ } m^2 \times 1{,}500 \text{ ml/day/}m^2$$
$$X = 1170 \text{ ml/day}$$

The child needs 1170 ml of fluid per day.

Quick quiz

1. While preparing to teach a class on child development, you review the works of a theorist who postulated that the personality is a structure with three parts called the id, the ego and the superego. This theorist is:
   A. Jean Piaget
   B. Erik Erikson
   C. Sigmund Freud
   D. Lawrence Kohlberg

Answer: C. Freud developed a theory that sexual energy is centred on specific parts of the body at certain ages: oral, anal and genital. He also viewed the personality as a structure with three parts: the id, ego and superego.

2. Which is the drug of choice for treating mild pain in children?
    A. Morphine
    B. Fentanyl
    C. Ibuprofen
    D. Paracetamol

Answer: D. Paracetamol is safe, even for neonates, and has the added benefit of helping reduce fever in addition to relieving mild pain. It also has few adverse effects or contraindications.

3. In an infant, which behaviour is the most common and consistent response to painful stimuli?
    A. Facial expression
    B. Vocalisation
    C. Body position
    D. Pattern of sleep

Answer: A. Facial expression may be the single best indicator of pain in an infant. Facial expressions that indicate pain include the mouth stretched open, the eyes tightly shut and grimacing.

Scoring

☆☆☆ If you answered all three items correctly, bravo! You've mastered the complex tasks in this chapter.

☆☆ If you answered two items correctly, good for you! You're on your way to a higher stage of functioning in CYP nursing.

☆ If you answered fewer than two items correctly, there's no need for a bruised ego! A second look at the chapter will be less painful.

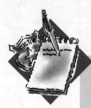

Just the facts

In this chapter, you'll learn:

♦ progression of system, physical and psychological development in infancy

♦ nutrition and sleep guidelines for infancy

♦ injury prevention strategies

♦ common infant health issues.

When reading the chapters on children's growth and development, children's and young people's (CYP) nurses should also refer to The Healthy Child Programme (DH, 2009), which emphasises the crucial periods of growth and development in childhood and identifies how every family should have access to a range of services that enable their child's well-being. The programme offers 'screening tests, immunisations, developmental reviews, and information and guidance to support parenting and healthy choices – all services that children and families need to receive if they are to achieve their optimum health and wellbeing' (DH, 2009).

The programme is based on the recommendations of the Royal College of Paediatrics and Child Health (RCPCH) reviews of child health surveillance and screening known as Health for all Children (Hall4). The programme not only enables the well-being of children but also helps to identify potential obesity issues as well as growth disorders. The role of the midwife and health visitor is crucial in supporting the health and development of the infant and so the CYP nurse should work collaboratively with a multidisciplinary team in meeting the needs of the family.

A closer look at the infant

Infancy, the period from birth to 1 year, is a time of many changes. During the first year of life, the infant progresses from a neonate, totally dependent on the world around them, to a baby who can interact and process change within his/her surroundings. Tremendous physiologic development also occurs.

System development

From birth to 1 year, remarkable changes occur in the infant's neurological, cardiovascular, respiratory and immune systems.

Neurological system

The central nervous system (CNS) is the fastest-growing system during the infancy stage, as brain cells continue to develop in both size and number. The effects of a poor environment, including nutritional deprivation, can't be reversed when experienced during this early stage.

Hold your head up!

Myelinisation refers to the development of a myelin sheath around nerve fibres. Myelin enables quick, efficient transmission of nerve impulses. Myelinisation of the neurons occurs in a cephalocaudal (head-to-toe) direction, although it takes up to 2 years for the entire process to be completed. Infants progress from being unable to hold their head up to being able to hold themselves in an upright position, sit and keep their head erect.

Extreme CNS makeover

As myelinisation reaches the extremities, the infant can put weight on his/her legs and use them to stand up. As the brain and CNS develop, more sophisticated cognitive and behavioural skills follow.

Converge, stare and search

Vision development is also tremendous. At 8 weeks, the baby is alert to moving objects and is attracted to bright colours and lighted objects, such as toys with flashing lights and an otoscope light. Convergence and following with the eyes are jerky and inexact. By ages 4 to 6 months, the baby has bifocal vision and can stare and search. By 1 year, distance vision and depth perception have markedly improved.

Cardiovascular and respiratory systems

The cardiovascular and respiratory systems undergo dramatic changes at birth. Because of placental oxygenation, the foetus shunts a majority of blood away from the lungs while in utero.

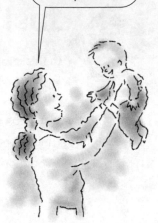

Before you know it, you'll be able to interact with others and notice the changes around you.

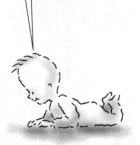

I think my neurons are starting to myelinate. Today, I hold my head up. Tomorrow, the world!

Cardiopulmonary drama

At birth, a cascade of physiological changes occur, and deoxygenated blood begins to circulate to the lungs, where it receives oxygen and is then pumped out to the rest of the body through the left ventricle of the heart. Within moments, the cardiovascular and respiratory systems are functioning at essentially the same level as those of an adult.

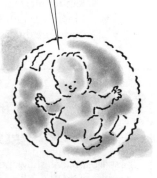

As soon as I get out of here, my heart and lungs will start to function just like my mom's!

Immune system

The immune system develops over the first year of life. The neonate depends on maternal antibodies for immunologic protection. By 6 to 8 weeks, an antigen–antibody response is present, and by 9 months, the infant is developing its own immunity.

Physical development

The physical growth and development that take place during infancy are astounding. Although patterns of growth and development will occur in a predictable order, it's important to remember that the rate at which they occur may vary among children of the same age. Also remember that the most reliable way to interpret growth measurements is to follow their trend over time.

Height, weight and head circumference

Intrauterine growth is assessed by measuring height, weight and head circumference. These parameters are also the basis of growth evaluation for the rest of childhood.

Height

Until the child is 24 months old, height, or length, is measured in the supine position, from the top of the head to the bottom of the heel. When measuring the infant, it's important to keep his/her body as straight as possible to achieve an accurate measurement.

Trunk first, legs to follow

At the end of the first year, the infant's birth length has increased by 50%, with growth of 2.5 cm per month for the first 6 months, followed by 1.3 cm per month for the second 6 months. Most of this growth occurs in the trunk rather than in the legs.

Height is the best indicator of growth failure caused by endocrine problems. For instance, short stature is typically a chief complaint in children with growth hormone deficiency or hypothyroidism.

Weight

Weight ideally is measured on an infant scale with a bucket-type area in which the infant can lie down or sit. Weight is the primary indicator of nutritional status; changes in weight can also be used to assess hydration status. The average infant will double his/her birth weight by 6 months of age, and triple it by 1 year.

Head circumference

Head circumference, or occipital frontal circumference, is measured by placing a measuring tape around the largest diameter of the head, from the frontal bone of the forehead to the occipital prominence at the back of the head.

Don't get a big head

A head circumference that's smaller, or lags behind the height and weight of an infant, may indicate inadequate brain growth. A head circumference that increases rapidly may indicate an increase in ventricular fluid and intracranial pressure (hydrocephalus). (See *Measuring height and head circumference*.)

Advice from the experts

Measuring height and head circumference

These illustrations show the correct (supine) positioning for measuring length and the proper location for measuring head circumference. Watch they don't get cold whilst measuring them!

Measuring height
Because of an infant's tendency to be flexed and curled up, these tips will help make assessing an infant's height (length) both easy and accurate:

- Using one hand, hold the infant's head in the midline position.
- Hold the knees together with your other hand and gently press them down towards the table until they're fully extended.
- Take the length measurement from the tip of the infant's head to his/her heels.

Measuring head circumference
To obtain an accurate head circumference measurement:

- Use a paper measuring tape to avoid stretching (as can happen with a cloth tape).
- Use landmarks – typically, place the tape just above the infant's eyebrows, and around the occipital prominence at the back of the head to measure the largest diameter of the head.
- Take into consideration the shape of the infant's head and make adjustments as needed to measure the largest diameter.

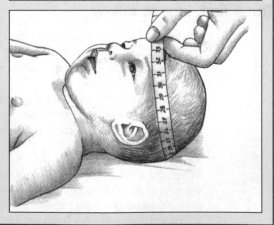

Locating the fontanelles

The locations of the anterior and posterior fontanelles are depicted in this illustration of the top of a neonatal skull.

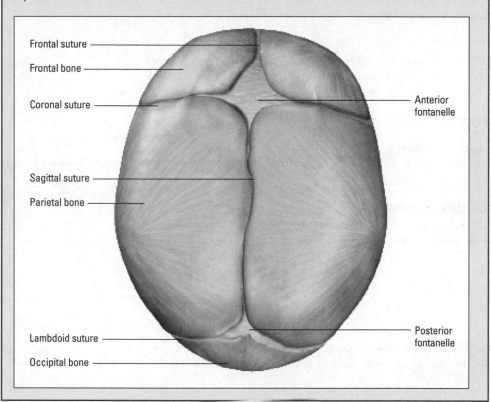

Frontal suture

Frontal bone

Coronal suture

Sagittal suture

Parietal bone

Lambdoid suture

Occipital bone

Anterior fontanelle

Posterior fontanelle

However, when measurements are plotted on a growth chart, a head circumference that persistently falls in a percentile larger than height and weight percentiles usually indicates that the baby simply has a parent with a large head.

Fontanelle changes

Fontanelles are the two openings between the bones in the neonate's skull. (See *Locating the fontanelles.*)

The anterior fontanelle is formed at the intersection of the sagittal, frontal and coronal suture lines. The average size of the anterior fontanelle is 2 cm × 2 cm at birth. It remains open for up to 18 months and gradually closes as the head grows.

The posterior fontanelle is formed at the intersection of the sagittal and lambdoid suture lines. The average size of the posterior fontanelle is 1 cm × 1 cm at birth. It's usually closed by 2 months of age.

Palpation and pulsation

In infancy, the fontanelles are assessed by palpation. The fontanelle should feel soft and flat. You may be able to see pulsations at the anterior fontanelle; this is a normal finding. A bulging or tense fontanelle may indicate increased intracranial pressure. A sunken fontanelle indicates dehydration.

Teeth

Most neonates don't have teeth. Occasionally, a 'natal tooth' will be present at birth. This tooth requires no intervention unless it's loose and poses a risk of aspiration.

A little drool, a big eruption

The average age at first tooth eruption is 8 months. Most infants start drooling and mouthing hard objects months beforehand. (See *Sequence of tooth eruption.*)

Gross motor development

Gross motor skills refer to the child's development of skills that require the use of large muscle groups. (See *Developmental milestones.*) They include:
- posture
- head control
- sitting
- crawling
- standing
- walking.

The infant will attain gross motor control in a cephalocaudal manner, progressing from the head to the toes. They can lift the head, then sit, stand and, eventually, walk.

Growing pains

Sequence of tooth eruption

A child's primary teeth will erupt in a predictable order, as described here:

Age	Tooth eruption
6 to 10 months	Central lower incisors
8 to 10 months	Central upper incisors
9 to 13 months	Lateral upper incisors
10 to 16 months	Lateral lower incisors

Growing pains

Developmental milestones

This chart shows the major gross and fine motor skills the infant should master when progressing through the first year of life.

Age	Gross motor skills	Fine motor skills
1 month	• Can hold head parallel momentarily but still has marked head lag • Back is rounded in sitting position, with no head control	• Strong grasp reflex • Hands remain mostly closed in a fist
2 months	• In prone position, can lift head 45 degrees off table • In sitting position, back is still rounded but with more head control	• Diminishing grasp reflex • Hands open more often
3 months	• Displays only slight head lag when pulled to a seated position • In prone position, can use forearms to lift head and shoulders 45 to 90 degrees off table • Can bear slight amount of weight on legs in standing position	• Grasp reflex now absent • Hands remain open • Can hold a rattle and clutch own hand
4 months	• No head lag • Holds head erect in sitting position, back less rounded • In prone position, can lift head and chest 90 degrees off table • Can roll from back to side	• Regards own hand • Can grasp objects with both hands • May try to reach for an object without success • Can move objects toward mouth
5 months	• No head lag • Holds head erect and steady when sitting • Back is straight • Can put feet to mouth when supine • Can roll from stomach to back	• Can voluntarily grasp objects • Can move objects directly to mouth
6 months	• Can lift chest and upper abdomen off table, bearing weight on hands • Can roll from back to stomach • Can bear almost all of weight on feet when held in standing position • Sits with support	• Can hold bottle • Can voluntarily grasp and release objects
7 months	• Can sit, leaning forward on hands for support • When in standing position, can bear full weight on legs and bounce	• Transfers objects from hand to hand • Rakes at objects • Can bang objects on table
8 months	• Can sit alone without assistance • Can move from sitting to kneeling position	• Has beginning pincer grasp • Reaches for objects out of reach

(continued)

Developmental milestones (continued)

Age	Gross motor skills	Fine motor skills
9 months	• Crawls on hands and knees with belly off floor • Pulls to standing position • Can stand, holding on to furniture	• Refining pincer grasp • Use of dominant hand evident
10 months	• Can move from prone to sitting position • Stands with support; may lift a foot as if to take a step	• Refining pincer grasp
11 months	• Can cruise (take side steps while holding on to furniture) or walk with both hands held	• Can move objects into containers • Deliberately drops object to have it picked up • Neat pincer grasp
12 months	• Cruises well, may walk with one hand held • May try to stand alone	• May attempt to build a two-block tower • Can crudely turn pages of a book • Feeds self with cup and spoon

Fine motor development

Fine motor skills refer to the infant's ability to use his/her hands and fingers to grasp an object. As the infant grows, he/she begins to refine fine motor skills to grab small objects and feed himself/herself.

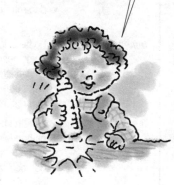

I'm 7 months old. Banging things on tables is my job.

Normal infant reflexes

All of a neonate's behaviour is controlled by reflex. At 4 to 8 weeks of age, these reflexes reach their peak – especially the sucking reflex, which affords nutrition (and, therefore, survival) and psychological pleasure.

At 3 months, the most primitive reflexes begin to disappear, except for the protective and postural reflexes (blink, parachute, cough, swallow and gag), which remain for life. (See *Infant reflexes*.)

Psychological development

Psychological development involves language development and socialisation as well as play and cognitive development.

Language development and socialisation

Language development and socialisation begin as soon as the neonate is born. Initially, the neonate communicates through crying and socialises through some of the reflexive behaviours such as the grasp reflex. However, tremendous strides are made in these areas during the first year of life.

Cry me a river

The infant cries to express needs. During the first 3 months, crying usually signals a physiological need such as hunger. As the infant grows, they may cry

Infant reflexes

This chart lists normal infant reflexes, how they're elicited and the age at which they disappear.

Reflex	How to elicit	Age at disappearance
Trunk incurvature	When a finger is run laterally down the neonate's spine, the trunk flexes and the pelvis swings towards the stimulated side.	2 months
Tonic neck (fencing position)	When the neonate's head is turned while he/she's lying supine, the extremities on the same side extend outward while those on the opposite side flex.	2 to 3 months
Grasping	When a finger is placed in each of the neonate's hands, the neonate's fingers grasp tightly enough to be pulled to a sitting position.	3 to 4 months
Rooting	When the cheek is stroked, the neonate turns his/her head in the direction of the stroke.	3 to 4 months
Moro (startle reflex)	When lifted above the crib and suddenly lowered (or in response to a loud noise), the arms and legs symmetrically extend and then abduct while the fingers spread to form a 'C'.	4 to 6 months
Sucking	Sucking motion begins when a nipple is placed in the neonate's mouth.	6 months
Babinski's	When the sole on the side of the small toe is stroked, the neonate's toes fan upward.	2 years
Stepping	When held upright with the feet touching a flat surface, the neonate exhibits dancing or stepping movements.	Variable

for attention, from fear or from frustration during the trials of mastering new skills. Parents usually become adept at translating their child's cry.

Infants who cry frequently and are difficult to console may be at increased risk of abuse. To help parents prepare for and effectively deal with crying infants, the CYP nurse should:

- reinforce that there are times when infants cry for no reason at all.
- assess how parents cope with fussy periods and offer support as needed.
- teach parents comforting techniques, such as holding, swaddling and massaging.
- help parents develop support networks.
- provide information on support groups such as Cry-sis (http://www.cry-sis.org.uk).

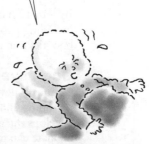

I cry, therefore I am ... expressing my needs; trying to get attention or feeling frustrated, afraid or just plain cranky.

Smile and say 'eh'

An infant's vocalisation develops from cries. By 2 months, the infant can produce single-vowel sounds, such as 'ah' and 'eh', and develops an instinctual smile. By 3 to 4 months, the infant can coo and gurgle, and develops a social smile.

The social smile is the infant's first social response; it initiates social relationships, signals the beginning of thought processes and further strengthens the bond between parent and child. At 4 months, the infant can laugh in response to his/her environment.

Stranger danger

By 6 months, the infant begins to experiment with sounds and attempts to imitate others. They can discern one face from another and exhibits stranger anxiety – being wary of strangers and clinging to or clutching parents. Separation anxiety may also develop at this period.

I'd like to buy a vowel

By 7 to 9 months, the infant can verbalise all vowels and most consonants but speaks no intelligible words. He/she'll focus intently on the mouth of someone speaking to him/her. Simple commands such as the word 'no' are understood. The infant may imitate the expressions of others, be able to play pat-a-cake and can recognise and respond to his/her own name.

Infant of few words

By ages 10 to 12 months, the infant can say about five words but understands up to 100 words by 12 months. They can wave good-bye and enjoy rhythm games. If the child experiences delays in vocalisation, they should be evaluated for hearing loss. (See *Language and social development*.)

Play

Play is an integral part of the socialisation process. From birth to 3 months, infants enjoy having their body parts touched and moved, and looking at objects with contrasting colours. They develop the ability to grasp objects and move them, so rattles are great toys at this time.

Mimicking Mommy

From 4 to 9 months, infants explore the world by using their senses: looking and touching. They tend to put everything within reach in their mouths. They enjoy being read to and will display more reciprocal play, such as talking back to and mimicking adult vocalisations.

Social butterfly

By 9 to 12 months, increased mobility allows infants to seek out new stimuli, including people, for interaction. They enjoy social games, such as peek-a-boo, tickling and swinging.

Cognitive development

Cognitive development refers to the intellectual abilities of a child – thinking, reasoning and ability to problem solve and understand. Cognitively, the infant develops the ability to perform very sophisticated mental operations. Even the neonate can process and react to stimuli in the surrounding environment.

Growing pains

Language and social development

This chart highlights the language and social development of an infant from birth to 1 year.

Age	Behaviours
0 to 2 months	• Listens to voices; quiets to soft music, singing or talking • Distinguishes mother's voice after 1 week, father's by 2 weeks • Prefers human voices to other sounds • Produces vowel sounds 'ah', 'eh' and 'oh'
3 to 4 months	• Coos and gurgles • Babbles in response to someone talking to him/her • Babbles for own pleasure with giggles, shrieks and laughs • Says 'da', 'ba', 'ma', 'pa' and 'ga' • Vocalises more to a real person than to a picture • Responds to caregiver with social smile by 3 months
5 to 6 months	• Notices how his/her speech influences actions of others • Makes 'raspberries' and smacks lips • Begins learning to take turns in conversation • Talks to toys and self in mirror • Recognises names and familiar sounds
7 to 9 months	• Tries to imitate more sounds; makes several sounds in one breath • Begins learning the meaning of 'no' by tone of voice and actions • Experiences early literacy; enjoys listening to simple books being read • Enjoys pat-a-cake • Recognises and responds to his/her name and names of familiar objects
10 to 12 months	• May have a few word approximations, such as 'bye-bye' and 'hi' • Follows one-step instructions such as 'go to daddy' • Recognises words as symbols for objects • Says 'ma-ma-ma' and 'da-da-da'

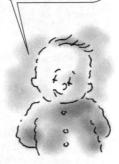

Da, ba, ma, pa, ga. That's all I've got. I'm 4 months old.

Over time, social skills are developed as well as a sense of object permanence (the realisation that objects continue to exist even when they can't be seen) and causality (understanding that a particular action, or cause, leads to an effect). (See *Cognitive development and play*, page 68.)

Trust begins to develop during this stage. Personality emerges as the infant displays the inborn characteristics that influence activity level, response to new people and situations and adaptability to change.

Growing pains

Cognitive development and play

This chart shows the infant's development of two cognitive skills, object permanence and causality. It includes play, an integral part of infant development.

Age	Object permanence	Causality	Play
0 to 4 months	• Objects out of sight are out of mind • Continues to look at hand after object is dropped out of it	• Creates bodily sensations by actions (e.g. thumbsucking)	• Grasps and moves objects such as a rattle • Looks at contrasting colours
4 to 8 months	• Can locate a partially hidden object • Visually tracks objects when dropped	• Uses causal behaviours to re-create accidentally discovered interesting effects (e.g. kicking the bed after the chance discovery that this will set in motion a mobile above the bed)	• Reaches and grasps an object and then will mouth, shake, bang and drop the object (in this order)
9 to 12 months	• Object permanence develops • Can find an object when hidden but can't retrieve an object that's moved in plain view from one hiding place to another • Knows parent still exists when out of view but can't imagine where they might be (separation anxiety may arise)	• Understanding of cause and effect leads to intentional behaviour aimed at getting specific results	• Manipulates objects to inspect with eyes and hands • Has ability to process information simultaneously instead of sequentially • Ability to play peek-a-boo demonstrates object permanence

This doesn't taste too bad – perhaps some food when I am older.

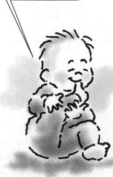

On stage with Piaget

According to Jean Piaget's stages of early cognitive development, infants are in the sensorimotor stage, which lasts from birth to 2 years. In this stage, infants are discovering relationships between their bodies and the environment. They rely on their senses to learn about the world around them, and they learn that the external world isn't an extension of themselves.

Maintaining health

Keeping an infant healthy involves:
• providing proper nutrition
• ensuring adequate sleep and rest
• providing dental hygiene.

Nutrition guidelines

Breast milk is recommended for the first 12 months of life. Human milk consumed through breastfeeding is considered optimal for neonates. Even so, not all mothers can or choose to breastfeed. Medical conditions, cultural background, anxiety, use of certain medications, substance misuse and other factors can prevent a woman from breastfeeding. Breast milk can be expressed and given via a bottle as an alternative. If feeding with breast or expressed milk is not possible then bottlefeeding with infant formula is an acceptable alternative.

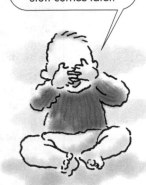

I can't see my mum, but I know she still exists. Where did she go? Hey, I'm only 9 months old – that stuff comes later.

Breast is best!

Breastfeeding is widely supported as the best start for the infant! The global 'Baby-Friendly Hospital Initiative' is a programme by UNICEF and the WHO to encourage the support for breastfeeding in all maternity units across the world and has been adopted by the UK Department of Health! Breastfeeding is recommended exclusively for the first 6 months, and then in combination with infant foods until age 1 year. (See *Advantages of breastfeeding*.)

I demand my 10 to 15!

How long a breastfed infant nurses at each feeding is very individual. In general, a neonate should nurse on demand, approximately 8 to 10 times per day for at least 10 to 15 minutes at each breast. The duration of feeding may increase and the frequency may decrease as the infant gets older and after solid foods are introduced.

Advantages of breastfeeding

It's a well-known fact that breastfeeding is best for an infant. Here are some of the reasons.

Passive immunity
Human milk provides passive immunity to the infant. *Colostrum* is the first fluid secreted from the breast (within the first few days after delivery) and provides immune factor and protein to the neonate. Many components of breast milk protect against infection – it contains antibodies (especially immunoglobulin A) and white blood cells that protect the infant from some forms of infection. Breastfed babies also experience fewer allergies and food intolerances.

Digestibility
Breast milk provides essential nutrients in an easily digestible form. It contains *lipase,* which breaks down dietary fat, making it easily available to the infant's system.

Brain development
The lipids in breast milk are high in linoleic acid and cholesterol, which are needed for brain development.

Low protein content
Cow's milk contains proportionally higher concentrations of electrolytes and protein than are needed by human infants. It must be cleared by the immature kidneys and thus isn't recommended until a baby is at least 12 months old.

Convenient and cost-free
The woman who breastfeeds saves the money and time that would be needed to buy and prepare formula.

It's all relative

Tips for preparing formula

Provide parents with these tips for properly preparing infant formula:

- Wash your hands before preparing formula.
- Boil water for 1 to 2 minutes, and then let it cool. Do not reboil.
- Wash utensils in warm, soapy water and rinse them well to ensure they're safe to use. Sterilise them between uses. Also, keep separate utensils for preparation.
- Avoid using microwave ovens; they fail to sterilise utensils and cause uneven heating, which increases the risk of burns.
- Discard a prepared bottle of formula after it's been offered to the infant or has sat at room temperature for longer than 1 hour.
- Cover and store opened liquid formula in the refrigerator; discard after 48 hours.

Parents should be assured that they can feel confident that their infant is receiving enough breast milk if he/she's growing appropriately. Keep in mind that intake is adequate if:
- weight loss after birth is normal (less than 10% of birth weight).
- there's a minimum weight gain of 15 g in the first 2 weeks of life.
- the infant has six to eight wet nappies or more per day.
- the infant regains the weight lost after birth by 2 weeks of age.

Formula feeding

Formula feeds can provide adequate nutrition when the mother shouldn't or can't breastfeed her infant. Some mothers may feel guilty about being unable to breastfeed or about making the decision not to breastfeed. The CYP nurse should support, and never judge, the mother who can't or who chooses not to breastfeed and should reassure her about the nutritional value of infant formulas.

Infant formulas are constituted to provide the proper variety and amount of carbohydrates, protein, fats and micronutrients needed for healthy growth and development. The composition and labelling of infant formula is tightly controlled to ensure infant safety. (See *Tips for preparing formula*.)

No moo cows, please

Women are strongly urged to use commercially prepared formulas rather than regular cow's milk because cow's milk:
- doesn't meet all of an infant's nutritional needs
- can be difficult to digest

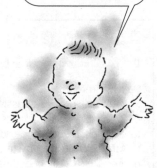

Oops! I think that was nappy number seven. I'm definitely getting enough breast milk.

- can strain the infant's renal system
- may increase the chance of allergies.

Unlocking the secret formula

Most formulas are based on cow's milk proteins, although preparations based on soy proteins and casein hydroxylate are available for infants who can't tolerate cow's milk–based preparations. There are also special formulas for infants with conditions such as phenylketonuria and other metabolic disorders.

Formula comes in powder form or premixed, ready-to-feed. Ready-to-feed formulas are convenient and prevent problems based on incorrect dilution and preparation but are more expensive.

Special care should be used so that formula is properly mixed or stored, to prevent harm to the infant.

Weaning

The Department of Health recommends that infants be weaned from the bottle to the cup by age 1 year. In preparation for weaning, and to promote the developmental step towards independent feeding, the cup should be introduced by 9 months in all infants. This is usually done gradually, by omitting one bottle at a time and replacing it with a cup over a period of several days to weeks.

Slow and steady to bottle-ready

How long a mother continues to breastfeed is an individual choice; however, there may be concrete reasons for weaning an infant from the breast to the bottle, such as a mother's return to work or severe illness. In such cases, the switch from breast to bottle is accomplished similarly to the weaning from bottle to cup. One breastfeeding session per day is replaced with a bottlefeeding until, over a period of days to weeks, the transition occurs.

This gradual weaning approach helps prevent engorgement in the mother and decreases her risk of mastitis. An infant can also be weaned from breastfeeding to a cup, eliminating the need for bottles.

Through these changes the mother should receive help and support so that she can effectively express her breast milk ready for the infant to then bottle feed on.

Introducing solid foods

Weaning should not usually commence before 6 months of age as before this the infants digestive system is too immature.

Rice is nice

Baby rice or other non-wheat–based grain mixed with breast or formula milk and offered to the infant once per day to start with. Pureed vegetables are another alternative. (See *Solid foods and infant age*, page 72.)

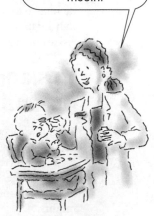

When an infant reaches 6 months of age, you can start feeding him/her a cereal mix. The trick is getting it in his/her mouth!

Solid foods and infant age

This table gives an overview of solid foods that are appropriate for the developing infant.

Age	Type of food	Rationale
4 months	Rice cereal mixed with breast milk or formula	Less likely than wheat to cause an allergic reaction
5 to 6 months	Pureed vegetables (offered first) and fruits	Vegetable offered first because they may be more readily accepted than if introduced after sweet fruits
7 to 8 months	Pureed meats, cheese, yogurt, rice, noodles, pudding	Provide an important source of iron and add variety to the diet
8 to 9 months	Finger foods (bananas)	Promote self-feeding
10 months	Mashed egg yolk (no whites until age 1); bite-size cooked food (no foods that may cause choking)	Use of bite-size pieces to decrease risk of choking (Avoiding foods that may cause choking is the safest option, even though the infant chews well.)
12 months	Foods from the adult table (chopped or mashed according to the infant's ability to chew foods)	Provides a nutritious and varied diet that should meet the infant's nutritional needs

Fingers before forks

By about 8 or 9 months, the infant should be able to sit up and grasp objects, so introducing finger foods at this time can help promote self-feeding. (See *Teaching points for feeding and nutrition.*)

Sleep and rest guidelines

The Department of Health, in common with other health organisations around the world recommend that all infants be positioned on their backs for sleep until they can roll over and determine their own sleeping position. Since its inception, this simple manoeuvre has significantly decreased the incidence of sudden infant death syndrome (SIDS). It is also recommended that infants are not put to sleep in the bed with parents as this increases the risk of inadvertent smothering.

To sleep, per chance to … wake up and eat!

Certain expectations for sleeping through the night can be made for each age group in infancy:
• From birth to 4 months, an infant will wake to feed at night from zero to three times. Because breast milk is digested faster than formula, breastfed infants commonly will wake up to feed more frequently than bottlefed infants.

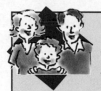

It's all relative

Teaching points for feeding and nutrition

Stress these feeding and nutrition points to the parents of an infant:

- Watch for behaviours that indicate feeding preferences. If the infant rejects a food initially, offer it again later.
- Keep the infant in an upright feeding position.
- Don't try to make the infant eat more to finish the serving or portion.
- Initially, offer iron-fortified rice cereal. Avoid wheat-based cereals for the first year.
- Introduce new foods one at a time, waiting 5 to 7 days between them.
- Avoid grapes and grape halves, until the infant has adequate chewing and swallowing skills.
- Avoid nuts
- Give regular, not sweetened, fruit juices.
- If the infant has a history of food allergies, delay offering eggs, wheat-based products and citrus fruits.
- Avoid honey, syrup and other unpasteurised products.

- From 4 to 6 months, infants are physiologically capable of sleeping (without feeding) for 6 to 8 hours at night. Infants may awaken during this sleep period but should be able to calm themselves and return to sleep. (See *Sleep requirements in infancy*.)

Napping

From birth to 3 months, infants may take many naps per day. However, an infant shouldn't be allowed to sleep longer than 4 hours at a time during the day, because this may lead to disrupted night sleeping and waking for more feeds.

From 4 to 9 months, the infant will have about two naps per day (one in the morning and one in the afternoon). Total naptime should add up to about 2 to 3 hours. By 9 to 12 months, most infants will have only one nap in the afternoon, for a total of 1 to 2 hours of napping time.

Dental hygiene

Gentle care can be given to the infant's gums and new teeth. Wiping the teeth and gums with a soft cloth and water alone provides adequate cleaning when the infant has only a few teeth.

Hold the paste

Once seven or eight teeth have erupted, they can be cleaned with a small, soft-bristled toothbrush and water. Toothpaste shouldn't be used, because the

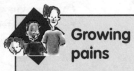

Growing pains

Sleep requirements in infancy

This chart shows the amount of sleep per 24 hours (including nighttime and naps) needed by infants from 1 week to 12 months.

Age	Hours of sleep per day
1 week	$16\tfrac{1}{42}$
1 month	$15\tfrac{1}{42}$
3 months	15
6 months	$14\tfrac{1}{42}$
9 months	14
12 months	$13\tfrac{3}{44}$

infant would swallow it. Ingesting fluoridated toothpaste can cause nausea and fluorosis, a grey discolouration of the permanent teeth.

Visits to the dentist can begin between 1 and 2 years. Although in most areas of the UK the water supply contains sufficient fluoride, supplements may be needed.

Preventing dental caries during infancy

To keep an infant's smile healthy, teach the parents how to avoid dental caries, with these tips:
- Don't put an infant to bed with a bottle either at night or naptime because pooling of sweet milk or other sweetened liquid around the infant's teeth can cause decay.
- Avoid fizzy drinks, fruit squashes, tea, coffee or drinks with artificial sweeteners.
- Don't allow the infant to carry a bottle filled with milk, formula, juice or other sweetened liquid to use as a pacifier throughout the day. Again, pooling around the teeth can occur, leading to decay. Bottles that contain milk or a liquid other than water should be offered only at mealtimes.
- Transition the infant to a cup around the time of his/her first birthday. Cup drinking doesn't permit pooling of liquids around the teeth.
- Don't offer the infant a dummy dipped in sugar or honey.
- Provide regular care of the infant's teeth and gums.

While pooling in here is fun, pooling around the teeth is no laughing matter.

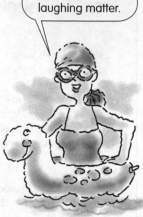

Injury prevention

Injury prevention during infancy is based on preventing aspiration and falls, and childproofing the infant's environment. This should be the basis for safeguarding children until they are old enough to be aware of any potential risks.

Aspiration

Because infants become adept at placing objects in their mouths for exploration, they're at risk for aspiration. To prevent aspiration:
- Feed infants in a slightly upright position.
- Burp infants in an upright or prone position.
- Cut solid foods into very small pieces when the infant starts eating solids.
- Avoid foods and other things that can be choking hazards. (See *Choking hazards*.)

Falls

Even a neonate is at risk for falling. As the child becomes mobile, the risk of falls increases. To prevent falls, encourage parents to:
- never leave an infant unattended, especially on a changing table, bed, sofa or counter

Choking hazards

These foods can easily cause choking and should be avoided during infancy:

- nuts
- popcorn
- hard sweets
- ice cubes
- grapes
- uncooked vegetable chunks

- ensure that cot sides are raised and locked in place
- place gates at the top and bottom of staircases
- put up window guards, if needed
- avoid placing infants in walkers because they can tumble over an uneven surface or the leg of a chair or table, or fall down stairs.

Childproofing

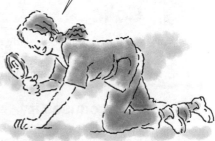

Here's a great strategy for childproofing. Get down on your hands and knees, crawl around a bit and see how much trouble you could get into!

After an infant is mobile, the risk for falls and injuries increases so childproofing takes on many dimensions! Here are some tips for childproofing, based on the infant's age.

At birth
- Turn down the thermostat on the water heater to 120° F (48.9° C) or lower. (See *Dangers of high temperature water*.)
- Add hot water to cold when pouring baths.
- To prevent an accidental scalding burn, never drink hot liquids while holding the infant.
- To prevent drowning, never leave the infant alone in the bath.
- Install smoke detectors.
- Install a carbon monoxide monitor outside the infant's room.
- Use flame-retardant night clothes.

From 4 months
- Cover all electrical outlets.
- Tape down all electrical cords (or place them behind furniture).
- Install childproof locks on all cabinets.
- Place all medicines and cleaning agents in high cabinets with locks.
- Remove all breakable items from tabletops and shelves within the infant's reach.
- Keep small toys and other small items off the floor.
- Keep hot drinks away from the edges of tables.
- Place gates into the danger areas such as kitchens.

Dangers of high temperature water

Teach the parents to cool it – the water heater thermostat, that is!

When the hot water temperature is set at 150° F (65.6° C), it takes only 2 seconds of exposure for an adult to suffer a full-thickness burn. Because infants have thin skin, it takes even less time for them to suffer a full-thickness burn.

By turning the water temperature down to a maximum of 120° F (48.9° C), parents can drastically reduce the risk of injury; at 120° F, it takes 10 minutes for a burn to occur.

Always run cold water first, add hot to raise the temperature.

Health problems

Health concerns during infancy include:
- colic
- faltering growth (FG)
- regurgitation
- SIDS.

Colic

Colic is defined as a daily period of crying for 3 hours or longer, during which the infant is virtually inconsolable. These episodes usually occur in the late afternoon or evening. About 10% to 20% of infants suffer from colic.

What causes it

No one knows for sure what causes this behaviour, but some possible causes include swallowing air from bottlefeedings and reactions to some foods.

How it happens

Although long thought to be related to the gastrointestinal (GI) tract, current theories about the origins of colic lean towards CNS maturation. The process of CNS maturation can cause intestinal spasms and pain as well as difficulties with the infant's ability to self-regulate (especially relating to overstimulation and an inability to self-calm).

What to look for

An infant is likely to have colic if they:
- cry and are inconsolable
- fail to calm in response to normal calming manoeuvres (holding, rocking)
- aren't hungry (refuses the breast or bottle)
- don't need changing (has a dry nappy)
- have no fever or other medical reason for crying.

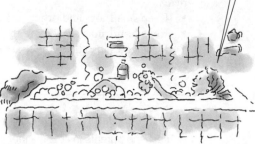

A warm bath can be very soothing. It works for an infant with colic, too!

Complications

Colic produces no complications unless a caregiver gets so frustrated that he/she harms the infant. Crying infants who are perceived to be difficult to care for may be at increased risk of harm.

How it's treated

No tests exist to help diagnose colic, and there's no medical cure for colic, except time. Most infants 'outgrow' it or sufficiently mature so that symptoms disappear or markedly improve by age 3 months.

What to do

Because this can be an incredibly stressful issue for parents and for some may lead to harming of the infant, the CYP nurse should make every effort to help parents deal effectively with an infant with colic.

Decreasing rapidly changing stimulation seems to be the most effective intervention for an infant with colic. Any strategy might work, but the key is to keep the stimulation consistent for at least 5 minutes so the infant can adjust to it. Rapidly trying different 'fixes' only increases stimulation and makes matters worse. (See *Tips for reducing colic*.)

When all else fails and parents are at their wits' end, suggest that they place the infant on their back in the bassinet or cot and leave the room. The infant will eventually fall asleep. The use of a baby monitor can help to alleviate parent's worries about leaving the infant for a short time, but the breathing space this gives can help avoid harm.

Faltering growth

FG (previously known as failure to thrive) is diagnosed when an infant isn't growing at the expected rate. FG is characterised by failure to maintain weight (and sometimes height) above the fifth percentile on age-appropriate growth charts. It can also be detected from a deviation in an already established growth curve.

What causes it

FG is divided into three types, according to cause:
• Organic FG results from an acute or chronic illness, such as GI reflux, malabsorption syndrome, congenital heart defects or cystic fibrosis.
• Nonorganic FG results from a psychological problem between the infant and the primary caregiver, such as failure to bond.
• Mixed FG results from a combination of organic and nonorganic causes.

How it happens

If caloric intake is less than that required for nutritional needs, growth and development suffer. The pathophysiology of organic FG depends on the physiologic disorder that's present.

Nonorganic and mixed FG represent a complex dynamic between parent and child. The parent may feel little emotional attachment to the child or may offer insufficient food. The child may sense parental detachment. In some cases, the child may inadvertently contribute to FG by being irritable, fussy or colicky.

What to look for

An absence of weight gain or a loss of weight is the first growth parameter to be affected; a drop in height percentile is the next sign, followed by a drop in head circumference. A drop in percentile over time or between visits warrants further investigation.

It's all relative

Tips for reducing colic

Providing parents with these tips may help them relieve their infant's colic behaviour.

Provide rhythmic movement

• Front-carrying sling
• Infant swing
• Car ride in approved safety seat
• Walking with the infant on your shoulder

Try alternative positioning

• Swaddling
• Prone position over parent's knees

Reduce environmental stimuli

• Quiet, soothing music
• No sudden, loud noises
• No smoking

Provide tactile stimuli

• Pacifier
• Warm bath
• Massage

The infant may exhibit altered body posture, may be stiff or floppy and may not cuddle. The infant may also be reluctant to smile or vocalise. History may reveal insufficient stimulation and inadequate parental knowledge of child development as well as inadequate feeding techniques, such as bottle propping and insufficient winding.

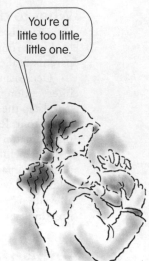

You're a little too little, little one.

What tests tell you
No definitive tests for FG exist. However, after taking a history and performing a comprehensive examination, it should be possible to determine whether medical causes are a possibility particularly Turner's syndrome or growth hormone deficiency.

Complications
Complications of FG can include developmental delay, growth retardation, impaired bonding and altered family relationships.

How it's treated
If a pathologic cause is determined, treatment focuses on the underlying disease process. If the cause is determined to be environmental, treatment is directed towards changing the surroundings. A change in the infant's environment might be as drastic as removing him/her from the home, or as simple as educating a caregiver on proper mixing of formula or reading the infant's cues more accurately.

What to do
When providing care to an infant with FG, the nurse should:
• weigh the child on admission to determine baseline weight and continue to weigh daily during treatment
• properly feed and interact with the child to promote nutrition and growth and development
• record weight and height on the appropriate centile chart
• provide the infant with visual and auditory stimulation to promote normal sensory development
• assess interaction between the parent and infant to determine whether FG is caused by the parent's inability to form an emotional attachment to the child
• teach the parents effective parenting skills to increase their knowledge of routine child care practices, such as comfort measures, age-appropriate developmental tasks and play activities
• praise the parents for positive interactions with the infant, and avoid judgemental statements and actions.

Posseting
Posseting, also referred to as regurgitation, is considered normal infant behaviour. Most infants will regurgitate at some time.

What causes it

Regurgitation in infants is most commonly caused by swallowing air or by overfeeding. However, it can also be caused by gastro-oesophageal reflux disease or pyloric stenosis.

How it happens

A posset involves either dribbling of undigested liquids from the mouth and oesophagus, or the expulsion of those liquids with the force of a burp.

What to look for

Regurgitation in infancy may be characterised by:
• white, curdled liquid plopping or running out of the corners of the mouth or, occasionally, coming from the nose
• a 'burp' of air that sometimes precedes the regurgitation
• projectile regurgitation that may land a few feet away from the infant.
The infant with regurgitation may:
• be fussy during feedings
• grimace, cry and pull away from the bottle or breast
• occasionally refuse to eat.

What tests tell you

Testing can rule out gastro-oesophageal reflux disease and pyloric stenosis, two common causes of regurgitation in infants.

Probing the problem

The definitive test for gastro-oesophageal reflux is called a pH probe. Because the pH of the stomach is so acidic (ph of 1 to 3), a probe placed in the oesophagus will demonstrate the presence of stomach acid if reflux is present.

Slow stomach

If pyloric stenosis is suspected then a test feed may be performed when the surgeon observes the infant taking the feed, palpates the abdomen for a swelling around the pyloric area and observes for visible peristalsis and how vomiting occurs. With pyloric stenosis vomiting is often forceful and projectile. An ultrasound of the area may demonstrate delayed or slowed stomach emptying, a thickened sphincter or complete closure of the sphincter.

Complications

Complications may include aspiration pneumonia, bronchiolitis, malnutrition or electrolyte imbalances.

How it's treated

If an infant is growing well, is generally happy and isn't bothered by posseting, regurgitation can be left to improve with time.

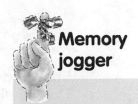

Memory jogger

When caring for an infant with regurgitation, remember to *BERP* him/her:

B – Burp the infant frequently
E – Evaluate feeding
R – Reassure parents that the condition will improve with time
P – Prevent aspiration.

If the infant isn't growing well, is refusing to feed, is unhappy or has been diagnosed with gastro-oesophageal reflux or pyloric stenosis, drug therapy or even surgery may be necessary.

What to do

When providing care to an infant with regurgitation:
• Evaluate feeding methods (amount of burping, air in nipple).
• Prevent aspiration by positioning the child on his/her side; maintain a patent airway.
• Wind the infant frequently; feed smaller amounts more frequently and don't overfeed.
• Reassure caregivers that posseting may improve with time. (The more time the infant spends in an upright position after feeding, the better the food will stay down.)

Sudden infant death syndrome

SIDS is the sudden death of a previously healthy infant when the cause of death isn't confirmed by a post-mortem examination. It is more likely to occur between 1 month and 1 year. However, the incidence of SIDS has declined dramatically by more than 40% since 1992, which is mostly attributed to the 1992 initiative to put babies on their backs, called the 'Back to Sleep Campaign'.

What causes it

Although the exact cause of SIDS is unknown, many factors have been shown to be associated with an increased risk of SIDS. (See *Risk factors for SIDS*.)

How it happens

Current theories focus on neurological immaturity related to the infant's inability to sense and regulate oxygenation status, ultimately leading to

---

Risk factors for SIDS

Risk factors for sudden infant death syndrome (SIDS) may be related to the infant (and his/her environment) or to the infant's mother.

Infant risk factors

• Prematurity
• Low birth weight
• Twin or triplet
• Male gender
• Aged between 2 and 4 months
• Winter months
• Passive smoke exposure
• History of respiratory compromise
• History of a sibling who died of SIDS

Maternal risk factors

• Maternal age below 20 years
• Smoking or illicit drug use
• Anaemia
• Multiple pregnancies with short intervals between them
• Low socioeconomic status, crowded living conditions
• Poor antenatal care and limited weight gain during pregnancy

respiratory arrest. The syndrome can't be prevented or explained; the infant usually dies during sleep without noise or struggle.

What to look for
When an infant dies of SIDS, evaluation may reveal history of:
- low birth weight
- sibling who died of SIDS.

What tests tell you
Post-mortem findings may show pulmonary oedema, intrathoracic petechiae and other minor changes suggesting chronic hypoxia.

Complications
Sudden death is the sole medical complication of SIDS. However, SIDS affects the family members of the infant who dies of SIDS.

Parents (and other caregivers) commonly have feelings of extreme guilt. This guilt can make the grieving process even more difficult and can sometimes lead to one parent blaming the other for the infant's death.

Parents may need counselling or some other form of help to cope with their loss and keep their relationship intact.

How it's treated
There is, of course, no way to treat a condition that, by its definition, is sudden death without warning. There are, however, measures that can be taken to prevent SIDS, including:
- putting the infant on his/her back to sleep
- not smoking anywhere near an infant
- removing pillows, quilts, stuffed toys or any other soft surfaces that may trap exhaled air from the infant's cot or sleeping environment
- using a firm mattress with a snug-fitting sheet
- making sure that the infant's head remains uncovered while sleeping
- keeping the infant warm while sleeping, but not overheated
- not allowing the infant to sleep in bed with parents.

What to do
When dealing with a family whose infant has just died of SIDS:
- Be aware that assessment, planning and implementation related to the parents' needs should begin as soon as they arrive in the emergency department.
- Provide the family with a room (for privacy) and a staff member who can stay with them.
- Stay calm and let the parents express their feelings. (In their need to blame someone or something for the tragedy, they may express anger at emergency department personnel, each other or anyone involved with the infant's care.)

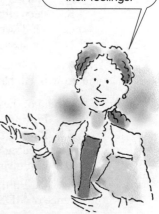

It's important to let the family of an infant who has died of SIDS express their feelings.

- Prepare the family for how the infant will look and feel.
- Explain to the family what will happen next.
  - Involvement of the Coroner or Procurator Fiscal in Scotland
  - Involvement of Police/Social Worker/Paediatrician in a multiagency assessment required for all sudden or unexplained child deaths
- Let the parents touch, hold and rock the infant, if desired. Allow them to say good-bye.
- Contact spiritual advisors, significant others, support systems and the local SIDS organisation.
- Provide literature on SIDS and support groups.

Quick quiz

1. A social milestone that infants should acquire by 2 to 3 months is:
    A. grasping at objects
    B. smiling
    C. vocalising 'mama'
    D. stranger anxiety

Answer: B. Smiling is a social communication milestone that should be reached by 2 to 3 months.

2. Which finger food is appropriate for an 8-month-old infant?
    A. Grapes
    B. Uncooked carrot sliced
    C. Banana
    D. Mixed nuts

Answer: C. Infants are developmentally ready to eat some solids by age 6 months, when they can maintain their posture in an upright position to decrease the risk of choking. Bananas are good because they are mushy and nice for the infant to mess with!

3. An infant is receiving enough formula or breast milk if they:
    A. don't cry after feeding
    B. sleep all night
    C. winds well
    D. has six to eight wet nappies or more per day

Answer: D. Infants receiving adequate formula or breast milk for hydration and growth will have six to eight wet nappies daily.

4. Which of these interventions decreases the risk of SIDS?
    A. Putting an infant on his/her back to sleep
    B. Raising the head of the cot
    C. Feeding the infant in an upright position
    D. Not giving a bottle in bed at night

Answer: A. Putting the infant on his/her back to sleep has decreased the prevalence of SIDS and will decrease the individual infant's risk as well.

Scoring

☆☆☆ If you answered all four items correctly, terrific! You've developed a strong sense of infant development.

☆☆ If you answered three items correctly, good job! Treat yourself to a play break and then read on.

☆ If you answered fewer than three items correctly, don't cry over spilled milk! Take a nap and review the chapter again.

Early childhood

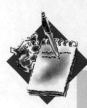

Just the facts

In this chapter, you'll learn:
- physical, psychological and cognitive development of toddlers
- developmental theories in the toddler and preschool years
- common concerns of parents of toddlers and preschoolers
- injury prevention for toddlers and preschoolers
- health problems of toddlers and preschoolers.

Toddlerhood

'Toddlerhood', from 1 to 3 years, is the stage in which children start displaying independence and pride in their accomplishments. They intensely explore their environment, trying to figure out how things work. It's also the time when they begin to display negative behaviour and have temper tantrums.

Physical development

During the toddler stage, physical growth is characterised by:
- growth rate that slows during the second year of life
- possible limited food intake, which may concern parents
- steady growth on a growth curve that's more step-like than linear, demonstrating growth 'spurts'.

Height, weight and head circumference

From 1 to 2 years:
- toddlers grow approximately 9 to 12.5 cm per year (with growth mostly in the legs, rather than in the trunk, like infants)

> The 'terrible two's' don't have to be terrible. 'No' may be a toddler's favourite word, but he'll also take pride in every little accomplishment.

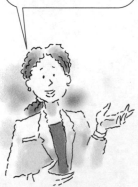

- toddlers gain about 227 g per month
- head circumference increases about 2.5 cm per year
- anterior fontanelle usually closes (between 12 and 18 months).

Two's take off

By age 2:
- birth weight has usually quadrupled; average weight is 12.3 kg
- head circumference is usually equal to chest circumference
- the child is about half of adult height, with an average height of 86.4 cm.

Three's relax

From ages 2 to 3, toddlers:
- grow 5 to 6.5 cm
- gain about 1.5 to 2.5 kg
- show slowed increases in head circumference 1.3 cm per year.

Teeth

By approximately 33 months, all deciduous teeth have erupted and the child has about 20 teeth. The child should already be brushing with a small, soft-bristled toothbrush (with parental supervision), and may use fluoride toothpaste or, if needed, fluoride supplements.

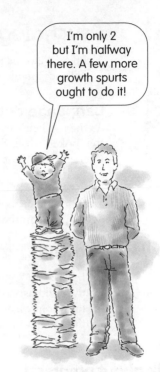

I'm only 2 but I'm halfway there. A few more growth spurts ought to do it!

Gross motor development

Gross motor activity develops rapidly in toddlers. 1-year-olds can:
- walk alone using a wide stance
- begin to run but fall easily.
  By 2 years, the toddler can:
- run without falling most of the time
- throw a ball overhand without losing their balance
- jump with both feet
- walk up and down stairs
- use push and pull toys.

Fine motor development

Fine motor development begins slowly; however, by 2 years the toddler has generally mastered some fairly complex fine motor skills.
  A 1-year-old can:
- grasp a very small object (but can't release it until about 15 months).
  A 2-year-old can:
- build a tower of four blocks
- scribble on paper
- drop a small object into a small, narrow container
- use a spoon well and drink well from a covered cup
- undress themselves.

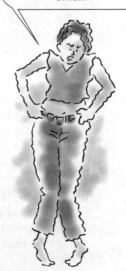

A toddler can undress themself, so what's my problem? I guess 2-year-olds are *too* smart *to* wear jeans that are *two* sizes *too* small.

Psychological development

A child develops a more elaborate vocabulary, a sense of autonomy and socially acceptable play skills during the toddler stage.

Language development and socialisation

As the toddler learns to understand and, ultimately, communicate with the spoken word, they develop the social skills that allow more effective interaction with others.

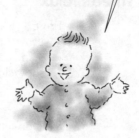

Foo, da-da, po-po, moop. Hey, I'm only 1. If you got 25% of that, I'm right on target.

Language

During toddlerhood, the ability to understand speech is much more developed than the ability to speak.

Now we're talking

By 1 year:
• the child uses one-word sentences or holophrases (real words that are meant to represent entire phrases or ideas)
• the toddler has learned about four words
• 25% of the 1-year-olds' vocalisation is understandable.

Talk about progress!

By 2 years:
• the number of words learned has increased from about four (at 1 year) to approximately 300
• the child uses multiword (two to three words) sentences
• 65% of speech is understandable
• frequent, repetitive naming of objects helps toddlers to learn appropriate words for objects.

Socialisation

During toddlerhood, children develop social skills that determine the way they interact with others. As the toddler develops psychologically, he can:
• differentiate himself from others
• tolerate being separated from a parent
• withstand delayed gratification
• control his bodily functions
• acquire socially acceptable behaviours
• communicate verbally
• become less egocentric.

Erikson's developmental theory

As discussed in Chapter 2, Erikson believed that each developmental stage is characterised by a particular psychosocial crisis (positive versus negative) that must be resolved before the child can master the task at-hand.

Putting the 'no' in autonomous

According to Erikson's developmental theory, autonomy versus doubt and shame is the developmental task of toddlerhood. In this context, Erikson maintains that:

• toddlers are in the final stages of developing a sense of trust (the task from infancy), and are ready to start asserting some control, independence and autonomy.

• negativism is displayed in the toddler's quest for autonomy.

• ritualism, a need to maintain sameness and reliability, gives the toddler a sense of comfort.

• the child's significant other is the 'paternal' person in his (or her) life.

• development of the ego creates a conflict for the child; specifically, how to deal with the impulses of the id (which requires immediate gratification), while learning socially acceptable ways to interact with the environment.

• development of the superego, or conscience, begins with the incorporation of the morals of society. (See *Toddler development*.)

Play

Play is the work of children. It's through play that the children learn about their capabilities and develop the skills needed to interact with others and their environment.

New rules, new game

During the toddler stage:

• Play changes considerably as the toddler's motor skills develop; physical skills are used to push and pull objects; to climb up, down, in, and out and to run or ride on toys.

• A short attention span requires frequent changes in toys and play media.

• Toddlers increase their cognitive abilities by manipulating objects and learning about their qualities, which makes tactile play (with water, sand, finger paints, clay) important. (See *Toddler toys*, page 88.)

• Many play activities involve imitating behaviours the child sees at home, which helps them learn new actions and skills.

• Play becomes more social but not necessarily interactive.

Parallel play

During the toddler stage, children commonly play with others without actually interacting. In this type of parallel play, children play side-by-side, commonly with similar objects. Interaction is limited to the occasional comment or trading of toys. This form of play helps the toddler develop the social skills needed to move into more interactive play.

Cognitive development

According to Piaget's developmental theory, a child moves from the sensorimotor stage of infancy and early toddlerhood (birth to 2 years) to the

Growing pains

Toddler development

At the toddler stage, children begin to master:

• individuation (differentiation of self from others)
• separation from parents
• control of body functions
• communication with words
• acquisition of socially acceptable behaviours
• lesser egocentricity when interacting with others.

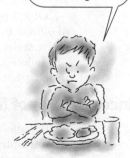

No! No! No! (I'm on a quest for my autonomy – whatever that means. How am I doing?)

Toddler toys

Safe toys that promote a toddler's exploration include:

- play dough and modelling clay
- big building blocks
- plastic, pretend housekeeping toys, such as pots, pans and play food
- stackable rings and blocks of varying sizes
- toy telephone
- wooden puzzles with big pieces
- textured or cloth books
- plastic musical instruments and noisemakers
- toys that roll, such as cars and trains
- tricycle or riding car
- fat crayons and colouring books
- stuffed animals with painted faces (button eyes can pose a choking hazard).

Always make sure they are safe to play with!

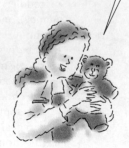

A toddler's favourite toy can change at the drop of a hat.

longer, pre-operational stage (2 to 7 years). Piaget made several observations about this transitional time in the young child's life.

- Tertiary circular reactions refer to the 13- to 18-month-old child's use of active experimentation (trial and error); they use newly acquired skills and knowledge to reach previously unattainable goals and discover new objects and areas.

Familiar at home, foreign at the shops

- The toddler may be aware of the relationship between two events (cause and effect) but may not be able to transfer that knowledge to a new situation. For example, a toddler might need to reinvestigate the function of a familiar object or the identity of a familiar person over and over again when encountering that object or person in a new, out-of-context setting.

That's using my head

From about 18 to 24 months, the toddler will look for new ways to accomplish tasks through mental calculations.

Object permanence advances as toddlers are more aware of the existence of objects that are out of sight, such as behind closed doors, in drawers and under tables.

Toddlers begin to use language and are able to think about objects or people when they aren't present.

Sincerest form of flattery

- Imitation displays deeper meaning and understanding of the toddlers role in the family, as the child observes and helps with household activities and identifies with the same-sex parent.

- Toddlers begin to use pre-operational thought, with increasing use of words as symbols.
- Problem-solving, creative thinking and some understanding of cause and effect begin during the toddler years.

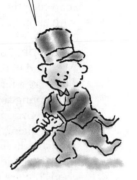

I'm hungry and I want my mom. If I make lots of noise, my mom will wake up and the toast is mine! How's that for problem solving?

Keys to health

Guidelines for nutrition, sleep and rest, and dental hygiene should be followed to maintain a toddler's good health. Reference should be made to the Healthy Child Programme (DH, 2009) when supporting parents and families in relation to the key health issues.

Nutrition
Nutrition guidelines for toddlers include:
- a decrease in protein requirements from infancy (to 1.2 g/kg/day)
- calorie requirement of approximately 100 kcal/kg/day
- considerable need for vitamins and minerals, such as iron, calcium and phosphorus.

A healthy start

Providing a good start to a balanced nutrition will help the young child to grow and develop; however, vitamin supplements may also be needed. At present, the UK departments of health (DH, 2007; NIHCE, 2008) recommend:
- breast-fed infants from 6 months (or from 1 month if the mother had a low vitamin status during pregnancy)
- formula-fed infants who are over 6 months and taking less than 500 ml infant formula per day
- children under 5 years of age.

In addition, supplements may also be needed for children who are picky or fussy eaters, those of Asian, African, Afro-Caribbean or Middle Eastern origin.

Developing healthy eating habits
The eating habits learned during the toddler years can set the stage for many years to come. Positive experiences with food and family meals are likely to set a foundation for a healthy, pleasurable 'relationship' with food. On the other hand, negative experiences such as power struggles, unpleasantness and food given or withheld to control behaviour may predispose the toddler to future food-related problems, such as overeating, extremely picky eating and even an increased risk for eating disorders.

You eat what you are

A toddler's developing eating habits are influenced by a range of factors, including:
- physiological anorexia, which occurs at approximately 18 months (when growth slows), and results in decreased appetite and a picky, fussy eater with strong taste preferences

- need to imitate family members (toddlers may refuse to eat a particular food that parents or siblings choose not to eat)
- being easily overwhelmed by large portions
- inability to sit through a long meal without becoming fidgety or disruptive at times
- food used as a reward or sign of approval (which may encourage overeating for non-nutritive reasons)
- food that's forced or mealtimes that are consistently unpleasant (which may keep the child from developing the sense of pleasure usually associated with eating).

Food preparation

Most toddlers eat the same food that's prepared for the rest of the family. Here are a few 'toddler truisms' to help make mealtime enjoyable:
- Serving size should be limited so as not to overwhelm the child with larger portions.
- Frequent, nutritious snacks are more likely to promote proper nutrition than are three large meals per day.
- Most toddlers prefer to feed themselves; they're skilful at handling finger foods but are still messy with soft foods as they're learning to use a spoon. But this is fun!

Sleep and rest

Parents are usually pleased to hear that most toddlers sleep through the night without awakening. A consistent routine, such as a set bedtime, a light snack, reading and a security object, helps toddlers prepare for sleep.

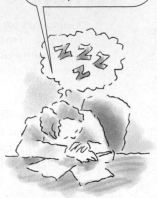

It's just about the time when toddlers stop taking naps (around 3 years) that their parents could really use them!

Good night, sleepyhead

Sleep requirements change slightly as a toddler grows and approaches the preschool stage.
- From 1 to 2 years, a toddler needs 10 to 15 hours of sleep every 24 hours.
- The 2- to 3-year-olds need 10 to 12 hours of sleep per night.
- During toddlerhood, naps gradually decrease to one per day; at 3 years, toddlers usually don't need a nap.

Dental hygiene

When teeth begin to break through the gum line, a child should begin brushing their teeth with a small, soft-bristled toothbrush (with parental assistance). Fluoride toothpaste should be avoided until the child is 2 years old; when used earlier, fluoride can discolour teeth.

Fluoride

Fluoride is a mineral that reduces the incidence of tooth decay. It's found naturally in water, certain foods and drinks made with fluoridated water.

Most of the water supply in the UK has adequate fluoride; however, where it doesn't, children aged 2 years and older may receive a daily fluoride supplement or have a fluoride gel applied to the teeth. However, it is recommended that a dentist is consulted about this. When administering supplements or teaching the caregiver to do so, keep in mind that:

• The supplement should be taken on an empty stomach, and the child shouldn't eat or drink for 30 minutes afterward.

• The supplement should remain in the child's mouth for 30 seconds before swallowing (if possible).

• Use of fluoride products can lead to accidental poisoning; fluoride-containing toothpastes, supplements and rinses must be stored out of the reach of young children.

Coping with concerns

A toddler is prone to developing troubling behaviours relating to toilet training, temper tantrums and discipline. Negativism and periods of separation anxiety may manifest through physical behaviours such as temper tantrums.

Toilet training

For toilet training to be successful, the child must display three signs of toilet training readiness:

First, the child must have control of the rectal and urethral sphincters.

Second, the child must have a cognitive understanding of what it means to hold their stool and urine until ready to go at a certain place at a certain time.

Third, the child must have a desire to delay immediate reward for a more socially accepted action.

It's in their head, too

Physical readiness for toilet training occurs between 18 and 24 months when myelinisation of pyramidal tracts and conditioned reflex sphincter control are intact. Despite physical readiness, however, many children aren't cognitively ready to begin toilet training until they're between 36 and 42 months of age.

Ready, set, go potty!

When physically and cognitively ready, the child can start toilet training. The process can take 2 weeks to 2 months to complete successfully. It's important to remember that there's considerable variability from one child to another. Other signs of readiness for toilet training include:

• periods of dryness for 2 hours or more, indicating bladder control
• child's ability to walk well and remove clothing
• cognitive ability to understand the task
• facial expression or words suggesting that the child knows when they're about to defecate.

Step by step

Steps to toilet training include:
- teaching words for voiding and defecating
- teaching the purpose of the toilet or potty
- changing the toddler's nappy frequently to give the experience of feeling dry and clean
- helping the toddler make the connection between dry pants and the toilet or potty
- placing the child on the potty or toilet for a few moments at regular intervals, and rewarding successes
- helping the toddler understand the physiological signals by pointing out behaviours they display when they need to void or defecate
- rewarding successes but not punishing failures.

Temper tantrums

As they assert their independence, toddlers demonstrate 'temper tantrums', or violent objections to rules or demands. These tantrums include such behaviours as lying on the floor and kicking feet, screaming and breath holding.

Hush little baby, don't throw a fit

Tantrums can occur at any time of the day but commonly occur before bedtime. The active toddler may have trouble slowing down and, when placed in bed, resists staying there.

Assessment of temper tantrums in a toddler should include the following questions:
- How often do tantrums occur?
- What circumstances provoke tantrums?
- How does the child behave during tantrums?
- How does the child behave between tantrums?
- Are expectations of the parent consistent with the child's developmental age?
- Have there been any recent changes in the home?
- Does the child have other behaviour problems?

Dealing with tantrums

Dealing with a child's temper tantrums can be a challenge for parents who may be frustrated, embarrassed and exhausted by their child's behaviour. If tantrums occur in public places, parents may feel as if they're being judged by others and viewed as inept at parenting and unable to control their child's behaviour.

Annoying but normal

The nurse should reassure parents that temper tantrums are a normal occurrence in toddlers, and that the child will outgrow them as they learn to express themselves in more productive ways. This type of reassurance should be accompanied by some concrete suggestions for dealing effectively with temper tantrums:

- Provide a safe and childproof environment.
- Hold the child to keep them safe if the behaviour is out of control.
- Give the toddler frequent opportunities to make developmentally appropriate choices.
- Give the child advance warning of a request to help prevent tantrums.
- Remain calm and be supportive of a child having a tantrum.
- Ignore tantrums when the toddler is seeking attention or trying to get something he/she wants.
- Help the toddler find acceptable ways to vent anger and frustration.

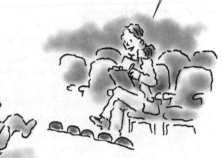

Sometimes, ignoring a temper tantrum is the best – and only – thing to do. I suggest a good pair of earplugs.

When to get help
Parents should be advised to seek help from a health care provider when problematic tantrums:

- persist beyond 5 years of age
- occur more than five times per day
- occur with a persistent negative mood
- cause property destruction
- cause harm to the child or others.

Negativism
Negativism refers to persistent negative responses to requests and is typical of toddlers as they strive for autonomy. 'No' and 'Me do' become the responses to almost everything, and the toddler's emotions are very strongly expressed with rapid mood swings.

No, non, nein!

Negativism commonly becomes exasperating for parents, who may find it easier to give in to the behaviour than to deal with it constructively. Unfortunately, this reinforces the child's negative ways of interacting with others.

Apple or orange?

Negativism can usually be reduced by giving the child appropriate choices. It's hard to say 'no' when the question is, 'Would you like apple juice or orange juice?'

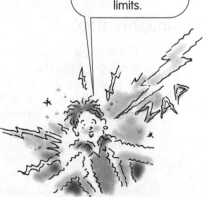

Stop the insanity! A toddler's negativism can push a parent's patience to the limits.

Discipline

Toddlers must be under direct supervision of a caregiver at all times. A childproof environment must be provided as they can move quickly and skillfully and are always exploring their surroundings.

Frustration-free zone

Most discipline for toddlers involves taking measures to make the environment safe and age-appropriate, which reduces the frequency of frustration-producing situations that require a 'no' from parents.

Tackle the triggers

Behaviour management for toddlers includes attending to their needs to reduce fatigue and hunger triggers, as most inappropriate behaviour occurs when the toddler is tired or hungry.

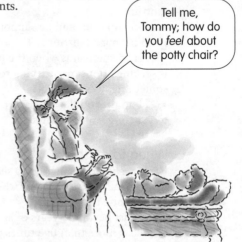

Tell me, Tommy; how do you *feel* about the potty chair?

Discipline guidelines include:
• setting up routines and creating and adhering to a consistent schedule
• providing an environment that limits opportunities for negative behaviour and giving positive feedback for good behaviour
• using behaviour modification, or positive reinforcement, for good behaviour and brief time-outs (with reasonable limits) for inappropriate behaviour
• recognising individuality in the toddler's temperament
• allowing toddlers to start attempting to solve some of their own problems
• understanding and recognising feelings of frustration, boredom and anger
• having the patience to allow toddlers to express themselves, and to provide distraction when they're bored
• avoiding physical punishment, threats and criticism (remembering that toddlers' behaviours are generally the result of normal development, such as exploring and experimenting with their environment).

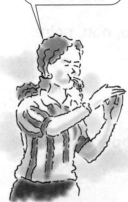

Time out! Unacceptable behavior – hitting sister. Penalty: 2 minutes in a neutral setting.

The 'naughty step'

When using the 'naughty step' in response to a toddler's inappropriate behaviour, keep these guidelines in mind:
• Make sure the child knows the rules ahead of the 'naughty step'.
• Give the child a simple explanation of why the behaviour requiring the 'naughty step' is unacceptable.
• Place the child in a neutral or uninteresting environment.
• Limit the time on the 'naughty step' to 1 minute per year of age (anything longer becomes frustrating and loses its intended effect).
• Reset the time if the child acts unacceptably.
• If the child is having trouble resolving the behaviour problem on their own, try discussing the offence calmly and constructively and, if appropriate,

helping the child determine ways to 'fix' the result of the bad behaviour (such as clean up a mess or apologise to a hurt friend).
• After a successful time-out, praise the child for their improved behaviour.
• Throughout, keep things simple and don't expect the toddler to understand things they can't understand!
• Remember some parents don't use or like the word naughty!

Separation anxiety

Stranger fear and separation anxiety are expected and normal reactions from an infant with a healthy parent–child attachment. As a child matures to toddler age, they may still protest when left with someone other than a parent, close friend or relative.

Parents should be reassured that separation anxiety is a normal, expected behaviour that is actually necessary for developmental growth and that children usually progress beyond these fears with time and support.

Anxiety antidote

The following information and advice will help parents deal with their toddler's separation anxiety:
• Toddlers should be allowed to explore at their own rate with close adult supervision. They're normally ready to venture away from their parents for short periods and are curious about strangers.
• A toddler should be allowed to 'warm' to a new person. To do so, the parent should hold or stand near the child at a 'safe' distance from the stranger, allowing the child to observe the new person from the safety of the parent's presence. (If the parent welcomes the new person, the toddler will likely do the same.)

Separation from parents can be a major stressor for toddlers, and this stress can be even more severe when a child is ill or hospitalised. To toddlers, nurses (and other health care professionals) are not only strangers, but also strangers in a strange environment.

Slow, low, small and clear

These measures can help a toddler who's hospitalised or undergoing a medical procedure:
• Start by talking to the parent in a soft voice while maintaining a safe distance from the child; avoid sudden movements or reaching for the child.
• Approach the child at eye level; you may be more likely to be accepted in a stance that makes you appear smaller and less threatening.
• Minimise separation between the child and parent to the extent possible. (A parent's presence during a painful or frightening procedure, such as an injection, venepuncture or cannula insertion, will reassure the child that nothing truly bad will happen to them.)

- If separation can't be helped (such as in the operating theatre or during a radiological examination), tell the child where the parent is, and reassure the child that their parent knows exactly where they are. This tends not to happen though as hospitals adopt family-centred approaches.
- If a child is hospitalised and the parents must leave the hospital, reassure the child that their parent will return, and tell them when they'll return in terms that are age-appropriate.

Preschool

During the preschool stage (3 to 5 years), children are gaining new initiative and independence and have well-developed language skills.

Physical development

Physical development is slow and steady during the preschool stage, with most growth occurring in the long bones of the arms and legs.

Height and weight
- Preschoolers grow about 6.5 to 7.5 cm per year; their average height is 94 cm.
- Weight gain is 1.5 to 2.5 kg per year; the average preschooler weighs 14.5 kg.

Teeth
By the preschool years, the development of the child's primary (or deciduous) teeth is complete. Prepare the child and parents for the loss of these temporary teeth and replacement with secondary (or permanent) teeth, which usually begins to occur from 6 years.

Gross motor development
A 3-year-old can:
- stand on one foot for a few seconds
- climb stairs with alternating feet
- jump in place
- perform a broad jump
- dance, but with somewhat poor balance
- kick a ball
- ride a tricycle.

Fabulous 4 and 5

A 4-year-old can:
- hop, jump and skip on one foot
- throw a ball overhand

- ride a tricycle or bicycle with stabiliser wheels.
  A 5-year-old can:
- skip, using alternate feet
- jump rope
- balance on each foot for 4 to 5 seconds.

Fine motor development

A 3-year-old can:
- build a tower of 9 to 10 blocks and a 3-block bridge
- copy a circle and a cross
- draw a circle with facial features (but often not a stick figure)
- use a fork well.
  A 4- or 5-year-old can:
- build a tower of 10 blocks
- copy a square and trace a cross and a diamond
- draw a person or stick figure with three or more parts
- use scissors to cut out a picture following an outline tie shoe laces (may be unable to tie a bow).

Psychological development

During the preschool years, the child functions more socially as he/she is able to learn and follow rules, and perhaps has entered nursery school, which enhances social development.

Many of the thought processes a preschooler will go through are essential to prepare them for nursery school and the school years ahead.

Psychosocial development

According to Erikson's psychosocial theory, children between 3 and 5 years have mastered a sense of autonomy and are now facing the task of initiative versus guilt. During this time:
- The child's significant other is the family.
- A conscience begins to develop, and dealing with the concept of right and wrong becomes a major task for preschoolers.
- A sense of guilt arises when the child feels that their imagination and activities are unacceptable or that they clash with his parents' expectations.
- The preschooler uses simple reasoning and can tolerate longer periods of delayed gratification.

Language development and socialisation

By the time a child reaches preschool age:
- vocabulary increases to about 900 words by 3 years and 2,100 words by 5 years.
- they may talk incessantly and ask many 'why' questions.
- they usually talk in three- or four-word sentences by 3 years; by 5, they can speak in longer sentences that contain all parts of speech.

> Why is the sky blue? Why do I have a baby brother? Why do I keep asking why?

Come one; come all

Socialisation continues to develop as the preschooler's world expands. Significant others now include grandparents, siblings and preschool staff (although parents remain central). Regular interaction with same-age children is necessary for the preschooler to further develop social skills.

Play

Play changes as children move into preschool years, and the parallel play of toddlerhood is essentially replaced by more interactive, cooperative play.

Ch-, ch-, ch-, ch-, changes!

Other changes in play include:
• more associative play, in which there's interaction between the children as they play together
• better understanding of the concept of sharing
• enjoyment of large motor activities, such as swinging, riding tricycles or bicycles and throwing balls
• more dramatic play, in which the child lives out the dramas of human life (in the context of the preschool years), and may have imaginary playmates. (See *Preschool play*.)

Cognitive development

Preschoolers exhibit pre-operational thought by using symbols or words to represent objects and people and by thinking about objects and people as well.

Piaget's cognitive theory divides the pre-operational phase into two stages during the preschool years: the preconceptual phase and the intuitive thought phase.

It's all about me!

The preconceptual phase, from 2 to 4 years, begins in the toddler stage and extends into the preschool stage. During this phase, the child is able to:
• form beginning concepts that aren't as complete or logical as an adult's are
• make simple classifications
• rationalise specific concepts but not the idea as a whole
• exhibit egocentric thinking (evaluating each situation based on his feelings or experiences, rather than the feelings of others).

Call it children's intuition

The intuitive thought phase begins at 4 years. During this phase, the child:
• can classify, quantify and relate objects (but can't yet understand the principles behind these operations)

Preschool play

Suggested play activities for preschoolers include:

• running and jumping in an open space
• creative play with dress-up clothes, pretend kitchens and dolls
• art activities with paints, paper, crayons, blunt scissors and markers
• trips to the museum, park, fire station, zoo, library and anywhere exciting
• swimming and other individual sports and activities to encourage gross motor development
• puzzles and toys to aid fine motor development and stimulate imagination.

- uses intuitive thought processes (but isn't able to fully see the viewpoints of others)
- uses many words appropriately (but without true understanding of their meaning).

Moral and spiritual development

Kohlberg's preconventional phase of moral development spans the preschool and school age stages, extending from 4 to 10 years. During this phase:
- Conscience emerges and emphasis is on external control.
- The preschooler's moral standards are those of others, and they understand that these standards must be followed to avoid punishment for inappropriate behaviour or gain rewards for good or desired behaviour.
- The preschooler behaves according to what freedom is given or what restriction is placed on their actions.
- Children of 4 to 7 years are more focused on meeting their own personal needs than on the desires of others.

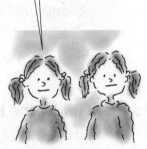

Today I learned a moral standard. It's wrong to put your sister's head in the toilet because your mom won't let you watch TV for a whole week if you do.

Spirituality

Children learn about faith and religion from significant people in their lives, such as their parents or religious teachers. The extent to which faith and religion influences the child more generally as well as their development will naturally depend on those they live with.

Friends at the top

Although preschoolers can imagine the physical characteristics of God, they commonly treat Him as an imaginary friend. They can understand the basic plot of simple religious stories but typically don't grasp the underlying meanings. Religious principles are best learned from concrete images in picture books and small statues such as those seen at a place of worship. The images and understanding will be influenced by the religion practised as well as the culture of the family.

During this stage, children may view an illness or hospitalisation as a punishment from God for some real or perceived bad behaviour.

Keys to health

Guidelines for nutrition, sleep and dental hygiene should be followed in order to maintain a preschooler's good health.

Nutrition

The daily caloric requirement for preschoolers is 85 to 90 kcal/kg/day, or about 1,700 to 1,800 calories per day. Daily fluid intake should average 100 ml/kg, depending on the preschooler's activity level.

Make pleasant conversation

By 5 years, the focus on the 'social' aspects of eating can begin. Parents should encourage table conversation, table manners and a willingness to try a variety of foods. Preschoolers are old enough to help with meal preparation and cleanup and usually enjoy this.

No food fights

Parents should be discouraged from using food as a bribe, reward or threat, which can set the stage for unhealthy attitudes towards food and eating.

Food preferences

Many 3- to 4-year-olds have strong taste preferences. The child may want to eat only one thing, or a narrow range of foods, over and over. Emphasis should be placed on the quality of the food eaten rather than the quantity to prevent emotional struggles over food.

To promote healthy eating habits, parents should encourage the child to eat fruits and vegetables (raw are usually preferred over cooked).

Sleep and rest

By the time a child reaches the preschool stage, sleep patterns have been established (during toddlerhood). Normal sleep patterns for preschoolers consist of 10 to 12 hours at night and, if not already stopped by 3 years, one daytime nap or rest period.

Monsters under the bed

Despite these well-established patterns, sleep-related problems may reappear during preschool years, including:
• Dreams and nightmares become more real as magical thinking increases and a vivid imagination develops.
• Problems falling asleep may occur due to overstimulation, separation anxiety, fear of the dark or monsters.
• Night-time waking may occur due to nightmares and night terrors as well as the child's inability to soothe and comfort themselves.
• Sleepwalking may occur if the child hasn't had enough sleep or is experiencing unusual stress.

Dental hygiene

Preschoolers have developed the fine motor skills needed to use a toothbrush properly and should be encouraged to brush two to three times daily. Parents should still supervise the child's brushing (assisting, as necessary) and perform flossing. As in toddlerhood, cariogenic foods should be avoided.

The preschool years are an excellent time to encourage good dental hygiene habits. Parents should administer fluoride supplements if the water supply isn't fluoridated. In addition, they should schedule a first dental visit so the child can become comfortable with the routine of preventive dental care. The child should then visit the dentist at 6 to 12-monthly intervals.

Coping with concerns

Parents may be concerned about their preschoolers in the areas of discipline and fears. They may also have concerns about their child's readiness to start formal schooling which may be from 4 years of age.

Discipline

Parents commonly have questions about how best to discipline young children. Here are some pointers about appropriate methods of discipline:
- Authority figures should administer discipline firmly, consistently and fairly.
- The child should be given simple explanations about why a certain behaviour isn't appropriate.
- Time-outs (generally 1 minute per year of age) can be used to help the child relieve intensity, regain control and think about his inappropriate behaviour.
- Discipline shouldn't be confused with punishment. Discipline refers to the process of managing behaviours – good and bad – to achieve desired outcomes. Punishment is a single action taken in response to a specific behaviour.
- Physical chastisement should be avoided.

Fears

Children experience more fears during the preschool years than at any other time. Common fears include:
- the dark
- ghosts
- being left alone
- animals (particularly large dogs)
- body mutilation, blood oozing out of cuts (children consider plasters very important to keep body contents inside)
- pain and objects or persons associated with painful experiences.

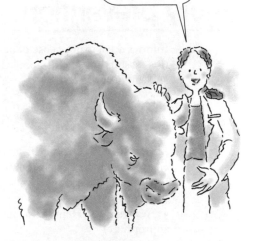

Preschoolers are commonly afraid of large animals.

Who you gonna call? Ghostbusters!

No amount of logical persuasion will help allay these fears, which leaves many parents perplexed about how to help. Parents can help their child overcome his fears by:
- actively involving him in finding practical solutions to dealing with fears, such as using a night light and keeping a door open or closed (to keep monsters under control)

• desensitising the child to the object of their fear by exposure to the object in a safe situation (for example, allowing them to watch a large dog interact with children who aren't fearful but never forcing the child to approach or touch one unless ready)
• giving it time (by 5 or 6 years, most children will have overcome these types of fears).

Preschool readiness

Factors to consider when assessing for preschool readiness include:
• visual, perceptual, cognitive, social and behavioural abilities (such as gross and fine motor skills, visual processing, spatial-body awareness, auditory language, memory, general knowledge, cognitive development, temperament, attention-activity and social readiness)
• physical, sensory, mental or emotional disabilities or problems.

Children now the have the opportunity to attend pre-school groups, pre-reception classes and can start school at earlier ages. This can help with separation anxiety for the child, and parents, as well promoting their development and learning.

All children are different and so may be able to undertake the above at different times so attending nursery can be a way of learning new skills and behaviours.

Injury prevention

Injuries are a major cause of death in toddler and preschool age-groups. For this reason, much continuing emphasis should be placed on injury prevention and safety awareness.

Aspiration

Aspiration can easily occur in toddlers because they're still exploring their environments with their mouths. Toddlers may ingest small objects, while the small size of their oral cavities increases the risk of aspiration while eating. Preventive measures include:
• learning the Heimlich manoeuvre (making sure the manoeuvre is age-appropriate)
• avoiding large, round chunks of meat to eat
• avoiding fruit with stones, fish with bones, hard sweets, chewing gum, nuts, popcorn, whole grapes and marshmallows
• keeping easily aspirated objects out of a toddler's environment
• being especially cautious about what toys the child plays with (choosing sturdy toys without small, removable parts). (See *Aspiration risks*.)

It's all relative

Aspiration risks

Toddlers explore their environment by putting things in their mouths. Foods and other items that can place a toddler at risk for aspiration include:

• small foods, such as popcorn, peanuts, whole grapes, cherry tomatoes, raw carrots, hard sweets, bubble and chewing gum, long noodles, dried beans and marshmallows
• small toys, such as balloons, button eyes, beaded necklaces and small wheels
• common household items, such as broken zips, tablets, bottle caps, and nails and screws.

Burns

Burns can easily occur in toddlers and preschoolers because they're tall enough to reach the top of the cooker and can walk to a fireplace to touch.

Hot stuff

Preventive measures include:
- setting the hot water heater thermostat at a temperature less than 120° F (49° C)
- checking water temperature before a child enters the bath
- keeping pan handles turned inward and using the back burners of the cooker
- keeping electric appliances towards the backs of counters
- placing burning candles, incense, hot foods and cigarettes (no smoking is better) out of reach
- avoiding the use of tablecloths so the curious toddler doesn't pull it to see what's on the table (possibly spilling hot foods or liquids on themselves).

Hot potato

- teaching the child what 'hot' means and stressing the danger of open flames
- storing matches and cigarette lighters in locked cabinets or out of reach
- burning fires in fireplaces with close and consistent supervision and always with the use a tight-fitting fire guard
- securing safety plugs in all unused electrical outlets and keeping electrical cables tucked out of reach.

The great escape

- practicing escapes from home and school with preschoolers
- visiting a fire station to reinforce learning
- teaching preschoolers how to call 999 (for emergency use only).

Drowning

Drowning can occur in a few inches of water, resulting from falls into buckets, baths, toilets, garden ponds and even fish tanks.

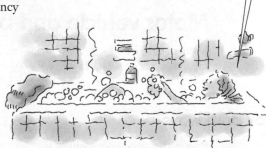

If it's too hot for you, it's too hot for the child. Always check the temperature *before* putting the child in the bath.

Water, water, everywhere

Preventive measures include:
- close adult supervision of any child near any water
- teaching children never to go into water without an adult and never to play near the water's edge

- using child-resistant pool covers and fences with self-closing gates around ponds
- emptying buckets when not in use and storing them upside-down.

Falls

Falls can easily occur as gross motor skills improve and the toddler and preschooler are able to move chairs to climb onto counters, climb ladders and open windows.

Movin' on up

Preventive measures include:
- providing close supervision at all times during play
- keeping cot rails up and the mattress at the lowest position
- placing gates across the tops and bottoms of stairways
- installing window locks on all windows to keep them from opening more than a few centimetres without adult supervision
- keeping doors locked or using child-proof doorknob covers at entries to stairs
- removing unsecured scatter rugs
- using a non-skid bath mat in the bath or shower
- avoiding the use of walkers, especially near stairs
- always restraining children in shopping trolleys and never leaving them unattended
- providing safe climbing toys and choosing play areas with soft ground cover and safe equipment
- teaching the difference between acceptable and unacceptable places for climbing.

Motor vehicle and bicycle injuries

Motor vehicle and bicycle injuries can easily occur in toddlers and preschoolers because they may be able to unbuckle seat belts, resist riding in a car seat or refuse to wear a bicycle helmet.

Look both ways

Preventive measures include:
- educating parents about the proper fit and use of bicycle helmets, and requiring the child to wear a helmet every time they ride a bicycle
- teaching the preschooler never to go into a road without an adult

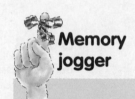

Memory jogger

Remember tips on preventing drowning when you think of the word WATER.

- *Wear life jackets*
- *Adult supervision*
- *Teach water safety*
- *Empty buckets*
- *Reinforce safety with pool covers.*

It's a dilemma. Medicines need to taste good so children will take them, but children need to learn that medicines aren't treats, no matter how good they taste.

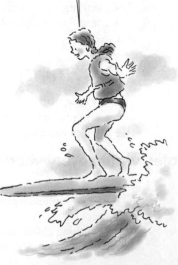

- not allowing a child to play on a curb or behind a parked car
- checking the area behind vehicles before backing out of the drive (small children may not be visible in rear-view mirrors because of blind spots, especially in larger vehicles)
- providing a safe, preferably enclosed, area for outdoor play (and keeping fences, gates and doors locked)
- educating parents on the use of child safety seats for all motor vehicle trips, and ensuring proper use by having the seats inspected.

Car safety seat guidelines

The law requires the use of correct child restraints until they are either 135 cm in height or the age of 12 (which ever they reach first). After this they must use an adult seat belt although it is the driver's responsibility to ensure children under the age of 14 years are restrained correctly in accordance with the law. Proper installation and use of a car safety seat are critical. The following guidelines for booster seat use will help ensure a child's safety while riding in a vehicle:

- Proper installation and regular checking of car safety seats are critical to protecting the child and other passengers
- Always make sure belt-positioning booster seats are used with both lap and shoulder belts
- Make sure the lap belt fits low and right across the lap/upper thigh area and the shoulder belt fits snug, crossing the chest and shoulder to avoid abdominal injuries
- Ensure the child is comfortable and that they have something age appropriate to keep them occupied
- Regularly check that they are secure and comfortable especially on long journeys

Poisoning

As toddlers gross motor skills improve, they are able to climb onto chairs and reach cabinets where medicines, cosmetics, cleaning products and other poisonous substances are stored.

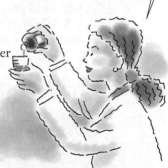

A delay in bonding, for whatever reason, may create a risk for abuse.

Please don't eat the daisies

Preventive measures include:
- keeping medicines and other toxic materials locked away in high cupboards, boxes or drawers
- using child-resistant containers and cupboard safety latches
- not storing a large supply of toxic agents

- teaching that medication is not a sweet or treat (even though it might taste good)
- teaching the child that plants outside aren't edible, and keeping houseplants (also explained as inedible) out of reach
- promptly discarding empty poison containers and never reusing them to store a food item or other poison
- always keeping original labels on containers of toxic substances
- if in doubt lock it away.

Suffocation

Suffocation can easily occur in toddlers and preschoolers exposed to objects that can occlude the airway. A child may place such an object over their head or get tangled in an object such as a cord or string. Suffocation can also occur if a child becomes enclosed in a small space with a limited oxygen supply.

Preventive measures are extremely important and include:
- storing plastic bags, balloons, strings and ribbons out of the child's reach
- keeping strings and cords (such as those on hooded clothing or window coverings) out of the child's reach
- discarding old appliances, such as refrigerators and ovens, or removing the doors from old appliances that must be stored (to prevent a child from becoming trapped)
- choosing safe toy boxes or chests without heavy, hinged lids.

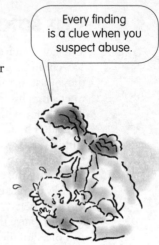

Every finding is a clue when you suspect abuse.

Health problems

Toddlers and preschoolers may suffer from a range of health problems, including lead poisoning. Unfortunately, they may also be subjected to harm through neglect and abuse.

Child abuse and neglect

Child abuse and neglect can occur as acts of commission or omission by a caregiver or those around them. These acts can prevent children from actualising their potential for growth and development.

What causes it
Risk factors that may predispose a child to abuse or neglect may involve the parent or the child.

Vicious cycle

Risk factors involving the parent include:
- history of being abused as a child
- substance abuse
- low self-esteem
- difficulty controlling aggressive impulses
- being a victim of domestic violence abuse
- youth or inexperience
- having limited support
- having unrealistic expectations of the child
- being overly demanding or overprotective.

It was an accident

Risk factors involving the child include:
- being unresponsive or overactive
- having frequent accidents, illnesses or slow recovery from illness
- being excessively negative
- being born prematurely.

Other risk factors include a history of abuse of the child's siblings and stressful environmental factors, such as divorce, poverty, unemployment and inadequate housing.

How it happens

Child abuse is a widespread problem and is part of a larger problem of violence. Many children die each day as a result of maltreatment:
- Between 250,000 and 350,00 children are affected by parental substance abuse.
- Estimated 2 million children are affected by parental alcohol abuse.
- One of every four parents who grew up in a violent home goes on to seriously injure a child.
- As domestic violence rates increase, the number of children who suffer from abuse will likely increase as well (children of women victims are at higher risk for abuse than other children).
- Many child abusers were abused as children and may not know healthier ways to discipline a child or to show love.

It's the law

If abuse is suspected, health care providers, including doctors, nurses and dentists, are legally and professionally required to report their concerns about a child in need or at risk of harm, through the appropriate channels and following the guidance Working Together to Safeguard Children (DCSF, 2010). CYP nurses are required by the NMC to protect the public, and as the Chief Nursing Officer (DH, 2004) stated it is the responsibility of all practitioners to safeguard vulnerable children.

What to look for

Physical indicators of abuse and neglect include:

- unexplained fractures (children younger than walking age rarely have fractures because their bones are still pliable)
- bruises with specific patterns, over soft tissue areas, back or genitals, in various stages of healing (because bruising caused by accidents most commonly occurs over bony prominences in children)
- bald spots (however, most infants normally have a bald spot over the occipital prominence of the skull since the inception of the 'Back to Sleep' campaign to prevent sudden infant death syndrome)
- welts from belt buckles or other distinctive instruments
- cigarette burns as well as 'glove', 'sock' or doughnut-shaped burns from dipping extremities in hot water or holding a child's bottom in hot water
- human bite marks larger than 19 (2.5 cm) (because they would not likely come from another child at that size)
- retinal haemorrhages indicating shaken baby syndrome
- inappropriate dress, poor hygiene or untreated medical needs
- faltering growth.

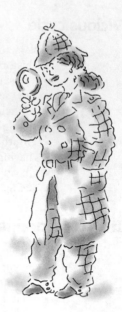

Acting it out

Behavioural indicators can include:
- withdrawn, passive, apathetic or depressed moods
- habit-related disorders such as excessive sucking or rocking.

When things don't add up

Other findings include:
- conflicting reports from caregiver and child about how injuries occurred
- inappropriate delay in seeking treatment for injuries
- inconsistency between the history of the injury and the child's developmental level
- inappropriate response of the child to the injuries.

What tests tell you

There's no definitive test to detect child abuse or neglect. However, many laboratory tests and X-rays may be indicated, such as:
- haemoglobin, because children who have been abused may not have had routine health care and are at higher risk for anaemia
- complete blood count to rule out any blood disorders
- laboratory studies to rule out sexually transmitted diseases whenever sexual abuse is suspected
- radiographic studies to diagnose suspicious injury or trauma

- skeletal X-ray survey to examine the entire body for evidence of fractures occurring at various times with various levels of healing. (X-rays may indicate previous non-accidental trauma that is ongoing and predate the incident that brought the child to the health care provider's attention.)

Calling in the cavalry

The CYP nurse should follow local safeguarding children procedures when referring a child they suspect to be at risk of harm. In addition, the Working Together to Safeguard Children (DCSF, 2010) document gives guidance on a wide range of issues including referral and this can be consulted.

All information, discussion and referrals should be documented.

Referral to Children's Services and/or the Police, in line with local safeguarding policy and procedures, is a requirement.

Complications
Complications of child abuse and neglect come in various forms depending on the severity and duration. Children can suffer a wide range of physical complications with lasting emotional effects.

How it's treated
Child abuse is treated by first identifying it as a problem. After the injury is treated, the child's safety must be assured if there is any concern about the child's welfare or if it is believed they are at risk of harm.

What to do
Dependent on the situation the CYP nurse should:
- assist in completing a thorough assessment of all body systems while comforting and reassuring the child to the extent possible
- carefully assess the child's emotional status
- document history, assessment and concerns objectively with clear descriptions
- report concerns following local safeguarding policies and procedures
- notify the parent that you're required by law to report your concerns and assessments – unless it places the child at immediate risk of doing so
- be alert to the possibility of domestic abuse and the potential risk to the accompanying adult
- work with the multi-agency team to safeguard the child
- ensure the safety of the child whilst in your care
- where the child discloses abuse then deal with this sensitively, in a non-judgemental manner and in line with procedures for managing such information.

Quick quiz

1. What Erikson psychosocial stage do toddlers try to master?
A. Trust versus mistrust
B. Autonomy versus doubt and shame
C. Initiative versus guilt
D. Industry versus inferiority

Answer: B. According to Erikson's developmental theory, autonomy versus doubt and shame is the developmental task of toddlerhood.

2. At mealtime, a toddler:
A. generally tries a variety of different foods willingly.
B. should only eat commercially prepared, pureed baby food.
C. can sit in the high chair for long periods of time.
D. should be served small portions of food.

Answer: D. Small so the child isn't overwhelmed with larger portions.

3. What's the average weight and height for a preschooler?
A. 3.6 kg and 55 cm
B. 8 kg and 68 cm
C. 14.5 kg and 94 cm
D. 24 kg and 116 cm

Answer: C. The average weight and height of a preschooler is 14.5 kg and 94 cm.

4. When a toddler is playing, they'll most likely:
A. play with similar objects near, rather than with, another child.
B. become more interactive with children around them.
C. willingly share toys with other children.
D. play with one toy for a while because of a long attention span.

Answer: A. During the toddler stage, children typically play with others without actually interacting. In this type of parallel play, children play side-by-side, usually with similar objects.

5. To help prevent aspiration of foods, toddlers and preschoolers should avoid which types of food?
A. Small pieces of cooked, lean meat
B. Round chunks of meat
C. Cooked vegetables, such as sweetcorn
D. Frozen desserts such as ice cream

Answer: B. To help prevent aspiration, avoiding large, round chunks of meat is advisable. (Slicing them into short, lengthwise pieces is a safer option.)

Scoring

☆☆☆   If you answered all five items correctly, hooray! You've mastered the tasks of early childhood.

☆☆   If you answered three or four items correctly, yippee! Buy yourself a new toy and read on.

☆   If you answered fewer than three items correctly, don't have a tantrum! Take a nap and give it another try.

Middle childhood and adolescence 5

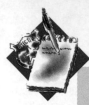

Just the facts

In this chapter, you'll learn:

♦ physical, psychosocial, cognitive and moral development of school-age children and adolescents

♦ keys to health maintenance in middle childhood and adolescence

♦ common concerns of school-age children and adolescents and their parents

♦ injury prevention for school-age children and adolescents

♦ common health problems during middle childhood and adolescence.

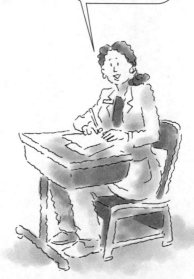

School can be joyful and yet physically and psychologically challenging.

School age

School age, or middle childhood, refers to the stage of a child's life between 6 and 12 years. The school-age years can be a spectacular journey filled with joys and successes as the child continues to grow and mature.

They can also be marked by challenges, as the child struggles to make sense of physical and psychological changes, an emerging identity, and the way they see themselves and are viewed by others (especially their peers).

Physical development

Physical growth at this time in a child's life is relatively slow and smooth.

Height and weight

Growth slows considerably during middle childhood. During this stage, height increases at an average of 5 cm per year, and weight increases at an average of 2.5 kg per year. However, during this time, the typical school-age child slims down and becomes more agile and graceful.

Ladies first

Girls tend to develop slightly faster than boys, although boys are, on average, taller and heavier than girls until the adolescent growth spurt.

Fine motor skills

By age 7, the brain has nearly completed its growth (at approximately 90%) and basic neuromuscular mechanisms are in place.

No more excuses

Development of small-muscle and eye-hand coordination increases, leading to the skilled handling of tools, such as pencils and papers for drawing and writing. The child can then spend the remainder of this period refining physical and motor skills and coordination.

Pubertal changes

The pubertal growth spurt begins in girls at about 10 years of age and in boys about 12 years.

Jumpin' in feet first

Different areas of the body reach their peak growth at different times. Changes are easily recognised in the feet, which are the first part of the body to experience a growth spurt. Increased foot size is followed by a rapid increase in leg length and then trunk growth.

Leggy and hippy

During this time, leg growth increases more dramatically than trunk growth in boys. In addition, although girls have a greater growth spurt in hip width, boys exceed girls in other areas of bone growth.

No turning back

In addition to bones, gonadal hormone levels increase and cause the sexual organs to mature.

Preparation for menses

In girls, the first menstruation, called menarche, can occur as early as 9 or as late as 17 years and still be considered normal. The menstrual cycle may be irregular at first.

Physical growth is slower during school age, but grace and agility make a stellar appearance.

My friends may call me a plodder today, but they'll call me a star when my legs hit their peak growth and it's nothing but net!

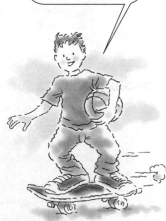

Secondary sexual characteristics may start to develop – including breasts, hips and pubic hair – and girls may experience a sudden increase in height. Nurses may find that this provides an excellent opportunity to educate school-age girls about breast self-examination and sexual responsibility.

Teeth

Loss of primary teeth and eruption of the first secondary teeth occur during the school-age years. Because of their size, secondary teeth may, for a while, appear disproportionately large in relation to the child's other, smaller facial features.

Psychological development

Attending school may mark an acceleration in the separation of the child from parents. It introduces the child to a new set of authority figures (particularly teachers) and strengthens the concept of peer relationships.

Psychosocial development

The school-age child enters Erikson's stage of industry versus inferiority. In this stage, the child wants to work and produce, accomplishing and achieving tasks. However, if too much is expected or they feel unable to measure up to set standards, the negative attributes of inadequacy and inferiority may prevail.

Language development and socialisation

The school-age child has an efficient vocabulary and begins to correct previous mistakes in usage. They begin to understand the double meanings of words and become proficient at giving others directions without using physical signals.

Pick a clique

In the early years at school, peers become increasingly significant to the child. A need to find a place within a group becomes important.

Same-sex cliques are established during this period, and competition becomes more common, as does bragging over accomplishments. The child may be overly concerned with peer rules; however, parental guidance continues to play an important role in the child's life.

Handle with care: Sensitive to ridicule

The child's world expands as interests and activities outside the home take on an expanded role in life. The child becomes more independent, inside and outside the home. They understand the reasons for rules and become more sensitive to criticism and ridicule.

Play

The child's personality has become structured, and is ready to be a partner in play with friends. The child in this age group typically has two to three best friends, who may change frequently. Most of their energy is devoted to school and his/her friends.

Cognitive development

School and learning are generally viewed by the school-age child as an exciting experience. The major developmental tasks at this time are achievement in school and acceptance by peers. Expectations in the classroom have intensified, and require concentration, attendance and complex auditory and visual processing.

The school-age child is in Piaget's concrete-operational period, a time in which the child uses thought processes to experience and understand events and actions. Children at this age are less egocentric and can see things from another's point of view.

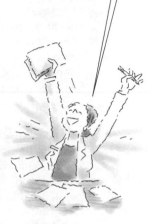

A school-aged child's enthusiasm for learning is contagious!

Try to remember

Reorganisation of the frontal brain, which is used for selective attention, occurs between 5 and 7 years. The ability to reason and memorise improves, and the child tends to use mnemonic strategies to remember new information. In addition, the following occurs:

• Magical thinking diminishes around this time, and the child has a much better understanding of cause and effect.
• The child begins to accept rules but may not necessarily understand them.
• Memory skills are continually improving, along with an increased attention span. The child is ready for basic reading, writing and arithmetic.
• Abstract thinking begins to develop during the middle primary school years.
• Parents remain very important during this time. Adult reassurance of the child's competence and basic self-worth is essential.

Moral and spiritual development

In general, the first level of moral thinking is put into practice at the primary school level, and the school-age child is in Kohlberg's conventional level. The child behaves according to socially acceptable norms because an authority figure tells him/her to do so. This obedience is compelled by the threat of punishment (external factors).

'Because I said so'

Between 11 and 12 years, as the child begins to approach adolescence, school and parental authority is questioned and, occasionally, even challenged or opposed. The importance of the peer group intensifies, and rough, bold or even brazen behaviour becomes increasingly common. The peer group becomes the source of behaviour standards and models.

Mum's still the bomb

Parental guidance, love and support are absolutely essential for the development of values during this time. The child at this age needs the opportunity to make decisions within defined boundaries. Ideally, those boundaries are set by responsible adults in the child's life.

Keys to health

During the school-age years, the child's understanding of cause and effect, coupled with the need for parental (and peer) approval, provides an excellent opportunity to continue teaching about the need to make healthy lifestyle choices. Parents should continue to teach their children about the importance of:
- proper nutrition
- sleep and rest
- exercise
- dental hygiene.

Parents and children can be advised with reference to key documents such as the supporting children and young people's health: from 5 to 19 years old (DCSF, 2010) which provides guidance on services and resources which can support children's health.

Nutrition

Children should be encouraged to eat a variety of healthy foods, such as lean meats, fruits, vegetables and grains, to ensure proper nutritional intake.

Developing healthy eating habits

Encouraging healthy eating habits now (during school age and, ideally, before) will lay a stable foundation for adolescence, when caloric needs increase. Childhood obesity is an increasing problem society wide, and measures should be taken to avoid high-fat, high-sugar and low-protein foods. (See *Encouraging proper nutrition*.)

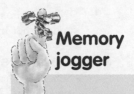

Memory jogger

When it comes to teaching children about being healthy, tell parents to remember these things to care for their PEDS:

- Proper nutrition
- Exercise
- Dental hygiene
- Sleep.

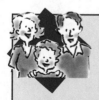

It's all relative

Encouraging proper nutrition

To ensure that children continue to develop and maintain healthy eating habits, encourage parents to:

- stock the cupboards and refrigerator with healthy choices for after-school snacks (raw vegetables, low-fat yogurts, fresh fruits)
- avoid taking children to fast-food outlets where high-fat foods are abundant
- teach children how to read nutrition labels while shopping
- involve children in planning and preparing meals for the family
- offer sweets as an infrequent privilege rather than a reward for good behaviour
- change their own eating habits to model good dietary habits for their children.

Be aware of maintaining healthy eating during specific religious periods such as Ramadan.

CYP nurses can advise parents and children about advice sources such as the '5 A Day' programme which can be viewed on the NHS Choices website http://www.nhs.uk/livewell/5aday/pages/5adayhome.aspx/.

Sleep and rest

Requirements for sleep and rest are unique and relate to the child's activity level and physical health. School-age children generally don't require an afternoon nap, and compliance at bedtime becomes easier.

Things that go bump in the night

Sleepwalking and sleeptalking may begin during this stage, and parents should take measures to ensure the child's physical safety during these episodes. Nightmares are usually related to a real event in the child's life and can usually be eradicated by resolving any underlying fears the child might have.

Exercise and activity

Exercise and other forms of physical activity should be encouraged to help the child begin healthy habits for a lifetime. Doing so may also prevent childhood obesity.

Children who are interested in sports should be encouraged to join sport teams or participate in sporting events. Sport teams and events are usually same-sex events at this age level, making them less intimidating.

Useful resources can be advised such as the Change 4 Life programme which aims to encourage healthy behaviour in all age groups.

Clicking the remote doesn't count

Parents should encourage physical exercise after school instead of more sedentary activities such as watching television or playing computer games, although this is a challenge! However, moderation is the key word here.

Dental hygiene

During the school-age years:
- Teeth should be brushed at least twice a day and, if possible, after meals.
- Drinking water should contain fluoride or fluoride supplements should be given.
- Flossing should be taught and parents should monitor for method and compliance until the child is 8 years old.
- Regular dental cleanings should be scheduled every 6 months.

Coping with concerns

During school age, the child's life revolves around home and family, school and peers. School-age children (and their parents) are commonly faced with concerns about school, after-school supervision and a limited understanding of ownership, which may lead to activities such as stealing.

School phobias

A child's refusal to go to school may be a sign of a separation anxiety, which occurs in families that are particularly close and caring or in a child who relies heavily on the support of his/her family. It may also occur after a particular trauma, such as the death of a pet, illness within the family or a move to a new school.

In these cases, children may be more fearful of leaving home than going to school. They may, for example, be afraid that something bad will happen to a parent, sibling or pet if they are not there to protect them.

Scary school

Refusal to go to school may also be related to fear of the school itself and what the child experiences there. Parents should talk to their child and try to determine the underlying cause of his/her fear. Possible reasons for school phobias include:
- being the target of a bully
- having an overly demanding teacher
- having problems adapting to the school structure.

Stealing

Stealing is attractive to the younger school-age child who simply wants items for themselves. The child has a limited sense of what belongs to someone else and will commonly lie to cover up the offence.

Low on cash?

A sense of responsibility for one's actions begins to take shape at the end of middle childhood. Stealing at the end of middle childhood is commonly a sign that something is lacking in that child's life. Possible causes include a lack of:
- financial means
- attention from a parent or caregiver
- limited boundaries and discipline at home
- sense of property rights
- peer or group pressure.

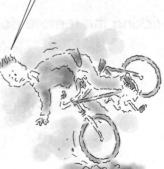

I know Mom will get upset because I'm not wearing a helmet, but at least I'm not stealing!

What's yours is mine

Parents should recognise the child's property rights and offer some privacy in this regard, when possible. A child who knows that their own property is respected is more likely to understand the importance of respecting the property of others.

Adolescence

Adolescence is defined as the developmental stage between 12 and 19 years (although legal age for adulthood is 18 years) and is the time that adolescents prefer to be called 'young people'!

Physical development

Adolescence is a time of change. As physical changes occur, young people struggle with the conflict between asserting their independence and still relying on their parents.

Terrible teens

Many adults view the changes that occur during adolescence with great fear and trepidation. It's commonly a turbulent time for the young person and their parents.

Height and weight

During this time, a young person's weight almost doubles and height increases by 15% to 20%. Girls may grow 7.5 to 15 cm per year until 16 years. Boys may grow 7.5 to 15 cm per year until 18 years. Major organs double in size; the exception is the lymphoid tissue, which decreases in mass.

Boys attain greater strength and muscle mass, but motor coordination lags behind growth in stature and musculature. Motor coordination catches up as strength improves.

Development of secondary sex characteristics

The pituitary gland is stimulated at puberty to produce androgen steroids responsible for secondary sex characteristics. (See *Beginning sexual maturity in girls* and *Beginning sexual maturity in boys*, pages 120–122.)

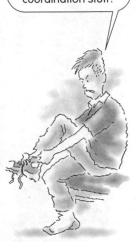

Sure, I have the strength and the muscles – so how much longer do I have to wait for this coordination stuff?

It's a girl thing

Female secondary sexual development during puberty involves increases in the size of the ovaries, uterus, vagina, labia and breasts. The first visible sign of sexual maturity is the appearance of breast buds. Body hair appears in the pubic area and under the arms, and menarche occurs. The ovaries, present at birth, remain inactive until puberty.

Boys will be boys ... until they're men

Male secondary sexual development consists of genital growth and the appearance of pubic and body hair.

Androgens and oestrogens

The trigger that starts puberty is unknown. What's clear is that, for some reason, the hypothalamus produces gonadotropin-releasing hormone, which

Growing pains

Beginning sexual maturity in girls

Breast development and pubic hair growth are the first signs of sexual maturity in girls. These illustrations show the development of the female breast and pubic hair in puberty.

Breast development

Stage 1
Only the papilla (nipple) elevates (not shown).

Stage 2
Breast buds appear; the areola is slightly widened and appears as a small mound.

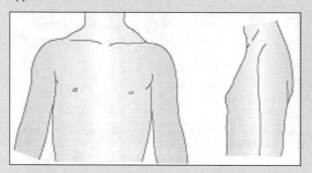

Stage 3
The entire breast enlarges; the nipple doesn't protrude.

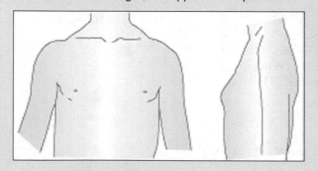

Stage 4
The breast enlarges; the nipple and the papilla protrude and appear as a secondary mound.

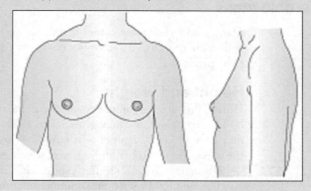

Stage 5
The adult breast has developed; the nipple protrudes and the areola no longer appears separate from the breast.

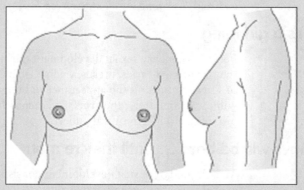

(continued)

Beginning sexual maturity in girls (continued)

Pubic hair development

Stage 1
No pubic hair is present.

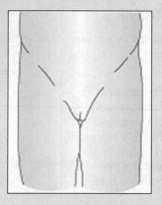

Stage 2
Straight hair begins to appear on the labia and extends between stages 2 and 3.

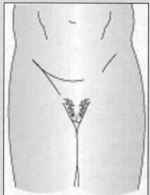

Stage 3
Pubic hair increases in quantity; it appears darker, curled and more dense and begins to form the typical (but smaller in quantity) female triangle.

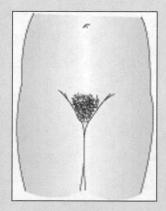

Stage 4
Pubic hair is more dense and curled; it's more adult in distribution, but less abundant than in an adult.

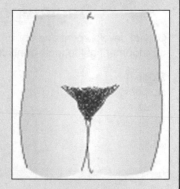

Stage 5
Pubic hair is abundant, appears in an adult female pattern, and may extend onto the medial part of the thighs.

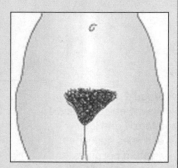

Growing pains

Beginning sexual maturity in boys

Genital development and pubic hair growth are the first signs of sexual maturity in boys. The illustrations below show the development of the male genitalia and pubic hair in puberty.

Stage 1
No pubic hair is present.

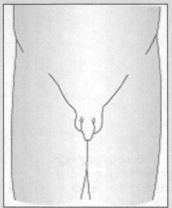

Stage 2
Downy hair develops laterally and later becomes dark; the scrotum becomes more textured and the penis and testes may become larger.

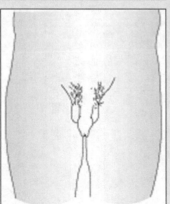

Stage 3
Pubic hair extends across the pubis; the scrotum and testes are larger; the penis enlarges in length.

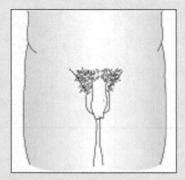

Stage 4
Pubic hair becomes more abundant and curls, and the genitalia resemble those of adults; the glans penis has become larger and broader and the scrotum becomes darker.

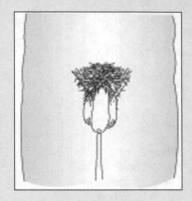

Stage 5
Pubic hair resembles an adult's in quality and pattern and the hair extends to the inner borders of the thighs; the testes and scrotum are adult in size.

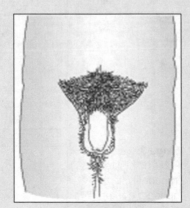

triggers the anterior pituitary gland to produce follicle-stimulating hormone (FSH) and luteinizing hormone (LH). FSH and LH initiate the ovulation cycle in girls and promote testicular maturation and sperm production in boys.

Tanner staging
The development of secondary sex characteristics occurs in an anticipated sequence for girls and boys, and is divided into distinct stages, called Tanner stages. While the timing of the stages is different for each individual, the sequence remains the same.

Menstruation and spermatogenesis
During early adolescence (11 to 14 years) most girls achieve menarche. Most boys achieve active spermatogenesis between 12 and 15 years.

Teeth
The secondary (permanent) teeth are all present during the early adolescent years. The four third molars (also called wisdom teeth) may need to be extracted if impaction occurs.

Psychological development

Psychological development during adolescence revolves around socialisation. As the young person ventures into the world outside their family and is exposed to other viewpoints, peers become increasingly important and independence is tested.

Psychosocial development
Adolescence is the period of identity development, according to Erikson, as the young person enters the stage of identity versus role confusion. Changes in the body are taking place rapidly, and there is a preoccupation with looks and how others view them. While trying to meet the expectations of peers, the young person is also trying to establish their own identity.

Early adolescence
During early adolescence, the young person begins to show more interest in the opposite sex, although the peer group usually consists of same-sex friends.

That's what friends are for

Friends become much more important and interest in family and family activities decreases.

Rebel with a question

Conformity to peer group standards is of utmost importance at this time. This may lead to rebellion and questioning of parental (and other adult) authority.

Middle adolescence

The young person becomes more self-assured during middle adolescence, and independent decision-making skills are tested.

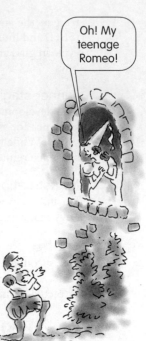

Oh! My teenage Romeo!

The young and the tasteless

Activities outside the home take on even greater importance, and the young person commonly defines themselves by whatever the peer group has defined, wearing what others in the group wear, speaking using the common language of the group and adjusting their taste in music and other preferences to go along with the crowd.

When girls suddenly become interesting

It's at this time that relationships with the opposite sex are established.

Now ... i'm not sure

Some young people develop a preference for and ultimately have relationships with the same sex. This can cause much confusion for the young person because of societal and family expectations about heterosexuality!

Later years

During the later years, rebellion has diminished. The young person has a fairly strong sense of who they are, but may not yet have committed to a particular occupation or role in life.

Cognitive development

During adolescence, the young person moves from the concrete thinking of childhood into Piaget's stage of formal operational thought. They can now reason logically about abstract concepts and derive conclusions from hypothetical premises.

I can see clearly now ...

They can imagine events in the future instead of focusing on the present (as in childhood). Because the future becomes a possibility, they may be more receptive to education that focuses on health promotion and can concentrate on future benefits as a result of current behaviours.

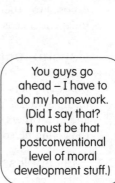

You guys go ahead – I have to do my homework. (Did I say that? It must be that postconventional level of moral development stuff.)

One step forward, two steps back

Although abstract thinking becomes more refined, the young person may revert back into concrete thinking during times of stress.

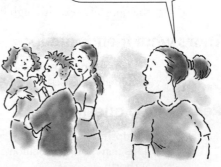

Moral and spiritual development

Kohlberg's conventional level of moral development continues into early adolescence. At this level, the child does what's right because it's the socially acceptable action. At this level, the child continues to advance in moral reasoning as cognition develops.

In with the in-crowd

The young person becomes increasingly dependent on the peer group for approval and associates good behaviour with 'fitting in' with the crowd. Morality may be dependent on the situation and relationship. Commonly, peer pressure will override individual own moral reasoning.

At long last – my own person

As the period of adolescence ends, the young person enters Kohlberg's postconventional, or principled, level of moral development. They start to question and discard the *status quo*, developing their own values, not necessarily what's dictated by peers. While the peer group's opinions are appreciated, the young person is now capable of forming a moral decision independent of the group.

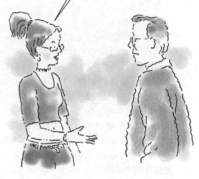

Hey, Dad. Can I have the car keys and £10 for petrol so I can be an adult and go vote?

What's the meaning of life?

The young person formulates questions about the larger world as they considers religion, philosophy and the values held by parents, friends and others. Young people may be suspicious about parental religious views, and curiosity about other religious beliefs is normal. They sort through and adopt those religious beliefs that are consistent with their moral character.

Look, I'm legal!

Their world view becomes solidified during this time. They may be considered a young adult and societal laws reinforce this. By 18, they can vote and, by age 21, is considered a full adult with all of the rights and responsibilities that go along with that status. (See *At what age can I?*, page 126.) Even so, the young person remains somewhat dependent on parents for finances and for help in meeting adult responsibilities.

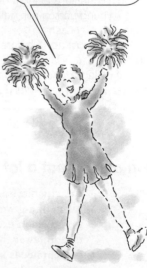

Iron, protein, keep me strong! I hope these cramps don't last too long!

Keys to health

Health issues during this period include nutrition, sleep and rest, exercise and dental hygiene.

Nutrition

Because physical changes are so drastic during adolescence, nutritional needs are greater than at any other time in a person's life.

At what age can I?

At 10

A young person has reached the age of criminal responsibility. This means that between the ages of 10 and 14, they can be convicted of a criminal offence if it can be proven that they knew what they were doing was seriously wrong.

At 13

A young person can have a part-time job, with some restrictions.

At 14

A young person is considered to be fully responsible for your actions, so if they commit a criminal offence, they will be treated the same as an adult (except from sentencing).

A young person can enter a pub, but they can't buy or drink alcohol there.

Between the ages of 10 and 14, a boy can be convicted of rape, assault with the intent to commit rape and unlawful sex with a girl if she is under 16, if it can be proven that he knew what he was doing was wrong.

At 16

A young person can have a full-time job once they have officially left school.

A young person can live independently, subject to certain conditions being met.

A young person can get married with their parents' or guardians' consent.

A girl must be 16 before she can legally have sex with a boy.

It is illegal for a boy or man to have sex with a girl under 16, even if she has agreed.

A male may consent to a homosexual act if he and his partner are both over 16.

A girl can have an abortion without her parents consent.

A boy can join the armed forces with his parents' or carers' consent.

A young person can have beer or cider whilst eating a meal in a restaurant or an eating area of a pub, but not in the bar.

At 17

A young person can hold a licence to drive most vehicles.

They can pilot a plane.

A young person can emigrate.

A care order can no longer be made on a young person.

At 18

A young person is legally seen as an adult in the eyes of the law.

A young person can vote in general and local elections.

A young person can get married.

A young person can buy cigarettes and tobacco.

A young person can open a bank account in their name without a parent or carer's signature.

A young person can buy and drink alcohol in a bar.

A young person can ask to see their birth certificate if they are adopted.

A young person can change their name.

A young person can be called to serve on a jury.

A young person can sue or be sued.

A young person can make a will.

A young person can place a bet.

A young person can have a tattoo.

A young person can buy fireworks and sparklers.

Run a little, eat a lot

Activity plays a large role in a young person's calorific requirements for maintaining weight. An active person playing sports for several hours per day may need in excess of 3,000 kcal per day, while an inactive girl may have to take in fewer than 2,000 kcal to prevent weight gain. In addition, iron and protein needs increase as girls begin the menstruation cycle and boys begin to develop lean muscle mass.

Got milk?

Because bone growth is so critical during adolescence, a proper intake of calcium and vitamin D is crucial. To achieve adequate levels, they need to consume at least three servings of calcium-fortified foods per day.

Watch out for the burgers!

Young people continue to select their own meals and form food preferences, making it even more important for parents to offer nutritionally balanced snacks and meals that will become lifelong choices. Peer and media pressure can be powerful at this time and influence eating habits so supportive information is crucial.

Sleep and rest

Sleep requirements increase slightly from the school-age years because of physical growth spurts and high activity levels in adolescents.

Use 'em or lose 'em

Sleep needs vary from person to person, but they usually require at least 8 hours of sleep each night and those 8 hours can't be made up or stored. Therefore, 'catch-up' sleep on the weekends isn't effective in replenishing their sleep store. But, with changes in hormonal levels, the young person will develop different sleep patterns to adults and this can be a challenge especially when it is time to get up in the morning!

Exercise

Physical fitness and exercise are important for several health related reasons. With obesity on the rise in the Western world, regular aerobic exercise can help maintain a healthy weight and prevent excessive gain. It also promotes a healthy cardiovascular system by reducing and preventing high blood pressure and hyperlipidemia.

Running from depression

Physical fitness may also help prevent periods of depression and help foster relationships between peers who have common sports activities. Some young people are not keen on sport and so alternative activities can be suggested which help them to keep healthy.

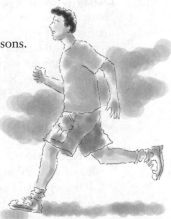

Physical fitness helps prevent depression, high blood pressure and parental nagging!

Dental hygiene

Good dental hygiene should consist of brushing at least twice daily, flossing once daily and professional cleanings twice per year. Snacks with high-sucrose levels and sweets that could cause dental caries should be avoided, but this is a challenge as the young person takes more responsibility for their personal hygiene.

Coping with concerns

Young people and their parents are typically faced with a range of concerns that may be intensified by the need for peer approval and the desire to assert independence.

Acne

During this period, acne is caused by blockage of follicles as a result of excessive sebum or bacteria. Acne has been associated with hormones due to the prevalence of flare-ups during a girl's premenstrual period.

Acne is found primarily on the face but can also appear on the chest and back. It's usually seen by the naked eye and treated with topical agents or antibiotics for inflammatory lesions.

No laughing matter

Acne can be devastating during this time of life when appearance is of the utmost concern. Even mild-to-moderate acne can have lasting negative effects on self-esteem and the young person's ability and willingness to develop friendships and other relationships. In severe cases, embarrassment and isolation can lead to depression.

For these reasons, acne should be considered a serious problem that warrants intervention, rather than a 'phase' that they should simply 'wait to grow out of'.

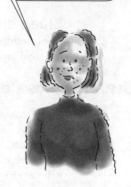

Adolescent acne should be taken seriously. Sometimes it makes me feel socially isolated and depressed.

Body piercings and tattoos

Young people may use body piercings and tattoos to make a 'statement' about their sense of style and to express their individuality. For health reasons, piercings and tattoos should be performed by an experienced, licensed person. It's important not to pass judgement on the individual who chooses to get a tattoo or piercing. Rather, consider their choice as an opportunity to provide education on the subject which, in turn, helps them make an informed decision.

Cigarette smoking

Cigarette smoking among young people continues to be a problem. The NHS reports that

> Almost a third of pupils (32 per cent) aged 11 to 15 in England in 2008 reported having tried smoking at least once and 6 per cent were regular smokers (smoking at least one cigarette a week). Girls were more likely to smoke than boys; 11 per cent of girls have smoked in the last week compared with 8 per cent of boys (http://www.ic.nhs.uk/pubs/smoking09).

Boys, however, consume more cigarettes than girls!

Dangling the bait

Peer influence and family practices have a tremendous influence on smoking. Young people may start smoking to 'look cool' or 'fit in' with their peer groups, despite their knowledge of the deadly health consequences. Tobacco use can be associated with increasingly risky behaviours, such as alcohol use, drug use and experimenting with sex.

Injury prevention

When children reach school age, they are no longer under parents' constant supervision. Because of this unfamiliar freedom, school-age children and young people can sustain a range of serious, sometimes life-threatening, injuries.

Motor vehicle accidents

Motor vehicle accidents are one of the leading causes of death among young people. During the later years, the young person is, by law, 'ready' to get a driver's license. However, with greater privilege comes increased responsibility. There has also been an increase in young people, oblivious to traffic whilst listening to music players or using mobile phones, being hit by vehicles.

The nurse's role

The nurse can help prevent motor vehicle accidents through education. Young people who are reluctant to listen to their parents may listen to another figure such as a nurse, particularly if they are non-judgemental.

Buckled up for safety

A young person should be shown that wearing a seat belt can drastically reduce the risk of life-threatening injuries in the event of an accident. They should also be encouraged to use a helmet when riding scooters, mopeds and motorcycle. This is of course a legal requirement in the UK; however, some young people still ignore it.

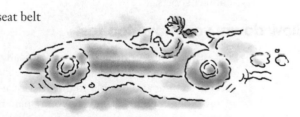

A deadly mix

Perhaps the greatest emphasis should be placed on educating the young person about the risks of mixing driving when under the influence of alcohol or drugs. This combination is not only illegal but also impairs the driver's judgement and could have deadly consequences.

Risk-taking behaviours

Young people are still maturing, both cognitively and emotionally. A lack of maturity may lead them to take unwise chances, in an attempt to be accepted by their peers.

Risky business

Young people have an 'it can't happen to me' attitude and feel they're invincible. They may take risks to seek attention from others because of failures in school, rejection by peers, neglect at home, or a combination of these factors. A young person tends to be less of a risk taker if they have established autonomy and respect their parents and other authority figures.

Sports injuries

While there's the potential for injury in any sport, most injuries occur during recreational sporting events rather than during organised competitions. Serious injuries are generally more common during recreational and individual sports.

There's safety in numbers. Sports injuries are less common in team sports.

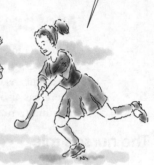

In any case, although injuries are usually random events, the risk of injury can be decreased by improving playing conditions, demanding compliance with rules and protective equipment and providing diligent coaching and supervision.

Injury protection

The nurse can help prevent sports injuries through education about safety equipment and potential risk. Younger people need to be encouraged to use helmets when riding bicycles and to wear appropriate protective equipment when playing contact sports.

Slow down, you move too fast

Because a young person's body is physically maturing, they will need to learn how to adjust in order to recognise limitations, avoid straining or overstretching and be able to then perform physically challenging activities. After experiencing an injury, a young person must be encouraged to follow rehabilitation instructions to prevent further injury or reinjury.

Health problems

Several serious health problems can affect school-age children and young people. Some of these problems may be life threatening.

Alcohol and drug abuse

Alcoholism is a chronic disorder most commonly described as the uncontrolled intake of alcoholic beverages. Psychoactive drug abuse and dependence is the use of illegal drugs or misuse of legal drugs, including narcotics, stimulants, depressants, anti-anxiety agents and hallucinogens. Alcoholism and drug abuse impair physical and mental heath, social and familial relationships and the ability to uphold responsibilities related to school and, later on, jobs.

Although the use of such substances can have severe consequences, recent data identifies that overall alcohol and drug usage amongst young people in the UK is decreasing. Those who need supportive services appear to receive them, and also the numbers of those needing specialist addiction treatment are very low.

What causes it

Numerous biological, psychological and socio-cultural factors may influence alcoholism and drug abuse. Family background may play a significant role, as the child of one alcoholic parent is seven to eight times more likely to become an alcoholic than a peer without such a parent.

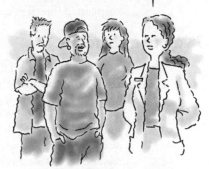

A positive adult role model is the best antidote for negative peer influences.

Psychologically speaking

Psychological factors that may influence alcohol or drug abuse may include:
• inadequate coping skills, leading to the urge to reduce anxiety and tension through the use of substances
• a desire to avoid responsibility
• an inability to deal effectively with loneliness or boredom
• a need to bolster self-esteem.

Socio-culturally speaking

Socio-cultural factors that may influence alcohol or drug abuse include:
• the availability of (cheap) alcohol and drugs
• group or peer pressure
• societal attitudes that condone alcohol or drug use.

What to look for

Substance abuse is defined as a maladaptive pattern of substance use (drug or alcohol) leading to clinically significant impairment or distress. This impairment or distress manifests as one or more of the following:
• recurrent substance use resulting in a failure to fulfil major role obligations at school, home or work
• recurrent substance use in situations in which using the substance is physically hazardous
• recurrent substance-related legal problems
• continued substance use despite persistent or recurrent social or interpersonal problems caused by or exacerbated by the effects of the substance.

Get in there first

Young people are often resistant to parental advice and education and so reference to other support can help avoid the use of substances. The FRANK campaign is a national resource which provides advice, support and information to young people in language and terms they use so as to understand the risk and dangers of drug use (http://talktofrank.com/).

Ups and downs

Chronic substance abusers may present with a variety of minor complaints, such as mood swings and depression, malaise and an increased incidence of infection.

Something smells fishy

The effects on personal appearance include poor personal hygiene, unexplained injuries (such as cigarette burns) and nutritional deficiencies.

I've got a secret

The young person or child may be secretive about their addiction and may engage in suspicious behaviours, such as lying and stealing money, to support the habit. The school may report multiple, unexplained absences, poor classroom performance and behaviour pattern changes. When confronted about this behaviour, they may deny the problem or become angry and violent towards others. The school should involve the School Health Nurse and the Education Welfare service where children and young people are demonstrating such ongoing problems. Equally a referral to Children's Services may be required if the child is considered to be a 'Child in Need' under section 17 of the Children Act 1989 and similarly with the Children (Scotland) Act 1995.

Acute intoxication

With acute alcohol or drug intoxication, look for one or any number of the following:
- decreased inhibitions
- euphoria followed by depression or hostility
- impaired judgement
- lack of coordination
- respiratory depression
- slurred speech
- unconsciousness
- vomiting.

What tests tell you

Urine, blood and saliva tests can confirm drug use and blood alcohol level, determine the amount and type of substance taken and reveal complications.

Complications of alcohol abuse

Alcohol can damage body tissues by its direct irritating effects, changes that take place in the body during its metabolism, aggravation of existing disease, accidents occurring during intoxication and interactions between the alcohol and drugs. Such tissue damage can lead to a range of complications, including those listed below:

Cardiopulmonary complications

- Cardiac arrhythmias
- Cardiomyopathy
- Chronic obstructive-pulmonary disease
- Essential hypertension
- Increased risk of tuberculosis
- Pneumonia

Hepatic complications

- Alcoholic hepatitis
- Cirrhosis
- Fatty liver

GI complications

- Chronic diarrhoea
- Oesophageal cancer
- Oesophageal varices
- Oesophagitis
- Gastric ulcers
- Gastritis
- GI bleeding
- Malabsorption
- Pancreatitis

Neurologic complications

- Alcoholic dementia
- Alcoholic hallucinosis
- Alcohol withdrawal delirium
- Korsakoff syndrome
- Peripheral neuropathy
- Seizure disorders
- Subdural hematoma
- Wernicke's encephalopathy

Psychiatric complications

- Amotivational syndrome
- Depression
- Fetal alcohol syndrome
- Impaired social and occupational functioning
- Abuse of multiple substances
- Suicide

Other complications

- Beriberi
- Hypoglycemia
- Leg and foot ulcers
- Prostatitis

Complications

Most body tissues can be adversely affected by the heavy intake of alcohol, and death can occur from abrupt alcohol withdrawal. (See *Complications of alcohol abuse*.)

Chronic drug abuse, especially IV use, can lead to life threatening complications, including:
- cardiac and respiratory arrest, subacute bacterial endocarditis, pulmonary emboli and respiratory infections
- intracranial haemorrhage
- vasculitis, thrombophlebitis and gangrene
- musculoskeletal dysfunction
- acquired immunodeficiency syndrome (AIDS) and hepatitis
- tetanus, septicaemia and malaria
- malnutrition
- trauma
- depression, psychosis and increased risk of suicide.

How it's treated

Treatment of alcoholism and drug abuse must be long term and requires the support of the child's parents and other significant people in their life.

Alcohol abuse

Total abstinence from alcohol is the only effective treatment of alcoholism. Participation in supportive programs, including Alcoholics Anonymous and Ala-Teen, may produce favourable long-term results, although failure and relapse rates are high. The recovering individual must also be able to fill the niche once occupied by alcohol with something constructive. In addition, there must be an assessment of alcohol use within the family as this might be a wider problem.

Symptom support

Acute intoxication is treated symptomatically by:
- supporting respiration
- preventing aspiration of vomit
- replacing fluids
- maintaining blood glucose levels
- initiating emergency treatment of trauma, infection and GI bleeding.

Drug abuse

Treatment of drug dependence commonly involves a triad of care: detoxification, short- and long-term rehabilitation and aftercare (meaning a lifetime of abstinence). Aftercare is usually aided by participation in self-help group programmes.

The NHS National Treatment Agency for Substance Abuse provides guidelines, resource information and evidence about helping young people who are substances abusers (see http://www.nta.nhs.uk/young-people.aspx).

Slowly but surely

The teen with acute drug intoxication should receive symptomatic treatment based on the drug ingested. Detoxification with the same drug or a pharmacologically similar drug may be necessary. Depending on the dosage and the time elapsed since ingestion, additional treatment may include gastric lavage, induced emesis, activated charcoal or forced diuresis.

What to do

- Be alert for potential alcohol and drug abuse problems. Ask the young person about their use of substances, and about their friends' usage. Ensure confidentiality, and ask questions and provide information in a straightforward manner to promote an open discussion.
- Be aware of signs and symptoms of intoxication with alcohol and commonly used drugs so you'll be prepared to identify them if seen in practice.

During an acute intoxication:
- Continuously monitor vital signs.
- Observe for complications of overdose and withdrawal, such as cardiopulmonary arrest, seizures and aspiration.
- Initiate advanced life-support measures as required by the situation.

When the party's over

After an acute intoxication and dependent on their age:
• Refer the young person to Child and Adolescent Mental Health services.
• Consider the need to refer the young person as in need or at risk of harm, following safeguarding procedures.
• Monitor the young person for immediate signs of depression or impending suicide.
• Encourage family members to seek professional help whether or not the young person does so.

Teenage pregnancy

Teenage pregnancy refers to those under the age of 18 years. The UK has had one of the highest rates of teenage pregnancy in Europe, although rates have decreased over the last decade. Despite this, the rates are still amongst the highest and particular for under-16-year-old young women. Contemporary data from 2008 shows that:
• In England there were 38,750 births in the under 18s
• In Wales 2575 births in the under 18s
• In Scotland 3857 births in the under 18s
• In NI there has been a reduction; however, measurement of data is different (TPIAG, 2009; DCSF, 2010; ISD Scotland, 2009; FPA, 2005).
    Also, in England and Wales, 20% of under-18 conceptions are repeat pregnancies which increases the rate even more and potentially puts the young women at risk of complications.

What causes it

Teenage pregnancy is a complex phenomenon and because of this attempts to reduce the incidence raise many challenges. Teenage pregnancies may occur because of:
• Lack of, or poor, knowledge about contraception
• Problems and barriers to accessing contraception
• Beliefs about avoiding getting pregnant (such as having sex whilst standing)
• Early sexual activity
• It just happened!
• Wanting a baby and the feeling of being a mother
• Seeking love and attention
• Deliberate decision through love and commitment
• Sexual abuse, rape or involvement in childhood prostitution.

What to look for

The signs of pregnancy are no different for the teenager; however, the young person may be unaware of or attempt to hide the pregnancy. Equally if their periods are not consistent, their absence may not lead to suspicions of a pregnancy. Often the discovery is accidental if the young person has been asked to undergo a pregnancy test when attending health care.

What tests tell you

A pregnancy test can be undertaken from the first day after the missed period. This measures the level of human chorionic gonadatrophin and if detected indicates a pregnancy. A negative result may need a further home test or a laboratory test via a health professional.

Complications

There are a range of physiological and social consequences of teenage pregnancy which impact upon the young person, including:
- Hypertension
- Anaemia
- Placental abruption
- Obstetric complications
- Depression
- Educational disruption and impaired academic achievement
- Social isolation
- Socio-economic disadvantage
- Babies have a 60% higher risk of dying in the first year of life.

How it's treated

Three options are available for the young person, including continuing the pregnancy, continuing and have the baby adopted or an abortion, all of which require advice, support and counselling in order to make an informed choice. For many, this will involve the family who can provide support and help; however, this may not always be the case. There may be occasions when decision-making will involve Children's Services, and the courts, particularly if the young person is in the care of the local authority.

What to do

- Be alert to the potential for pregnancy in young girls.
- Follow guidelines for offering pregnancy tests prior to health care interventions.
- Consider pregnancy in young girls who seek non-specific health care advice and seem reluctant to discuss particular topics.
- Need to maintain confidentiality for the young person when discussing pregnancy tests, results and implications unless there is a risk of harm in which safeguarding procedures must be adhered to.
- Follow local safeguarding children procedures and refer the young person at any stage if harm is suspected or an illegal act has been perpetrated.
- Ensure maternity services are involved in the young person's antenatal and general health care.

Anorexia nervosa

Anorexia nervosa is a disorder that involves voluntary refusal to eat, accompanied by a severe loss of body weight without an organic cause. It

Bulimia

Bulimia is defined as regular episodes of binge eating, followed by self-induced vomiting, strict dieting or fasting, vigorous exercise or taking laxatives or diuretics. The condition usually begins in adolescence or early childhood and may coexist with anorexia nervosa. The exact cause of bulimia is unknown.

Signs and symptoms

- Alternating episodes of binge eating and purging
- Thin or slightly overweight build
- Use of diuretics or laxatives
- Vomiting
- Reports of abdominal and epigastric pain, amenorrhea and painless swelling of the salivary glands
- Hoarse and irritated voice
- Calluses on the knuckles from vomiting (Russell's sign)
- Anxiety and avoidance of conflict
- Extreme need for approval
- Guilt and self-disgust
- Constant preoccupation with food
- Preoccupation with exercise (and excessive exercise)

Key test findings

The Beck Depression Inventory may reveal depression; an eating attitudes test suggests an eating disorder. Metabolic acidosis may occur from diarrhoea caused by enemas and excessive laxative use. Metabolic alkalosis (the most common metabolic complication) may occur from frequent vomiting. Laboratory tests revel elevated bicarbonate, decreased potassium and decreased sodium levels.

Bulimia complications

- Dental caries
- Erosion of tooth enamel and gum infections
- Increased risk of oesophageal tears, gastric rupture and mucosal damage to the intestines
- Life-threatening cardiac arrhythmias, cardiac failure or sudden death

Treating bulimia

- Inpatient or outpatient therapy
- Self-help groups
- Selective serotonin reuptake inhibitors, such as paroxetine and fluoxetine

---

results from a distorted, unrealistic perception of body size, weight and food intake. It may coexist with bulimia. (See *Bulimia*.)

The skinny on being skinny

These perceptions override feelings of hunger, family members' threats or pleas to eat, and an intellectual (but not emotional) acknowledgement of the problem.

Girl power?

Although more than 90% of those with anorexia nervosa are young girls and young women, the condition is increasingly appearing in males and has been diagnosed in children as young as 7 years.

By conservative estimates, 0.5% to 1% of females in late adolescence and early adulthood meet the diagnostic criteria. Over their entire lifetime, an estimated 0.5% to 3.75% of females suffer from anorexia. The ratio of girls to boys is 10:1.

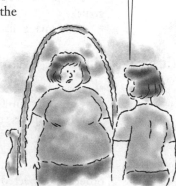

It doesn't matter how thin they say I am. There's always a fat person in my mirror.

What causes it

The exact cause of anorexia nervosa is unknown; however, a number of external and internal influences are thought to contribute to the disorder. These influences include:

- societal attitudes that equate slimness with beauty
- excessive pressure to achieve
- dependence and independence issues
- control issues
- stress due to multiple responsibilities.

Related risks

Anorexia nervosa is a subconscious effort to exert personal control over life or to protect oneself from dealing with issues surrounding sexuality. Several risk factors have been identified, including:

- low self-esteem
- compulsive personality
- history of sexual abuse
- high, sometimes unrealistic, achievement goals (set by the person at risk or by parents or other authority figures).

How it happens

Decreased calorific intake depletes body fat and protein stores. In adolescent girls and women, oestrogen deficiency occurs because the stress on the body diminishes the production of LH and FSH, resulting in amenorrhea.

In adolescent boys and men, testosterone levels fluctuate, resulting in reduced erectile function and a reduction in sperm count. Ketoacidosis occurs from increased use of body fat as energy.

What to look for

When anorexia nervosa is suspected, look for:

- emaciated or skeleton-like appearance, not regarded by the teen as being abnormal or undesirable
- evidence of secret dieting
- lack of satisfaction with weight loss (constantly setting new, lower weight goals)
- body image distortion (weight, size, shape).

Cold, constipated, weak and absent

- possible reported symptoms, including cold intolerance, low blood pressure, low pulse rate and abdominal pain
- GI symptoms such as constipation or laxative dependence
- muscle weakness, seizures or cardiac arrhythmias
- emaciated appearance with dry skin and lanugo hair over back and extremities
- amenorrhea (absence of at least three consecutive menstrual cycles when otherwise expected to occur), fatigue, loss of libido and infertility

- cognitive distortions, such as overgeneralisation, or dichotomous thinking (black or white, good or bad, all or nothing)
- compulsive behaviour such as excessive exercising
- dependency on others for self-worth.

Guilty, impaired and needing to please

- guilt associated with eating
- impaired decision-making
- need to achieve and please others
- overly compliant attitude
- perfectionist attitude
- obsessive rituals concerning food and a preoccupation with food preparation
- refusal to eat and to maintain or achieve normal weight for age and height
- intense fear of gaining weight or becoming fat, even though underweight.

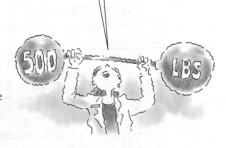

A child or young person with anorexia nervosa may exercise to excess.

What tests tell you

All criteria described in the *Diagnostic and Statistical Manual of Mental Disorders*, Fourth Edition, Text Revision must be met for a diagnosis of anorexia nervosa. (See *Diagnosing anorexia nervosa*.)

In addition, findings from an eating attitude test performed on a person with anorexia nervosa suggest an eating disorder, and an electrocardiogram (ECG)

Diagnosing anorexia nervosa

The diagnosis of anorexia nervosa is confirmed when the individual meets the following criteria from the *Diagnostic and Statistical Manual of Mental Disorders*, Fourth Edition, Text Revision.

Abnormally low weight and body image distortion

- The young person refuses to maintain weight at or above a minimally normal weight for age and height (e.g. weight loss leading to maintenance of body weight that's less than 85% of the expected weight) or fails to achieve expected weight gain during a growth period, resulting in a weight less than 85% of that expected.
- Even though underweight, the young person has an intense fear of gaining weight or becoming fat.
- The young person has a distorted perception of body weight, size or shape; their weight or shape has an undue influence on self-evaluation; or they deny the seriousness of the underweight condition.

- If the young person is of menstruating age, she has missed at least three consecutive menstrual cycles (excluding menses induced by hormone administration).

Subtypes of anorexia nervosa

There are two subtypes of anorexia nervosa:

restricting, in which a young person hasn't regularly engaged in binge-eating or purging (self-induced vomiting or misuse of laxatives, diuretics or enemas) during the current episode of the disorder

binge-eating or purging, in which the young person has regularly engaged in binge-eating or purging during the current episode.

reveals non-specific ST interval, prolonged PR interval and T wave changes. Other findings include:

- low oestrogen levels in female patients
- low testosterone levels in male patients
- low haemoglobin levels and low platelet and white blood cell counts
- elevated blood urea nitrogen
- electrolyte imbalances.

Complications

Complications of anorexia nervosa include:

- electrolyte imbalances
- chronic malnutrition
- acute dehydration
- oesophageal erosion, ulcers, tears and bleeding
- tooth and gum erosion and dental caries
- decreased left ventricular muscle mass and chamber size
- decreased cardiac output and hypotension
- ECG changes
- increased susceptibility to infection
- anaemia.

How it's treated

Medical management includes behaviour modification and group, family or individual psychotherapy. Young people should be helped to achieve a well-balanced diet with a normal eating pattern and vitamin supplements. However, a rapid weight gain should be avoided due to the potential for severe metabolic abnormalities.

Bring out the troops

Drug therapy may include anti-anxiety agents, such as lorazepam; antidepressants, such as amitriptyline and imipramine and selective serotonin reuptake inhibitors, such as paroxetine and fluoxetine. Despite all the above, the evidence that they effectively influence core symptoms is not strong.

The involvement of the Child and Adolescent Mental Health Team is crucial in effectively managing the care of the young person, however hospitalisation may also be required and this should be in a specialist centre. Support in the community can be effective as long as the young person is not detiorating or their behaviour poses a risk to themselves or others.

What to do

Early recognition is key. Young people need to be aware of the seriousness of this type of self-imposed disease. Positive, early interventions include:

- teaching coaches, teachers and parents to recognise early signs
- supporting the young person's efforts to achieve their target weight

and helping to negotiate adequate food intake in a relaxed, non-punitive treatment atmosphere.

Express for success

Long-term success involves helping the young person identify coping mechanisms for dealing with anxiety and encouraging them to express feelings without fear of reprisal or judgement.

In addition, the nurse should:
• Provide a specific goal-oriented plan that can be followed consistently.
• Encourage early family therapy, which is most effective when it's started soon after the diagnosis is made.
• Foster an open, honest therapeutic relationship with the adolescent, yet be firm to counteract manipulative behaviour; behaviour modification therapy may be helpful to decrease the young person's manipulative behaviour.

Attention deficit hyperactivity disorder

Attention deficit hyperactivity disorder (ADHD) is a behaviour problem characterised by difficulty in focusing attention; difficulty engaging in quiet, passive activities or both. It's possible to have attention deficit without hyperactivity.

One in every classroom ...

ADHD affects roughly 3% to 5% of school-age children in the UK – an average of one in every classroom. It affects at least twice as many boys as girls.

... and in the office, too

Until recently, experts thought that children outgrew ADHD by adolescence. We now know that many symptoms continue into adulthood. In fact, the disorder affects approximately 2% to 4% of adults.

To be diagnosed with ADHD, a child's behaviours must:
• be present in two or more settings
• begin before the age of 7
• result in significant impairment in social or academic functioning.

What causes it

The underlying causes are unknown. There's limited evidence of a genetic component, and some studies suggest that it may result from altered neurotransmitter levels in the brain. Other theories point to a deficit within the right hemisphere of the brain or an alteration of the reticular activating system of the midbrain that causes the child to react to all stimulation, not just selected stimuli.

How it happens

Alleles of dopamine genes may alter dopamine transmission in the neural networks. During foetal development, bouts of hypoxia and hypotension could selectively damage neurons located in some of the critical regions of the anatomic networks.

What to look for

A child or adolescent with ADHD may exhibit several behaviours and difficulties, including:
- climbing, running or talking excessively
- decreased attention span
- difficulty organising tasks and activities
- difficulty waiting for turns or playing quietly
- being easily distracted; failing to give close attention to schoolwork or to finish an activity
- failing to listen when spoken to directly.

So many things to do ...

- fidgeting or squirming in their chair (being disruptive in the classroom)
- frequent periods of forgetfulness (frequently losing things needed for tasks)
- impulsive behaviour
- losing their temper easily
- inability to follow directions.

What tests tell you

Complete psychological, medical and neurological evaluations must rule out other problems before an ADHD diagnosis can be made. To make the diagnosis, the findings are combined with data from several sources, including parents, teachers and the child. (See *Diagnosing ADHD*.)

Complications

Complications of ADHD include emotional and social difficulties (which may be extreme) and poor nutrition. Children with ADHD may also be at increased risk of abuse because parents may become exasperated with the child's behaviour and may become abusive out of frustration and exhaustion. The child's behaviour may also bring them into conflict with the police, ending with involvement of the Youth Justice system.

Looking for the label

In addition, the child may experience long-term difficulties at school because of being 'labelled' with an ADHD diagnosis, although services are often not provided until the label is given! Children with ADHD may also have adverse reactions to medications used to treat the disorder.

How it's treated

Medical management starts with behaviour modification and psychological therapy. Interdisciplinary interventions include a pathologic assessment and diagnosis of specific learning needs. Drug therapy may include amphetamines, such as methylphenidate or dextroamphetamine, to help the child concentrate. Nutritional therapy by the addition of substances considered to be deficient or excluding potentially harmful ones has been

Diagnosing ADHD

The *Diagnostic and Statistical Manual of Mental Disorders*, Fourth Edition, Text Revision groups a selection of symptoms into inattention and hyperactivity-impulsivity categories. To be diagnosed with attention deficit hyperactivity disorder (ADHD), the child must have at least six symptoms from the inattention group or at least six from the hyperactivity-impulsivity group. Symptoms must have persisted for at least 6 months and to a degree that's maladaptive and inconsistent with the child's developmental level.

Symptoms of inattention

The child manifesting *inattention* will commonly:

- fail to pay close attention to details or make careless mistakes in school or other activities
- have trouble sustaining attention in tasks or play activities
- seem not to listen when spoken to directly
- demonstrate forgetfulness in daily activities
- fail to follow through on instructions or to finish schoolwork or tasks (not because of oppositional behaviour or failure to understand instructions)
- have trouble organising tasks and activities
- avoid, dislike or be reluctant to engage in tasks that require sustained mental effort (such as schoolwork or homework)
- lose things necessary for tasks or activities (toys, school assignments, pencils, books)
- become distracted by extraneous stimuli.

Symptoms of hyperactivity-impulsivity

The child manifesting *hyperactivity* will commonly:

- fidget with their hands or feet or squirm in their seat
- leave their seat in the classroom or in other situations in which remaining seated is expected
- run about or climb excessively in inappropriate situations
- have trouble playing or engaging in leisure activities quietly
- be described as 'always on the go'
- talk excessively.
- The child manifesting *impulsivity* will commonly:
- blurt out answers before questions have been completed
- have difficulty waiting their turn
- interrupt or intrude on others in conversations or games.

Additional features

- Some symptoms causing impairment appear before the age of 7 years.
- Impairment from the symptoms is present in two or more settings (at school and at home).
- Clinically significant impairment in social, academic and job-related functioning is clearly evident.

used; however, the evidence for this is very limited. Where there is a link between a specific dietary substance and the young person's behaviour then exclusion may be helpful.

What to do

The child with ADHD and their parents need information and ongoing support:
- Monitor the child's growth, especially if receiving methylphenidate (as growth may be slowed).
- Give one simple instruction at a time so the child can successfully complete the task (which promotes self-esteem).

Meals matter

- Educate parents to give medications in the morning and at lunch to avoid interfering with sleep.

- Encourage adequate nutrition as medications and hyperactivity may increase nutrient needs.
- Suggest that parents reduce environmental stimuli to decrease distraction, and formulate a schedule for the child to provide consistency and routine.

Report and support

- Suggest that teachers provide a daily report on the child's progress to ensure that rules given at the home are being reinforced in other environments.
- Involvement of the SEN (Special Educational Needs) teacher and Education Welfare Officers to develop plans.
- Provide parents with information about support groups, such as local organisations and online groups.
    Up-to-date guidance on the management of this disorder can be found at: http://www.nice.org.uk/nicemedia/pdf/ADHDFullGuideline.pdf

Obesity

Obesity is an excess of body fat that's generally 20% or more above ideal body weight for a person's age and height. Obesity rates in school-age children rocketed from 6.5% in the 1970s to more than 15% in 2000. Adolescent obesity rates in the same period increased even more dramatically, from 5% to 15.5%.

Equality of the sexes

In addition, boys and girls seem equally at risk for obesity in both age groups (school-age boys, 16%; school-age girls, 14.5%; adolescent girls and boys, 15.5%).

What causes it

Obesity results when a person takes in or consumes more calories than they are expending. Simply put, the child eats more calories then the body burns.
    Obesity in childhood and adolescence can be related to these factors:
- sedentary lifestyle (couch-potato children due to increased television viewing, computer usage and decreased physical activity)
- overeating
- poor eating habits
- stressful changes or life events, such as divorce, death, moving or abuse
- low self-esteem
- depression
- family problems or problems with peers.

How it happens

The aetiology of obesity is complex and usually multifactorial. Theories to explain this condition include:

- genetic predisposition
- biological factors
- psychological factors.

Genetic predisposition

Obesity in parents increases the probability of obesity in children. In fact, a child of parents with obesity has an 80% chance of having obesity as a child. A child who's obese between 10 and 13 years has an 80% chance of becoming obese as an adult.

Some contributors to the genetic disposition towards obesity include:
- a body type that's predisposed to the accumulation of subcutaneous fat (such as those with a rounded, soft body shape)
- an inherited defect that interferes with the metabolic break-down of fat
- familial and cultural eating patterns and behaviours.

Biological factors

Certain diseases and endocrine and metabolic problems can contribute to childhood obesity. Underlying disease is attributed to only 5% of cases of childhood obesity. Such conditions as hypothyroidism, muscular dystrophy, Down's syndrome and spina bifida can cause accumulation of fat due to decreased metabolism or limited mobility.

Endocrine and metabolic factors are complex. The relationships between feelings of hunger and satiety, the central nervous system and the body's ability to metabolise carbohydrates, protein and fat are still under investigation.

Psychological factors

Many children, as well as adults, eat in response to how they're feeling. Eating gives older children and adolescents a sense of well-being, satiety and security – feelings that were developed when they ate during infancy.

However, for a child who's bored, tired, depressed, sad or lonely, eating is a way of obtaining those warm, nurturing feelings; it becomes a comfort. In addition, parents may use food as a reward, or withhold it as punishment, furthering the child's misuse of food.

What to look for

Observation and comparison of height and weight to a standard table indicate obesity. Measurement of the thickness of subcutaneous fat folds with callipers provides an approximation of total body fat.

What tests tell you

Body mass index can be calculated by dividing a person's weight by the square of his/her height. This number can be compared to normal values on standardised graphs to diagnose progressive levels of obesity; however, it does not fully account for changes in muscle mass or adipose levels with age. Therefore, body mass index percentiles are better used to define obesity in childhood.

Complications

Obesity may lead to serious complications, such as respiratory difficulties, hypertension, cardiovascular disease, diabetes mellitus and renal disease as well as psychosocial difficulties, including emotional taunts from peers.

How it's treated

Weight-loss diets are not the answer for children and young people because of their nutritional needs during a time of rapid growth. Instead, it's recommended that the child be helped to maintain current weight while allowing for stature to continue growing. The child, in effect, outgrows their obesity (this isn't necessarily the case with adolescents).

While restrictive diets aren't the normal treatment, dietary changes can have significant results. Suggestions include:
- avoiding fast food establishments
- providing low-fat alternatives for after-school snacks
- switching from whole milk to skimmed milk
- exchanging fresh vegetables for fried snack foods
- offering a variety of fresh and dried fruits.

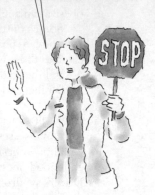

Weight-loss diets and children aren't a good mix. Instead, the emphasis needs to be on maintaining current weight because they'll 'grow into it'.

What to do

When providing care to a child or young person with obesity:
- Obtain an accurate dietary history to identify the child's eating patterns and determine the importance of food to their lifestyle.
- Work in partnership with the child and parents to develop a plan of action
- Encourage the child and parents to adhere to the agreed dietary meal plan to help ensure a successful outcome.
- Suggest low-calorie, low-fat snacks, such as fresh fruits and vegetables.
- Encourage parents to avoid overfeeding their children and discourage the use of food as a reward for good behaviour.
- Promote physical activities, such as involvement in organised sports teams and individual events and a personalised exercise program.

Vim and vigour

Children with obesity or normal weight should be encouraged to participate in some type of daily, vigorous, aerobic activity to help reduce or prevent childhood obesity and to promote a habit of daily exercise that will last a lifetime. This requires a sensitive approach as the child may feel embarrassed, awkward and thus reluctant to exercise with others!

Sexually transmitted diseases

An important group of sex-related disorders results from infection that's transmitted through sexual contact. These sexually transmitted diseases (STDs) include:
- AIDS
- chlamydia infections

- genital herpes
- genital warts
- gonorrhoea
- syphilis
- trichomoniasis.

They're everywhere

STDs are among the most prevalent infections around the world. Gonorrhoea, chlamydial infections and genital warts continue to increase in incidence in the UK. In the past 10 years, between one-fifth and one-third of all reported cases of chlamydia, gonorrhea and syphilis affect adolescents and young adults up to 24 years of age.

What causes it

The cause of an STD may be bacterial, viral or parasitic. (See *Common STDs*, page 148.)

How it happens

STDs are passed from one person to another through anal, oral or vaginal sexual contact. The rate of transmission and, therefore, the incidence of these diseases are rising because of societal attitudes towards sex (such as those who condone multiple sexual partners), a lack of effective health promotion (for condom use or abstinence) and increased reporting of new cases.

When STDs are diagnosed in children who are school-age or younger, child abuse must be considered and local safeguarding procedures followed. There may be instances where a neonate displays signs of infection for example gonorrhoea, and this has been acquired during delivery.

What to look for

Symptoms vary depending on the infectious organism, and symptoms of a particular STD may vary by gender. Some classic symptoms of STDs include:
- pain during urination
- vaginal or penile discharge
- growths that appear on the genitalia and sores on the mouth or genitalia
- evidence of sexual abuse, such as vaginal tears, vaginal bruising, blood in the child's underwear and difficulties voiding. (Never assume that a child of any age has acquired an STD by consensual sexual contact.)

What tests tell you

A sexual history provides the basis for prevention, diagnosis and treatment of an STD. The physical assessment, primarily a diagnostic tool, can also serve as an excellent opportunity for prevention.

I.D. the STD

To help identify the infectious organism, the suspected lesion is cultured with the appropriate culture method:

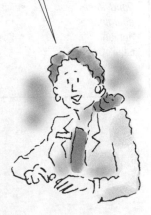

Reassure the child that you're there to help, and that nothing that has happened is his fault.

Common STDs

This chart lists several sexually transmitted diseases (STDs) along with their causative organisms, assessment findings and appropriate treatments (including those used in pregnant patients).

STD	Assessment findings	Treatment
Chlamydia *Chlamydia trachomatis*	• Asymptomatic (commonly); suspicion should be raised if partner has been treated for nongonococcal urethritis • Heavy, grey-white vaginal discharge • Painful urination • Positive vaginal culture using special chlamydial test kit	• Amoxicillin
Syphilis *Treponema pallidum*	• Painless ulcer on vulva or vagina (primary syphilis) • Hepatic and splenic enlargement, headache, anorexia and maculopapular rash on the palms of the hands and soles of the feet (secondary syphilis; occurring about 2 months after initial infection) • Cardiac, vascular and central nervous system changes (tertiary syphilis; occurring after an undetermined latent phase) • Positive Venereal Disease Research Laboratory serum test; confirmed with positive rapid plasma reagin and fluorescent treponemal antibody absorption tests • Dark-field microscopy positive for spirochete	• Penicillin G I.M. (single dose)
Genital herpes Herpes simplex virus, type 2	• Painful, small vesicles with erythematous base on vulva or vagina, rupturing within 1 to 7 days to form ulcers • Low-grade fever • Dyspareunia • Positive viral culture of vesicular fluid • Positive enzyme-linked immunosorbent assay	• Acyclovir orally or in ointment form
Gonorrhea *Neisseria gonorrhoeae*	• May not produce symptoms • Yellow-green vaginal discharge • Male partner who experiences severe pain on urination and purulent yellow penile discharge • Positive culture of vaginal, rectal or urethral secretions	• Cefixime as a one-time IM injection
Condyloma acuminata Human papillomavirus	• Discrete papillary structures that spread, enlarge and coalesce to form large lesions; increasing in size during pregnancy • Possible secondary ulceration and infection with foul odour	• Topical application of trichloroacetic acid or bichloracetic acid to lesions • Lesion removal with laser therapy, cryocautery or knife excision

- A genital tract specimen from a male should contain urethral discharge or prostatic fluid.
- From a female, the specimen should contain urethral or cervical specimens.
- Two swabs should always be collected simultaneously.

Privacy is paramount

Keep in mind that examinations of this kind can be extremely difficult and embarrassing for school-age children and young people. Procedures should be explained thoroughly and as much privacy as possible should be provided.

The privacy problems

Encouraging children and young people to access sexual health services can be problematic and when they do so it brings the challenge of respecting their privacy and need for confidentiality versus the practitioner's responsibility to uphold the law and operate within safeguarding policies and procedures. Each service must have clear guidelines about sharing of information and breaching confidentiality; but in all cases the welfare of the child is the paramount issue!

Within the UK, contact tracing takes place in an effort to identify those with specific STDs and enable them to gain treatment. This can be a problem when the young person refuses to identify whom they have had sexual contact with because:
- they are embarrassed and frightened about the consequences
- they feel they are to blame
- they are being sexually abused
- they are involved in prostitution.

Complications
Complications that are common to all STDs include emotional stress, male or female infertility, ectopic pregnancies and even death.

How it's treated
STDs may be treated with antibiotic or antiviral medication. They're also treated symptomatically with analgesics and antipyretics. Some diseases, such as herpes and AIDS, have no known cure.

What to do
Protection of the child as well as protection against and prevention of STDs should be the foci of nursing education. This information should be kept in mind when educating about STDs:
- Although sex education and handing out condoms in schools remain controversial, the use of latex condoms for those who are sexually active could protect a young person from a disease.
- Young people should be strongly encouraged to seek medical treatment immediately if they suspect that they have contracted an STD.

- If approached by a young person about treatment, remain non-judgmental and try to address all of their concerns.
- Urge the young person to inform sexual contacts of the infection so they can receive medical treatment, and stress the importance of remaining abstinent until the completion of treatment.

Suicide and attempted suicide

Suicide is the third leading cause of death among 15- to 24-year-olds. The rate of attempted suicides is higher in females, but males are three times as successful as females in their attempts.

What causes it

One-third of those attempting suicide wish to die, while others seek to gain attention, communicate love or anger or escape a difficult or painful situation.

What to look for

Risk factors include:
- interpersonal conflict or loss
- family discord
- legal or disciplinary problems
- chronic drug or alcohol abuse
- history of physical or sexual abuse
- recent failure or disappointment
- preoccupation with death
- previous suicide attempt. (See *Suicide warning signs*.)

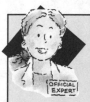

Advice from the experts

Suicide warning signs

During an assessment of the young person, be alert for these signs of suicidal behaviour:

- overwhelming anxiety (the most frequent precipitant of a suicide attempt)
- withdrawal and social isolation
- signs and symptoms of depression, including crying, fatigue, helplessness, poor concentration, reduced interest in previously enjoyable activities, sadness, constipation and weight loss
- goodbyes expressed to friends and family members
- giving away prized possessions
- covert suicide messages and death wishes
- obvious suicide messages such as 'I'd be better off dead'.

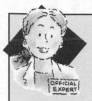

Advice from the experts

Suicide prevention guidelines

To help deter potential suicide in the individual with major depression, keep the following guidelines in mind. Some will naturally depend on the young person's age, for example with the need to shave. Also young people will be cared for in a specialist Child and Adolescent Mental Health Unit.

Assess for clues

Watch for such clues as:

- communicating suicidal thoughts, threats and messages and talking about death and feelings of futility
- hoarding medication
- giving away prized possessions
- describing a suicide plan
- changing behaviour, especially as depression begins to lift.

Provide a safe environment

Check areas and correct dangerous conditions, such as:

- windows without safety glass
- access to the roof or open balconies.

Remove dangerous objects

Remove potentially dangerous objects from the young person's environment, such as:

- belts
- light and window blind cords
- glass
- knives
- nail files and clippers.

Consult with staff

Include the child and adolescent mental health care team in aspects of care and be sure to:

- recognise and document both verbal and nonverbal suicidal behaviours
- keep the medical staff informed and share data with all staff
- clarify the young person's specific restrictions
- assess the young person's risk and plan for observation
- clarify day and night staff responsibilities and frequency of consultation.

Observe the suicidal young person

Take some steps for easy observation of a suicidal young person, including:

- being alert when the young person is using a sharp object (shaving), taking medication or using the bathroom (to prevent hanging or other injury)
- assigning the young person to a room near the nurses' station and with another young person
- continuously monitoring the acutely suicidal young person.

Maintain personal contact

Help the young person remain in contact with his environment by:

- reassuring the suicidal young person that they are not alone or without resources or hope
- encouraging continuity of care and consistency of primary nurses
- helping the young person build emotional ties to others (the ultimate technique for preventing suicide).

Complications

After a young person or school-age child (although rare under 12 years) attempts suicide, they are at risk for another attempt. Existing emotional problems may be compounded through stigmatisation by peers or even by adults.

The parents of a young person or child who commits suicide must deal with a range of emotions, including intense grief and guilt. Parents are also likely to feel guilty when an attempt is unsuccessful. They may become excessively protective of the child who made the attempt and of their other children.

How it's treated

Treatment of a suicide attempt is based on the underlying psychiatric, emotional or physical difficulty that led the child or young person to feel suicide was the only option.

Immediate hospitalisation without consent, with use of the Mental Health Act, is warranted if threat of self-harm still exists. Treatment might also involve therapy (both group and individual), medications (such as tricyclic antidepressants), remediation of social and problem solving deficits and family conflict resolution. May also need to consider referring the young person to social services as in need of help and support.

What to do

To help deter potential suicide in the child or adolescent with major depression, the nurse should keep certain guidelines in mind. (See *Suicide prevention guidelines*, page 151.)

Quick quiz

1. What's the first area of the body that's easily recognised as the beginning of the growth spurt in puberty?
   A. Hands, followed by lengthening of the arms
   B. Feet, followed by lengthening of the legs
   C. Shoulder width
   D. Abdominal girth

Answer: B. Different areas of the body reach their peak growth at different times. Changes are easily recognised in the feet, which are the first part of the body to experience a growth spurt. Increased foot size is followed by a rapid increase in leg length and then trunk growth.

2. Which statement by a young female reveals an early sign of anorexia nervosa?
   A. 'I have my menstrual period every 28 days'.
   B. 'I go out to eat with my friends at least 3 times per week'.
   C. 'I jog three times a day for a total of 5 hours per day'.
   D. 'I try to maintain my weight around 115 lb for my height of 5 ft'.

Answer: C. Excessive exercise, consumption of very small amounts of food and food rituals are all signs of anorexia nervosa. Menstruation commonly stops, and the girl's weight is below normal.

3. Which statement is true about physical growth during adolescence?
   A. Boys will typically grow much faster than girls.
   B. Girls will typically continue their growth in height until age 21.
   C. Most major organs will double in size.
   D. Motor coordination is even with growth in stature and musculature.

Answer: C. Major organs double in size during adolescence; the exception is the lymphoid tissue, which decreases in mass.

4. Because of the effects of menstruation, a girl should increase her dietary intake of:
   A. calcium.
   B. iron.
   C. carbohydrates.
   D. fats.

Answer: B. Iron is needed in the production of the protein haemoglobin, which is vital to carrying oxygen in the blood and is lost during menses.

5. Russell's sign is one way to assess for:
   A. anorexia nervosa.
   B. bulimia.
   C. obesity.
   D. attempted suicide.

Answer: B. Russell's sign includes calluses on the knuckles or abrasions and scars on the dorsum of the hand due to induced vomiting with bulimia.

Scoring

☆☆☆ If you answered all five items correctly, call your parents! They'll be proud of the abstract thinking and formal operational thought it took to master the tasks in this chapter.

☆☆ If you answered three or four items correctly, tell your peers! They'll say your understanding of middle childhood and adolescence is 'way cool'.

☆ If you answered fewer than three items correctly, don't get depressed! Your knowledge of middle childhood and adolescence is due for a growth spurt.

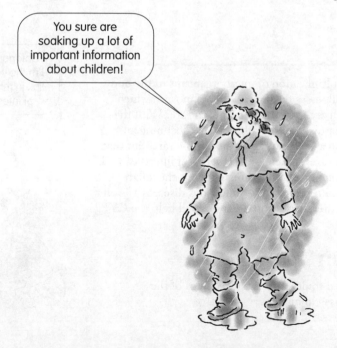

You sure are soaking up a lot of important information about children!

Communicable and infectious diseases

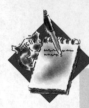

Just the facts

In this chapter, you'll learn:

♦ the chain of infection

♦ recommended immunisation practices for infants and children

♦ common childhood infectious diseases of viral and bacterial aetiology

♦ nursing interventions for the care of children with viral and bacterial illnesses.

Infection

Infection is the invasion and multiplication of microorganisms in the body. Infection can cause numerous illnesses during childhood, most of which are common, but some of which are less common or even rare. With the introduction of vaccinations, many childhood illnesses are declining and so what may have been common a few years ago is now quite rare, but that doesn't mean we shouldn't be aware of them! The severity of illness caused by infection can range from subclinical to life threatening. A thorough understanding of the aetiology and symptoms of infectious diseases as well as the appropriate diagnostic and therapeutic interventions will help the CYP nurse provide optimal care.

Chain of infection

Chain of infection is a term used to describe the three links of the transmission of infectious diseases in humans.

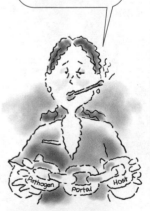

Unfortunately, I'm the weakest link in this chain of infection.

The chain begins with a pathogen that's capable of producing disease in humans.

The second link in the chain is the portal of entry (the site where disease transmission occurs), through which a pathogen can enter the body by penetrating the skin or a mucous membrane barrier by direct contact or ingestion.

The third link is the host; a susceptible host is necessary for an infectious disease to be transmitted.

Immature immunity

Infants and children are susceptible to infectious diseases because their immune systems are immature. As children mature and grow, their exposure to infectious agents increases and they develop antibodies naturally. Subsequent infections with the same pathogen may be less severe or avoided completely.

Stages of infection

Infections follow a predictable sequence of events during transmission that results in five distinct stages of disease.

The incubation period is the phase during which the pathogenic organism begins active reproduction in the host; the child has no clinical symptoms but may be contagious to others during this time.

The prodromal phase is the initial appearance of clinical symptoms in the host; common symptoms include fever, malaise, headache, sore throat, cough and rhinitis.

During the acute stage, maximum symptoms are experienced by the host; toxins deposited by the pathogenic organism can produce tissue damage. (Inflammatory changes and tissue damage can also occur as a result of the immune response of the host.)

The convalescent stage is characterised by progressive elimination of the infection (or elimination of the pathogen), healing of damaged tissue and symptom resolution.

The resolution stage is the host's recovery from the infection without residual signs or symptoms of disease.

Cover your mouth, please

The period of communicability is the time when the infectious organism may move from the infected host to another person. It varies with different disease states but usually begins during the incubation phase.

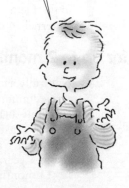

I may look healthy during the incubation period, but I'm already giving my infection to my mom, my brother and my bratty little sister.

Immune protection

Children receive protection from communicable diseases naturally and artificially.

Methods of obtaining immune protection

There are five different methods in which immune protection can be obtained: natural immunity, naturally acquired active immunity, naturally acquired passive immunity, artificially acquired active immunity and artificially acquired passive immunity.

Natural (innate) immunity

Innate immunity is a combination of natural and non-specific immunity that can protect the human body from pathogens and foreign agents. For example, the phagocytic action of white blood cells (macrophages) may be triggered by the body's innate ability to recognise and distinguish normal cells from foreign cells. The body's ability to distinguish self from non-self is natural, or innate, immunity.

Naturally acquired active immunity

Naturally acquired active immunity is obtained when the body's immune system responds to a specific pathogen. Antibodies and memory cells prevent or reduce the severity of subsequent infection with that specific pathogen. Naturally acquired active immunity persists for many years.

Naturally acquired passive immunity

Naturally acquired passive immunity involves mother-to-foetus transmission of maternal antibodies.

A gift that keeps on giving ...

The mother's immunoglobulin G crosses the placenta and is transmitted to the foetus. After birth, the infant can receive passive immunity through maternal antibodies in breast milk.

... for up to 2 months

Naturally acquired passive immunity differs from active immunity. While active immunity lasts many years, or even a lifetime, passive immunity lasts only as long as the antibodies remain in the blood of the foetus or infant (usually from a few weeks to about 2 months). Even so, some antibodies transferred across the placenta have been isolated up to the age of 1 year, which is why the measles immunisation is delayed until 12–13 months.

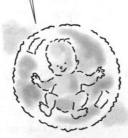

Hey, Mom – got milk? If you do, I'll have at least a few more weeks of passive immunity once I get out of here.

Artificially acquired active immunity

Artificially acquired active immunity is achieved by deliberate administration of a vaccine or toxoid. The vaccine or toxoid stimulates the immune system's production of antibodies against a specific antigen but symptoms of the disease aren't produced in the person receiving the vaccine.

Artificially acquired passive immunity

Artificially acquired passive immunity is conferred when antibodies developed in another person or animal donor are injected into an individual. In children, this transfer usually involves IV administration of a specific immunoglobulin. Examples include:
- gamma globulin (a mixture of antibodies against prevalent community diseases, pooled from 1,000 human plasma donors)
- hyperimmune or convalescent serum globulin (such as tetanus antitoxin, hepatitis B immune globulin and varicella zoster immune globulin)

Types of immunisations

Various immunisations are given at specific times to protect children from certain diseases. These vaccines fall into two general categories:
- live, attenuated vaccines
- inactivated vaccines.

Live, attenuated

Live, attenuated vaccines are created from a live organism that's grown under suboptimal conditions to produce a live vaccine with reduced virulence.

Weak but stimulating

Thus, an attenuated immunisation contains weakened microorganisms and stimulates immune response and production of antibodies in the host. The vaccine confers 90% to 95% protection for more than 20 years with a single dose.

Measles, mumps and rubella – itch, ouch

Examples of live, attenuated vaccines include the measles, mumps and rubella (MMR) vaccine and the varicella vaccine (not routinely offered).

Inactivated

- An inactivated, or killed, vaccine confers a weaker response than a live vaccine, necessitating frequent boosters.
- An inactivated vaccine doesn't promote replication and provides 40% to 70% protection.

Toxoids

Some bacteria, such as diphtheria, produce toxins, which cause disease. The vaccine to prevent a disease caused by a toxin is called a toxoid. A toxoid:

- is another form of an inactivated vaccine
- is a toxin that has been specially treated with formalin or heat to weaken its toxic effect but retain its antigenicity
- provides 90% to 100% protection by stimulating the production of antibodies.

Inactive but popular

Examples of inactivated vaccines include:
- diphtheria and tetanus toxoids
- inactivated poliovirus vaccine (IPV)
- pertussis vaccine
- hepatitis B vaccine.

Immunisation schedule

Childhood immunisations include diphtheria and tetanus toxoids and acellular pertussis vaccine (DTaP), *Haemophilus influenzae* type B (Hib) vaccine, IPV, MMR vaccine, varicella virus vaccine and pneumococcal 7-valent conjugate vaccine (PCV). These immunisations are given according to a predetermined schedule. (See *Immunisation schedule for children*.)

See also NHS information (http://www.hpa.org.uk/web/ HPAweb&Page&HPAwebAutoListDate/Page/1204031508623).

Baby's first ouch

Hepatitis B vaccine is only given to babies whose mother is hepatitis B positive The vaccine is given IM at birth (or before hospital discharge). Where babies have a high risk of coming into contact with tuberculosis (TB) the BCG may also be given at this stage.

Adverse reactions

Common reactions are pain and redness at the site of injection and elevated liver enzymes. Mild-to-moderate fever may occur (more common in children and adolescents than in adults). Anaphylaxis is rare.

DTaP vaccine

The DTaP vaccine is given to protect infants and young children from acquiring diphtheria, tetanus and pertussis. The bacterium that causes diphtheria can create a toxin that damages tissue and attacks the heart and nerves. Such an attack can be fatal. Tetanus can cause muscle spasms that can interfere with breathing, which can lead to death. Pertussis is particularly dangerous for young children, especially infants younger than age of 1 year, who are most at risk for complications and death.

Adverse reactions

Fever, fussiness and anorexia are common adverse reactions as well as redness, pain and swelling at the injection site. Redness, pain and swelling at

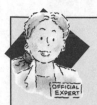

Advice from the experts

Recommended immunisation schedule for children

In addition to following the recommended immunisation schedule for children in the table below, considering these simple steps will help ensure the child's safety.

Before immunisation

- Obtain a history of allergic responses, especially life-threatening anaphylactic reactions to antibiotics or past vaccinations (certain vaccinations may be contraindicated in these children).
- Assess the child for moderate or severe illness. Vaccinations may be delayed in these children until they recover. However, a child with a minor illness, such as a cold, may receive immunisations.
- Keep in mind that children receiving corticosteroids for longer than 2 weeks, chemotherapy, or radiation therapy; those with human immunodeficiency virus infection, acquired immunodeficiency syndrome or another disease that affects the immune system and those with cancer will need special consideration for vaccination. (They may not be able to receive live virus vaccines, such as MMR or varicella.)

After immunisation

- Tell the parents to watch for and report reactions other than local swelling and pain and mild temperature elevation.
- Give parents the child's immunisation record.

Age	Immunisation
At 2 months	Diphtheria + Tetanus + Pertussis + Polio + Hib – One injection Pneumococcal – One injection
At 3 months	Diphtheria + Tetanus + Pertussis + Polio + Hib – One injection Meningitis C – One injection
At 4 months	Diphtheria + Tetanus + Pertussis + Polio + Hib – One injection Pneumococcal – One injection Meningitis C – One injection
Between 12 and 13 months	Hib + Meningitis C – One injection Measles + Mumps + Rubella – One injection Pneumococcal – One injection
At 3–5 years (usually before child starts school)	Diphtheria + Tetanus + Pertussis + Polio – One injection Measles + Mumps + Rubella – One injection
At 12–13 years (girls only)	Human papillomavirus (HPV) – Three injections given over six months
School leavers (At 13–18 years)	Tetanus + Diphtheria + Polio – One injection

the injection site occur more commonly after the fourth or fifth dose in the DTaP series. Anaphylaxis, fever above 38.9° C, persistent crying for 3 hours or longer and seizures are rare but severe reactions that require emergency treatment.

Hib vaccine

The Hib vaccine is used to prevent infection with Hib. This infection can lead to severe invasive illnesses, including meningitis, epiglottitis and pneumonia. Until recently, Hib was the most common cause of meningitis in children older than 1 month, but vaccination with the Hib vaccine has drastically reduced the incidence.

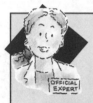

Advice from the experts

Tips for giving injections to children

When giving a child an injection, the major goals should be minimising trauma and discomfort while providing safe, efficient administration of a necessary medicine or vaccination.

Be their advocate

- Always ensure that the most appropriate method of giving any medication has been discussed and where possible IM injections are avoided. This may mean advocated on the child's behalf to ensure their needs are considered and that they are not just another 'patient.'
- Always ensure that prescribed local anaesthetic is used to reduce the discomfort from injections.

Minimising trauma

- To most toddlers and preschoolers, and to many older children, the prospect of getting an injection is the most frightening part of any treatment.
- Many strategies, including those outlined below, can be used to reduce the trauma of receiving an injection, while establishing trust between the child and the health care team and making future injections easier for the child (and for the nurse who's giving the injection).

Medicine to keep you healthy

- Give the child a simple, age-appropriate explanation for why the injection is being given. When a child is being vaccinated, that explanation might be, 'This will give you medicine to stop you from getting poorly'. (Young children may think an injection is being given as a punishment and may not even realise that medication is being given.)
- Allow the child to give an 'injection' to a doll or stuffed animal; this gives a sense of control, let them see that the injection has a beginning and an end and gives a concrete understanding of what will happen.

The best policy

- Be honest; tell the child that it will hurt for a moment but that it will be over quickly. (Honesty promotes trust; if a nurse is honest about the potential for pain, the child will believe them when told something won't hurt.)

Coping and comfort

- Give the child a coping strategy, such as squeezing mother's hand, counting to five, singing a song and looking away.

- Have a parent hold and comfort the child while the injection is being given. A parent's presence reassures the child that nothing truly bad will happen. (The child may actually cry more when a parent is present, but this is because they feel safe enough to do so.)
- Older children may still need lots of comfort and support so bear this in mind when performing injections. They may have also developed a fear or phobia towards needles and so will need help in coping with this.

Praise and cover

- When the injection has been given, tell the child that 'the hurting part' is over, and praise them for what a good job they did (regardless of how they reacted). Never tell a child to 'be brave', to 'be a big boy', or not to cry, as these requests will set the child up for failure.
- Give the child a plaster. (A young child may not believe the 'hurting part' is over until a plaster has been applied.)
- Always give injections in a designated area. Avoid performing painful procedures in a playroom or, if possible, in the child's hospital room because they need to know there are places where they can feel completely safe.
- Many immunisations are given at school and so privacy and respect of the young person must be considered. At the same time it is important to treat the young person as an individual and not just another immunisation!

Giving the injection

- Apply firm pressure at the site for 10 to 15 seconds immediately before giving the injection to decrease discomfort (a numbing patch may be used).
- When two or more injections are needed, give them simultaneously in different extremities; have two or more nurses to assist (and provide manual restraint if needed but following local guidelines) during the procedures. (The child has only one painful experience when multiple injections are given simultaneously; this is believed to be less traumatic than receiving painful injections one after the other.)
- Apply a plaster to each site, and immediately comfort and console the child following the injections.
- Always keep resuscitation equipment and adrenaline readily available in case of an anaphylactic response to an immunisation.

Adverse reactions

Hib is one of the safest vaccines available because it causes only mild reactions, if any. Common adverse reactions are low-grade fever, localised pain, redness and swelling at the injection site. Anaphylaxis is rare.

IPV vaccine

IPV is now recommended for use in all polio vaccine doses to prevent vaccine-associated polio, a rare infection that was associated with the oral polio vaccine, which contained live virus and is no longer used.

Adverse reactions

Localised pain, redness and swelling at the injection site are common adverse reactions, although IPV is safe and usually well tolerated. Anaphylaxis is rare.

MMR vaccine

The MMR vaccine stimulates immunity against measles, mumps and rubella. Because the vaccine contains live virus, it's contraindicated during pregnancy. Females shouldn't become pregnant within 3 months of immunisation.

Intact immunity required

Live virus shouldn't be administered to anyone receiving immunosuppressive therapy or to those with immunodeficiency diseases.

Adverse reactions

Common adverse reactions to the MMR vaccine are low-grade fever for 1 week after immunisation; localised pain, redness and swelling at the injection site; rash and joint pain. Severe reactions are rare but include viral encephalopathy and anaphylaxis.

Varicella virus vaccine

Varicella virus vaccine is used to stimulate immunity to varicella (chickenpox). The vaccine contains live virus and is contraindicated during pregnancy. It's also contraindicated in individuals receiving immunosuppressive therapy and in those with immunodeficiency diseases. It is not routinely offered.

Adverse reactions

Common adverse reactions to the varicella virus vaccine are pain, redness, localised swelling and varicella-like rash at the injection site. Low-grade fever and irritability for 1 week after vaccine administration are also common. Anaphylaxis is rare.

PCV

PCV is recommended for preventing and decreasing the severity of pneumococcal infections caused by *Streptococcus pneumoniae*. These invasive infections can result in otitis media, pneumonia, meningitis and sepsis, with the most serious illness occurring in children younger than 2 years.

Some adverse reactions to the DTaP vaccine require emergency treatment.

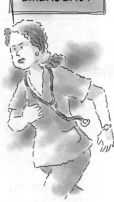

Immunisation with live vaccines is contraindicated in children with any type of immune deficiency.

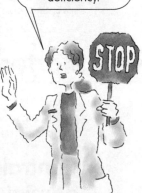

Adverse reactions

So far, this vaccine has been found to cause only mild reactions. Common adverse reactions from PCV are drowsiness, irritability, restless sleep, diarrhoea, vomiting, decreased appetite and injection site reactions (including swelling, redness, inflammation, skin discoloration and tenderness).

Influenza vaccine

Also known as the flu shot, the influenza vaccine is an inactivated or killed vaccine. Because the influenza virus changes each year, the vaccine gets updated every year in an attempt to prevent the most common strains that are circulating at that time. Therefore, the influenza vaccine needs to be given yearly.

Protection from the influenza virus should begin 2 weeks after the vaccination, and may last for up to 1 year.

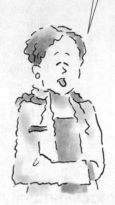

The influenza virus changes every year ... which is why you need to get a flu jab every year!

Who gets it?

The influenza vaccine is recommended for children older than age 6 months with risk factors such as, but not limited to, asthma, diabetes, cardiac problems and human immunodeficiency virus infection and healthy children aged 6 to 23 months who are at high risk for serious illness. Household contacts and caretakers of children younger than 2 years are also encouraged to have the vaccine.

Dosing

The inactivated vaccine is administered IM once per year, and is most effective when given early in the flu season, typically in October or November. For children younger than 9 years who are receiving the influenza vaccine for the first time, two doses are necessary and should be given 1 month apart.

Adverse reactions

The influenza vaccine typically produces only mild adverse reactions, such as soreness, redness or swelling at the injection site; fever or body aches. Such severe adverse effects as a life-threatening allergic reaction rarely occur.

New starter

Since 2008 there has been the addition of a vaccine against human papillomavirus (HPV) for 12 to 13-year-old girls, which protects against two particular strains of HPV virus that can cause cervical cancer.

Contraindications to vaccine administration

Mild illnesses and low-grade fevers that are common in children aren't contraindications to vaccine administration. However, there are several reasons to withhold or delay vaccine administration:

- Vaccination is contraindicated in children with moderate-to-severe illness or a history of allergic response or anaphylaxis to the vaccine or certain antibiotics.
- Vaccination with preparations containing live or attenuated viruses shouldn't be performed in children who are pregnant, have an immunodeficiency disease or are receiving immunosuppressive therapy.
- The DTaP vaccine shouldn't be given to a child who has a progressive and active central nervous system (CNS) problem. However, a child with cerebral palsy can receive immunisations.
- The measles vaccine shouldn't be given at the same time as a tuberculin purified protein derivative test. The measles vaccine can make person who's positive for tuberculosis (TB) appear to be TB-negative.
- The connection between the MMR vaccine and autism has been shown not to exist.

However, parents may require extra information and reassurance before this vaccination is given.

Bacterial infections

Bacteria are single-celled microorganisms that break down dead tissue. They have no true nucleus and reproduce by cell division. Pathogenic bacteria contain cell-damaging proteins that cause infection. These proteins come in two forms:
- exotoxins – released during cell growth
- endotoxins – released when the bacterial cell wall decomposes. These endotoxins cause fever and aren't affected by antibiotics. (See *How bacteria damage tissue*, page 164.)

A class by any other class

Bacteria are classified several other ways, such as by their shape, growth requirements, motility and whether they're aerobic (requiring oxygen) or anaerobic (not requiring oxygen).

The young and the susceptible

Bacterial infections are common in infants and young children who haven't achieved active immunity because their immune systems haven't been challenged by many pathogens. Such infections in infants include diphtheria, tetanus, pertussis and Hib. Most of these are rare in the UK; however, should always be considered and particularly if the child/family have been or come from abroad, or have been in contact with infected persons. Antibiotic therapy is the usual treatment of bacterial infection, although some organisms are become resistant to certain drugs.

How bacteria damage tissue

The human body is constantly infected by bacteria and other infectious organisms. Some are beneficial, such as the intestinal bacteria that produce vitamins, and others are harmful, causing illnesses ranging from the common cold to life-threatening septic shock.

Invading forces

To infect a host, bacteria must first enter it. They do this by adhering to the mucosal surface and directly invading the host cell or attaching to epithelial cells and producing toxins, which invade host cells.

I will survive

To survive and multiply within a host, bacteria or their toxins adversely affect biochemical reactions in cells.

The result is a disruption of normal cell function, or cell death (shown below left). For example, the diphtheria toxin damages heart muscle by inhibiting protein synthesis. In addition, as some organisms multiply, they extend into deeper tissue and eventually gain access to the bloodstream.

Clot and deprive

Some toxins cause blood to clot in small blood vessels. The tissues supplied by these vessels may be deprived of blood and may be damaged (shown below center).

Bring down the walls

Other toxins can damage the cell walls of small blood vessels, causing leakage. This fluid loss results in decreased blood pressure, which, in turn, impairs the heart's ability to pump enough blood to vital organs (shown below right).

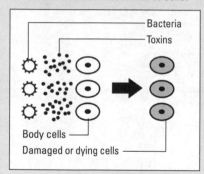

Bacteria
Toxins
Body cells
Damaged or dying cells

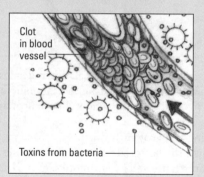

Clot in blood vessel
Toxins from bacteria

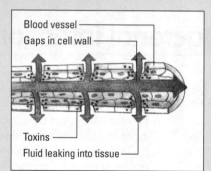

Blood vessel
Gaps in cell wall
Toxins
Fluid leaking into tissue

Diphtheria

Diphtheria is an acute, highly contagious, toxin-mediated infection that's preventable by vaccine. Diphtheria is rare in the UK but remains a serious problem in some other parts of the world. There have only been eight cases since 1986, and all of those have returned from abroad.

What causes it

Diphtheria is caused by an infection of *Corynebacterium diphtheriae*, a gram-positive rod that usually infects the respiratory tract (primarily the tonsils, nasopharynx and larynx). It's more serious when it occurs in infants because they have smaller airways, which are more susceptible to obstruction because of their size.

How it happens
The infection is transmitted by:
- contact with an infected patient's or carrier's nasal, pharyngeal, eye or skin lesion discharge
- contact with articles contaminated with the bacteria
- ingestion of unpasteurised milk.

Incubation and communicability
The diphtheria incubation period is 2 to 7 days. The period of communicability is 2 to 4 weeks after the onset of symptoms, or until 4 days after the initiation of antibiotic therapy.

What to look for
Symptoms of diphtheria include:
- fever
- malaise
- purulent rhinitis
- cough, hoarseness and stridor
- cervical lymphadenopathy
- pharyngitis.

Obstruction production
The infection, localised to the tonsils and posterior pharynx, is characterised by a thick, patchy, greyish green, membranous lesion that can lead to airway obstruction. Some children also exhibit infectious, ulcerated skin lesions as a manifestation of the disease.

What tests tell you
- Culture specimens from the nose, throat and skin lesions reveal the presence of coryneform organisms.
- Sensitivity tests determine the optimal antibiotic therapy.
- Serologic testing will identify the presence of diphtheria toxin.

Complications
Infection with the toxin can result in myocarditis, thrombocytopoenia, peripheral neuropathy or an ascending paralysis with symptoms similar to Guillain–Barré syndrome. Renal, cardiac and peripheral CNS damage may also occur.

It's a cover-up
The membranous lesion that covers the tonsils can spread to cover the posterior pharynx, which can result in airway obstruction. Removal of the membrane may be indicated, but attempting to do so can cause bleeding. Left untreated, however, it can result in death.

How it's treated
Diphtheria is treated with antitoxin and antibiotics.

No time to waste

IV administration of diphtheria antitoxin and antibiotic therapy must begin within 3 days of the onset of symptoms. The patient should be tested for allergy to horse serum before administering the antitoxin. The antibiotic of choice is usually penicillin G or erythromycin for those allergic to penicillin.

Too close for comfort

Close contacts of the infected child should be identified, monitored for signs of illness and treated with prophylactic antibiotic therapy (oral erythromycin for 7 to 10 days). Cultures of the nose, the throat and skin lesions should be obtained.

What to do

Diphtheria is a preventable disease. The immunisation series is designed to begin at age of 2 months. The vaccine confers immunity for 10 years, after which boosters should be given every 10 years throughout the lifespan. Passive immunity conferred from the presence of maternal antibodies lasts as long as 6 months after birth.

Diagnose, then act

When the disease is diagnosed, follow these steps:
• Report the infection to the local public health department.
• Place the infected child in droplet isolation to prevent respiratory transmission. (Show the child isolation gowns, masks and gloves that will be worn and provide a simple explanation such as, 'your parents, nurses and doctors are going to wear these so everyone stays healthy'.)
• Institute contact isolation precautions if skin lesions are present.
• Maintain infection precautions until after two consecutive negative nasopharyngeal cultures to prevent spread of the disease.
• Closely monitor the child for signs of airway obstruction. Provide humidified oxygen, if oxygen is ordered, to reduce airway inflammation.
• Administer antitoxin and antibiotics as ordered. Monitor for allergic or anaphylactic reaction.
• Maintain the child on complete bed rest to prevent myocarditis. Provide age-appropriate activities to prevent boredom.

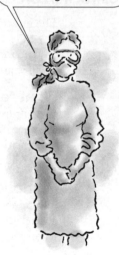

To avoid frightening a child, explain why masks and gowns are worn, and tell the child your name every time you enter the room (because they might not recognise you).

Haemophilus influenzae type B

Hib is a bacterium with several serotypes, but type B is the particularly virulent one. Bacterial infection can result in invasive and devastating illnesses in the child population.

What causes it

Infection is caused by the coccobacillus *H. influenzae*, which is a gram-negative, pleomorphic, aerobic bacillus.

How it happens

Hib can be isolated as part of normal upper respiratory flora in healthy children and adults. However, in some instances, it breaks through the body's natural defence system and causes infection. Infectious symptoms typically begin with a viral upper respiratory infection.

The invasion begins

The pathogenic organisms can invade mucosal tissues and reach the bloodstream, resulting in bacteraemia.

All systems aren't go

Systemic bacteraemia can cause:
- meningitis
- cellulitis
- epiglottitis
- pneumonia
- septic arthritis
- sepsis.

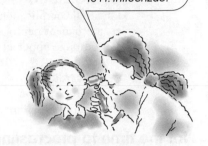

Sometimes there's more to an earache that meets the eye. Otitis media can be secondary to *H. influenzae*.

Not-so-honourable mention

Otitis media, sinusitis and conjunctivitis are examples of localised, non-invasive diseases secondary to *H. influenzae* infection.

Incubation and communicability

The incubation period of *H. influenzae* infection isn't known. The period of communicability begins 3 days after transmission and lasts until the development of symptoms.

What to look for

H. influenzae infections are a common cause of epiglottitis, laryngotracheo-bronchitis, pneumonia, bronchiolitis, otitis media and meningitis.

You'd be irritable too

Symptoms vary according to the disease state and whether it's localised (non-invasive) or invasive. For example, a child with *H. influenzae* meningitis might complain of headache, fever, neck stiffness and photophobia. Infants may be irritable, and demonstrate signs of increased intracranial pressure (ICP), such as a bulging fontanelle and a high-pitched cry.

Tender to the touch

When cellulitis develops as a complication of *H. influenzae*, there's usually no history of trauma. A localised area of soft-tissue oedema and erythema with indistinct margins is present. The area is tender to touch, and the child usually has a high temperature.

What tests tell you
- Culture and sensitivity tests positively identify *H. influenzae*.
- Peripheral blood smear may reveal leukocytosis as the body responds to the bacterial infection.

Complications
Potential complications of Hib include:
- permanent neurological sequelae from meningitis
- complete upper airway obstruction from epiglottitis
- cellulitis
- pericarditis
- pleural effusion
- respiratory failure from pneumonia.

Not the time to procrastinate

Complications are rare with non-invasive disease. In invasive disease, complications are less likely when the disease is diagnosed promptly and appropriate antibiotic therapy is begun early. How complications develop also depends on the disease caused by the infecting organism; for example, hearing impairment can result from meningitis. When appropriate treatment is delayed, the potential for serious and life-threatening complications is greater.

How it's treated
IV administration of broad-spectrum antibiotics (in particular, antibiotics that are effective against penicillin-resistant strains) is indicated for invasive disease. Cephalosporins, such as cefotaxime (Claforan), and chloramphenicol (Chloromycetin) are effective.

Non-invasive disease, such as sinusitis and otitis media, can be treated effectively with oral antibiotics.

Stamp out colonisation

Rifampicin may be given prophylactically to close contacts of the infected child. Rifampicin is effective in eliminating colonisation of the organism.

What to do
- Use droplet isolation precautions with the infected child until 24 hours after antibiotic therapy has been initiated.
- Maintain adequate respiratory function through cool humidification, oxygen as needed and a croup or face tent.
- In children with meningitis, continually monitor level of consciousness.
- Advocate active immunisation at the recommended times.

Pertussis

Pertussis, also known as whooping cough, is an extremely contagious acute respiratory tract infection. It typically produces an irritating cough that becomes paroxysmal and commonly ends in a high-pitched inspiratory whoop.

Less than 500 cases occur in the UK every year. Children who are too young to have been fully immunised and those who haven't completed the immunisation series are at highest risk for serious illness.

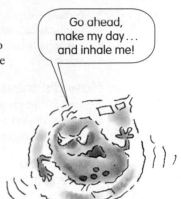

Go ahead, make my day... and inhale me!

What causes it

The pertussis infection is usually caused by the non-motile, gram-negative *coccobacillus Bordetella pertussis* and, occasionally, by the related, similar bacterium *B. parapertussis* and *B. bronchiseptica*.

How it happens

The disease is transmitted through inhalation of contaminated respiratory droplets or by direct contact with contaminated articles such as soiled bed linens.

Incubation and communicability

The incubation period ranges from 3 to 12 days. The period of communicability begins about 1 week after exposure and lasts for 5 to 7 days after antibiotic therapy has begun.

What to look for

Symptoms of rhinorrhoea and nasal congestion begin insidiously, followed by a non-productive cough. These symptoms are commonly accompanied by a low-grade fever, sneezing and watery eyes.

The cough of the giant crane

The coughing becomes increasingly more severe. Spasms of paroxysmal coughing followed by stridor on inspiration produce the characteristic 'whooping' sound.

Flushing and draining

Flushing, cyanosis and watery drainage from the nose, eyes and mouth may accompany the coughing. Infants can have symptoms of choking and gasping for air, and vomiting may occur if the they choke on mucus.

What tests tell you

Isolation of *B. pertussis* in laboratory culture of respiratory secretions remains the gold standard for confirming pertussis infection. A peripheral blood smear may demonstrate leukocytosis caused by the body's response to the bacterial infection.

Complications

Complications from pertussis infection are most severe and death rates are highest in infants younger than 6 months. Complications include:
- secondary infection, such as pneumonia and otitis media
- increased venous pressure
- anterior eye chamber haemorrhage, detached retina and blindness

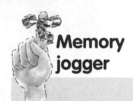

Memory jogger

To remember the complications from pertussis, just remember that the disease is highly contagious so it IS SHARED:

- *Increased venous pressure*
- *Seizures*
- *Secondary infection*
- *Hernia*
- *Anterior eye chamber haemorrhage*
- *Rectal prolapse*
- *Encephalopathy*
- *Death.*

- rectal prolapse
- inguinal or umbilical hernia
- encephalopathy
- seizures.

How it's treated

Erythromycin given orally in four divided doses for 14 days is standard treatment of pertussis infection. Co-trimoxazole may be used for those who can't tolerate erythromycin.

What to do

To prevent pertussis, nurses should advocate active immunisation according to the recommended schedule. When providing care for a child with pertussis, follow these steps:
• Use droplet isolation for those with suspected or documented infection, until 5–7 days after antibiotic therapy has been initiated.
• Closely monitor cardiorespiratory function and oxygen saturation. Maintain a patent airway; keep suctioning equipment readily available.
• Create a quiet environment to decrease coughing stimulation.
• Offer the child a small amount of fluids frequently to prevent dehydration.
• Report diagnosed disease to the local public health department.
• Treat close contacts of the infected child prophylactically with oral erythromycin.

Tetanus

Tetanus is a vaccine-preventable disease caused by an acute exotoxin-mediated infection that's usually systemic but may also be localised.

Tetanus causes painful muscle rigidity and spasms all over the body, tightening the muscles of the jaw (lockjaw), which makes opening the mouth for breathing or swallowing impossible. Tetanus is a rare disease with all recent cases being adult injecting-drug users.

What causes it

Tetanus is caused by *Clostridium tetani*, a spore-forming anaerobic bacterium. Because *C. tetani* spores exist everywhere, tetanus is still a global health problem. However, the disease occurs primarily in those who are unvaccinated or inadequately immunised.

How it happens

The tetanus bacterium is transmitted through penetrating wounds; burns; open wounds in the skin or contact with contaminated soil, dust, animal excreta or surgical instruments.

Axon reaction

The infection reaches the axons of the nerves, causing involuntary muscle contraction, muscle rigidity and painful paroxysmal seizures.

Incubation and communicability

The incubation period averages 2 to 14 days. The disease isn't communicable, except through contact with infected skin wounds.

What to look for

History will reveal an injury or wound in an unimmunised child. Clinical manifestations of the disease include:

- stiffness of the neck and jaw
- dysphagia
- painful facial muscle spasms that progress to involve the respiratory muscles as well as the muscles of the abdomen, hips and thighs
- irregular heartbeat and tachycardia
- hyperactive deep tendon reflexes
- high sensitivity to external stimuli
- profuse sweating
- low-grade fever.

The child remains alert throughout the disease process because consciousness is unaffected.

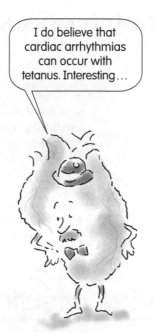

I do believe that cardiac arrhythmias can occur with tetanus. Interesting…

What tests tell you

Diagnosis is based on the history and symptoms of muscle rigidity in a neurologically intact child. There's also no history of previous tetanus immunisation. Serum laboratory studies are usually normal. An increase in leukocytes on the peripheral blood smear may be noted from a wound infection or from the stress of tetanic muscle contractions.

Complications

Tetanic seizures and severe, sustained tetanic contractions as well as rigid muscle paralysis produce many complications. Laryngospasm, respiratory muscle spasms and respiratory distress can lead to asphyxia and death. Autonomic instability, unstable blood pressure and cardiac arrhythmias may also occur.

How it's treated

Treatment of tetanus is multifaceted and includes:

- tetanus immune globulin (used to neutralise tetanus toxin) administered simultaneously with tetanus toxoid (Td) injected at a different site
- penicillin G, the antibiotic of choice, administered IV (or metronidazole, erythromycin or tetracycline for patients with penicillin allergy)
- surgical wound excision or debridement, if needed
- muscle relaxants and sedatives, if necessary, to treat muscle spasms
- intensive care and careful monitoring of cardiorespiratory status, if needed.

What to do

Active immunisation begins at age 2 months with DTaP. The series continues with immunisations at ages 3 & 4 months and 4 years, for a total of five doses.

Ten-year reunion

After the completion of the series, the Td vaccine should be administered at 10-year intervals and should continue throughout adulthood.

Close encounter with a rusty nail

Td vaccine is given to any person with any potentially contaminated wound if the tetanus immunisation status isn't known, or if it has been more than 5 years since the last immunisation.

Child care essentials

For the child with tetanus, follow these steps:
• Maintain a patent airway and adequate ventilation; keep emergency airway equipment readily available. Closely monitor vital signs.
• Maintain a quiet environment, reducing external stimuli from light, sound and touch. Schedule care to reduce handling of the child and allow for extended periods of rest.
• Remember that the child's consciousness is unaffected, and so will be frightened of the muscle spasms and rigidity. If potent muscle relaxants are used, the resulting paralysis can make it impossible for the child to communicate clearly. Thoroughly explain procedures to the child, and observe closely for changes in vital signs, which can indicate pain or anxiety, particularly if the child can't communicate. Stay with the child as much as possible, and use a calm and reassuring tone to reduce the child's fear and anxiety.

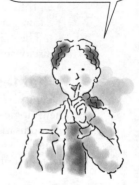

Make sure you create a quiet environment for the child with tetanus.

Viral infections

Viruses are the smallest known organisms; they're visible only with an electron microscope. Independent of host cells, viruses can't replicate; instead, they invade a host cell and stimulate it to participate in forming additional virus particles.

Supportive therapy is the treatment of viral infections. Antiviral medications are sometimes used. Antibiotic therapy isn't indicated for illnesses caused by viral infection but may be appropriate if a secondary bacterial infection has complicated the clinical course of the viral illness.

Rash of rashes

Common childhood rash-producing viruses include:
• fifth disease (slapped cheek syndrome or erythema infectiosum)
• roseola infantum
• german measles (rubella)
• measles (rubeola)
• chicken pox (varicella). (See *Common rash-producing infections.*)

Common rash-producing infections

Infection	Incubation (days)	Duration (days)
Fifth disease	6 to 14	7 to 21
Roseola infantum	10 to 15	3 to 6
Rubella	14 to 21	3
Rubeola	8 to 14	5
Varicella	14 to 17	7 to 14

Not so rash

Common viral infections without rash include:
- mumps
- poliomyelitis.

Fifth disease (slapped cheek syndrome or erythema infectiosum)

Fifth disease is a contagious viral disease characterised by rose-coloured eruptions diffused over the skin, usually starting on the cheeks.

The fifth dimension

Fifth disease got its unusual name when it was counted as the fifth of the classic, rash-producing infections of children. The other rash-producing infections referred to in this chronology were measles, scarlet fever, rubella and another rash that's unknown to doctors today but was referred to as 'the fourth disease'.

What causes it

Fifth disease is caused by human parvovirus B19.

How it happens

The virus is transmitted through infected respiratory droplet secretions and through infected blood.

Incubation and communicability

The incubation period for fifth disease is 6 to 14 days. The period of communicability lasts from several days before the appearance of a rash until the appearance of the rash.

It occurs in a 3 to 4 year epidemic cycle and peaks in the first half of each year.

What to look for

Clinical manifestations in the prodromal phase are mild, including low-grade fever, headache and symptoms of upper respiratory infection.

A slap in the face

The typical rash in the initial stage is described as a red facial flushing, or a 'slapped-cheek' appearance. The macular rash spreads rapidly to the truck and proximal extremities. The centres of the macules fade, which give the rash a lacy appearance.

Spare the hands, spoil the feet

The rash isn't present on the palms or soles. It resolves spontaneously in 1 to 3 weeks. (See *Fifth disease rash*.)

What tests tell you

Diagnosis of fifth disease is usually based on reviewing the clinical presentation of the child, observing the rash and excluding other differential diagnoses. Methods to detect the virus in laboratory studies are available, though not routinely used.

Complications

Complications of fifth disease are rare. Children with chronic haematological conditions may experience transient anaemia. Arthritis and joint symptoms may occur in adults but are rare in children.

Pregnant? Watch out!

Infection of a pregnant woman is associated with foetal disease and may result in foetal death. Even so, risk of infection is minimal in pregnant women who come into contact with affected children.

How it's treated

No specific treatment or cure for fifth disease exists. Nursing care is supportive. No vaccine is available to prevent the illness.

What to do

Treatment is supportive and directed towards relief of symptoms:
• Antipyretics, such as paracetamol or ibuprofen (as appropriate), are given to relieve fever.
• Soothing baths or antipruritics can be used to alleviate itching.

Don't fence me in

Fifth disease is benign and self-limiting. Because the child isn't infectious to others when the rash appears, there's no reason to isolate the child.

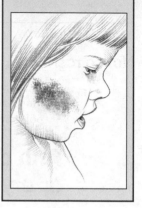

Fifth disease rash

The rash that appears on the face of a child with fifth disease makes it look as if the child has been slapped.

Mumps

Mumps, also called parotitis, is an acute inflammation of one or both parotid glands and sometimes the sublingual or submaxillary glands. Painful swelling of the salivary glands is a common presenting symptom.

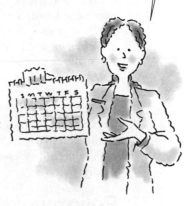

Mark your calendars! The incubation period for mumps is 12 to 25 days.

What causes it

Mumps is caused by paramyxovirus found in the saliva of an infected person.

How it happens

Mumps is spread by contaminated airborne respiratory droplets or by direct contact with the saliva of an infected person.

Incubation and communicability

The incubation period is 12 to 25 days. The period of communicability is from 7 days before the parotid gland enlargement until 9 days after the glandular swelling has resolved.

What to look for

During the prodromal phase of the illness, symptoms include:
- headache
- neck pain
- fever
- malaise
- painful chewing
- anorexia.
  These symptoms are followed by acute and painful swelling of the parotid glands.

What tests tell you

- Peripheral blood smear may reveal leukocytosis and lymphocytosis.
- Serum amylase may be elevated when the parotid glands are enlarged.

Complications

Complications of mumps include:
- epididymitis
- oophoritis
- pancreatitis
- meningoencephalitis
- deafness
- orchitis (most common in adolescent boys and rare in prepubescent boys).

How it's treated

Mumps is treated symptomatically. The child should be on bed rest during the acute phase of the illness, and diet should be adjusted according to their ability to chew.

Orchitis should be treated with scrotal support and bed rest. Corticosteroids or non-steroidal anti-inflammatory drugs (NSAIDs) may be given for arthritis symptoms.

What to do

Most children with mumps are uncomfortable but not seriously ill and are usually cared for at home.
• If a child with mumps is hospitalised, droplet precautions should be maintained until the period of communicability has passed.
• Paracetamol and NSAIDs, such as ibuprofen, may be administered to control pain and fever.
• A soft or puréed diet may be needed.
• Warm, moist or cool compresses may be offered to place on the swollen areas.
• The child should be monitored for such signs of complications as meningeal signs (positive Kernig's and Brudzinski's signs) and testicular swelling in males.
• Confirmed cases should be reported to the local public health department.

Tell parents to be creative! Just about any food a child craves can go in a blender – and makes mumps a little easier to stomach.

Poliomyelitis

Poliomyelitis, or polio, is a viral illness distributed worldwide. In countries where vaccines aren't readily available and economic conditions are poor, it remains a significant disease among infants and children.

It is many years since the last reported case of polio in the UK, with the most recent being as a result of the live vaccine used.

Oral is ousted

For that reason, oral polio vaccine is no longer used in the UK; it was replaced with IPV in 2000.

Poliomyelitis may range in severity from unapparent infection to fatal paralytic illness.

What causes it

Polio is caused by polioviruses type 1, type 2 and type 3.

What's in a name?

The three types of poliovirus were named for the first people known to have the disease:

 Type 1 is also called *Brunhilde*.

 Type 2 is also called *Lansing*.

 Type 3 is also called *Leon*.

How it happens

Transmission of the virus occurs by direct contact with infected oropharyngeal secretions or stool, infecting the GI tract. When a susceptible person is infected with the poliovirus, the responses may range from a brief, febrile, minor illness to a major illness with CNS involvement and paralysis.

Incubation and communicability

The incubation period is usually 7 to 10 days. The period of communicability isn't completely understood. The infected child can infect others for weeks before the development of symptoms. The virus is shed in respiratory secretions for a few days, and in stool for several weeks.

What to look for

Children with poliomyelitis have a wide range of symptoms. In subclinical cases, the child may report or show no symptoms at all. Clinical manifestations of a mild infection include fever, headache, nausea, vomiting and pharyngitis. Major infections may be non-paralytic or paralytic.

Non-paralytic

Clinical manifestations of non-paralytic poliomyelitis include:
- irritability
- moderate fever
- headache
- vomiting
- lethargy
- pains in the neck, back, arms and legs; abdominal muscle tenderness and weakness and spasms in the extensors of the neck and back.

Paralytic

Clinical manifestations of paralytic poliomyelitis are similar to those of non-paralytic poliomyelitis. In addition, patients may have:
- asymmetric weakness of various muscles
- loss of superficial and deep reflexes
- paraesthesia
- hypersensitivity to touch
- urine retention
- constipation
- abdominal distension.

What tests tell you

Diagnosis is usually based on the patient's clinical history and presentation. The virus can be detected in specimens from the pharynx and stool. Rising antibody titres in the blood can also indicate recent infection.

Complications

Complications include hypertension, urinary tract infection, urolithiasis, atelectasis, pneumonia, myocarditis, skeletal and soft-tissue deformities, paralytic ileus, permanent paralysis, respiratory arrest and death.

How it's treated

No cure for polio exists. Treatment is supportive and is directed at symptom relief. Lifesaving measures may be necessary in cases of respiratory distress or failure. In general, the more extensive the paralysis, the greater the resulting disability.

What to do

Passive antibodies transferred across the placenta from mother to foetus persist for about 6 months. Vaccination is the only effective method of disease prevention.

Children should be vaccinated with the IPV according to the recommended schedule The vaccine provides lifelong immunity to polio. When providing care to a child who's hospitalised with polio, follow these steps:
• Consider the child infectious and institute droplet precautions.
• Allow direct patient contact with only his/her family members and facility personnel who have been vaccinated against poliomyelitis.
• Ensure good body positioning and range of motion to prevent contractures.
• Provide continuous, vigilant monitoring of respiratory function.
• Monitor for all complications of immobility, including skin breakdown, bone demineralisation and pneumonia.
• Report confirmed cases to local public health department.

Roseola infantum

Roseola is a common, acute, benign, presumably viral illness characterised by fever with subsequent rash. Children with roseola usually present with a high fever of an unknown origin.

What causes it

Roseola is caused by the human herpes virus 6.

How it happens

Transmission of roseola isn't completely understood. The virus is detected in human saliva and is believed to be passed by oral viral shedding.

Incubation and communicability

The incubation period for roseola is 5 to 15 days. The period of communicability is unknown.

What to look for

The onset of symptoms occurs with a sudden, high fever. Children can have temperatures 39.4° to 41.1° C. Other than the unexplained fever, the child appears well, behaving normally. Most cases occur in infants and children younger than age 2 years, with peak incidence in children ages 6 to 12 months. The fever resolves on the third or fourth day of the illness.

Don't be rash

The febrile phase is typically followed by the development of a body rash that begins on the trunk and spreads to the neck, face, arms and legs. The rash fades within 3 days. Some children, however, don't develop a rash.

What tests tell you

Diagnostic laboratory tests aren't usually performed. It's possible to perform antibody titres to detect the virus.

Complications

Complications of roseola are rare but include extreme hyperthermia, persistent seizures, encephalitis and hepatitis.

How it's treated

Treatment is supportive and directed at relief of symptoms. Antipyretics, such as paracetamol, are given to relieve fever. Treating fever is important to prevent febrile seizures.

What to do

Roseola is benign and self-limiting. In addition to treatment of fever, care of a child with roseola should include:
* observation for the development of complications
* replacement of fluids and electrolytes as needed
* investigation of other common causes of high fever in young children such as otitis media.

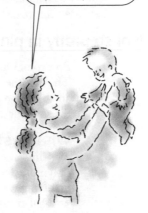

At the onset of roseola, appearances can be deceiving. Aside from a sudden, high fever, the child can appear perfectly well.

Rubella

Rubella, also known as German measles or 3-day measles, causes a distinctive maculopapular rash (resembling that of rubeola or scarlet fever) and lymphadenopathy. Cases of rubella having been declining for some years and provisional data for 2009 showed only 3 cases in under 15-year-olds in England and Wales.

What causes it

Rubella is caused by a viral infection with rubella virus (a toga-virus).

How it happens

Rubella is a mild viral illness transmitted by airborne respiratory droplets, direct contact with an infected person or direct contact with contaminated articles. The virus then enters the bloodstream.

Incubation and communicability

The incubation period of rubella is 14 to 21 days. The period of communicability is from 1 week before the onset of the rash until about 4 days after the appearance of the rash.

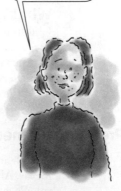

I hope they named it 3-day measles for a reason! Of course, 1-day measles would have been even better.

What to look for
Prodromal symptoms include:
- fever
- malaise
- headache
- purulent nasal drainage
- sore throat
- lymphadenopathy
- anorexia.

Not so pretty in pink

Prodromal symptoms occur for about 1 to 5 days before the onset of a pink rash. The exanthematous, maculopapular, mildly pruritic rash appears first on the face and then spreads to the neck, trunk and legs. Small, red, petechial macules on the soft palate (Forchheimer spots) usually precede or accompany the rash.

What tests tell you
- Clinical presentation usually confirms diagnosis of rubella. The presence of lymphadenopathy helps to distinguish rubella from other illnesses involving rashes.
- Cell cultures of the throat, blood, urine and cerebrospinal fluid, as well as convalescent serum that shows a fourfold rise in antibody titres, also confirm the diagnosis.

Complications
Complications of rubella are rare but can occur. Neuritis, arthritis, encephalitis and thrombocytopenic purpura can complicate the disease. In foetal infection (rare after 20 weeks' gestation), intrauterine death, spontaneous abortion and congenital malformations of major organ systems can occur.

How it's treated
Rubella is a mild, self-limiting illness. Treatment is supportive and directed at relief of symptoms. Antipyretic medications are used to control fever, and fluid intake is encouraged to promote and maintain adequate hydration.

What to do
Children with rubella are rarely hospitalised; they're usually treated at home because rubella is generally a mild, self-limiting viral illness:
- During the period of communicability, the child shouldn't attend school or nursery and should be isolated from pregnant women.
- If the child is hospitalised, droplet precautions should be instituted until 5 days after the rash disappears.

Pregnant women, beware

Rubella in early pregnancy may cause severe congenital anomalies of the foetus. All females of childbearing age should be immunised to prevent rubella and the potential for congenital rubella syndrome in their offspring. When caring for a child with rubella:

• Make sure that the child receives care only from non-pregnant hospital workers who aren't at risk for contracting rubella.
• Make sure that all health care providers have documented immunity to rubella through a positive rubella titre.
• Report confirmed rubella cases to the local public health department.

Rubeola

Rubeola, also known as measles, is a highly contagious viral disease that causes a characteristic maculopapular rash.

What causes it
Rubeola infection is caused by the rubeola virus. Outbreaks of illness occur mostly in unimmunised children or in those with compromised immune systems.

How it happens
Rubeola is transmitted by airborne respiratory droplets or by direct contact with contaminated articles.

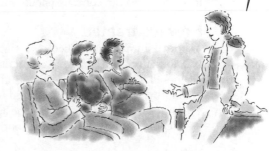

Better safe than sorry. Pregnant health care workers at risk for rubella should leave the care of children with the virus to someone else.

Incubation and communicability
The incubation period for rubeola is 8 to 12 days. The period of communicability begins several days before the appearance of the red rash and continues until 5 days after the rash has resolved.

What to look for
Symptoms of the prodromal phase include:
• fever
• malaise
• lethargy
• cough
• periorbital oedema
• conjunctivitis
• profuse drainage from the nose
• Koplik's spots, which are tiny grey-white specks surrounded by red halos that may be noted on the buccal mucosa opposite the molars about 2 days before the appearance of the body rash. (See *Spotting Koplik's spots*, page 182.)

You look acute

During the acute phase of the illness, a red, blotchy, flat rash begins on the face and spreads to the trunk and extremities. The rash and other symptoms (severe cough, rhinorrhoea and lymphadenopathy) gradually subside in 5 to 7 days.

What tests tell you
Diagnosis of rubeola is usually based on clinical presentation. Laboratory tests are rarely needed.

Complications
Potential complications include:
- pneumonia
- otitis media
- encephalitis
- seizures
- secondary bacterial infections
- autoimmune reactions.

The infection can be severe or fatal in patients with impaired cell-mediated immunity; mortality is highest in children younger than 2 years and in adults, who can contract pneumonia secondary to the disease.

How it's treated
Maternal immunity to rubeola is active in the infant for about 1 year after birth. Immunisation with MMR vaccine induces active immunity. After the disease is diagnosed, treatment is supportive and is directed at the relief of symptoms:
- Antipyretic medications are used to control fever.
- Antipruritic medications may be administered for itching.
- A cool mist vaporiser may be soothing to inflamed mucous membranes.

What to do
In addition to providing supportive treatment:
- monitor breathing to detect adventitious sounds
- encourage fluid intake to promote hydration and decrease the viscosity of secretions
- in the hospitalised child, maintain droplet precautions during the period of communicability
- report measles cases to the local public health department.

Varicella

Varicella, also called chickenpox, is an acute, highly contagious viral infection that can occur at any age.

What causes it
Infection with varicella zoster virus (VZV) causes chickenpox. The virus remains latent in dorsal root ganglia. Reactivation of the virus can cause herpes zoster infection (shingles) later in life.

How it happens
Airborne spread of respiratory secretions or, less commonly, direct contact with lesions of an infected person can cause infection in a susceptible child.

Incubation and communicability
The incubation period for chickenpox is 10 to 21 days. The period of communicability begins up to 5 days before the appearance of the body rash and continues until all lesions on the skin are crusted over.

Spotting Koplik's spots

Koplik's spots differentiate rubeola from other rash-producing viruses. The spots appear on the buccal mucosa opposite the molars and then extend to the entire buccal surface. The raised base of the spots may join together so that the blue-white centres stand out (looking like grains of salt) on the erythematous membrane.

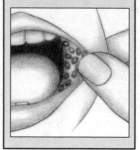

What to look for

The onset of symptoms usually occurs 14 to 16 days after exposure. Prodromal symptoms of fever, malaise and anorexia occur 24 to 48 hours before the development of the rash.

The clinical picture is one of a child with lesions in all stages of evolution present on the skin. The rash is pruritic. In addition:
- the rash begins as itchy red macules on the face, scalp or trunk that progress to papules
- papules develop into clear vesicles on an erythematous base (called 'dewdrops on rose petals')
- vesicles become cloudy and break easily; then scabs form
- as initial lesions are crusting over, new lesions form on the trunk and extremities.

What tests tell you

VZV antibody tests and titres may be useful in establishing a diagnosis. Most commonly, diagnosis is based on the clinical history and presentation of a child with the characteristic vesicular rash.

Complications

Complications of varicella are rare. The disease can have significant, life-threatening complications in children who are immunocompromised.

Complications of varicella include secondary bacterial infections, such as cellulitis, lymphadenitis, abscesses and sepsis. Other potential complications include encephalitis and meningoencephalitis, hepatitis, acute thrombocytopenia and pneumonia.

Quick quiz

1. Which sexually transmitted disease is preventable through vaccination?
    A. Syphilis
    B. Gonorrhea
    C. Hepatitis A
    D. Hepatitis B

Answer: D. The hepatitis B vaccine is given IM at birth (or before hospital discharge), at ages 1 to 4 months, and again at ages 6 to 18 months, for a total of three doses. For older children and adolescents, the initial IM dose is given, the second dose is given 1 month later, and the third dose is given 6 months after the first dose.

2. The mother of a child with varicella asks the nurse when the child may return to nursery. The nurse correctly responds by telling the mother that the child can return:
    A. when the fever is resolved.
    B. 24 hours after the appearance of the rash.
    C. when all lesions are crusted over.
    D. after receiving the first dose of diphenhydramine.

Answer: C. The period of communicability for varicella (chickenpox) begins up to 5 days before the appearance of the body rash. The period of communicability continues until all lesions on the skin are crusted over.

3.   What's an early symptom of roseola infantum?
    A.   High, unexplained fever
    B.   Vomiting
    C.   Development of a body rash
    D.   Behavioural changes and anorexia

Answer: A. The onset of symptoms of illness occurs with sudden, high fever. Fevers of 39.4° to 41.1° C can occur. Other than the unexplained fever, the child appears well, with normal behaviours.

Scoring

☆☆☆   If you answered all three items correctly, bravo! Go forth and spread your understanding of viral and bacterial illnesses.

☆☆   If you answered two items correctly, excellent work! Your knowledge of communicable disease is infectious.

☆   If you answered fewer than two items correctly, don't go into isolation! Take another look at the chapter, and forge ahead.

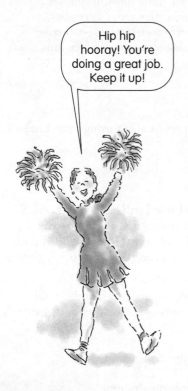

Hip hip hooray! You're doing a great job. Keep it up!

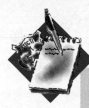

7 Neurological problems

Just the facts

In this chapter, you'll learn:

♦ structures of the neurological system

♦ assessment of patients with problems involving the neurological system

♦ diagnostic tests for neurological problems

♦ treatments and nursing interventions for children with neurological disorders.

Anatomy and physiology

The neurological system consists of the central nervous system (CNS), the peripheral nervous system and the autonomic (involuntary) nervous system (ANS). Through complex and coordinated interactions, these three parts integrate all physical, intellectual and emotional activities. Understanding how each part works is essential to conducting an accurate neurological assessment.

Central nervous system

The CNS is composed of the brain and all its component parts and the spinal cord. Structurally, the CNS is contained within the skull and the vertebral column.

Central command

Integration among all parts of the nervous system enables normal functioning of body parts, both voluntary and involuntary. A person's perception of himself and his environment, his reactions and interactions with the environment

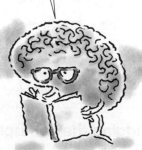

I like to think of myself as an intellectual. Seems like I'm the brains in this operation.

and his adjustment to development and environmental changes are greatly influenced by the proper integration and functioning of the nervous system.

Brain

The brain, the centre of the CNS, collects, integrates and interprets stimuli and initiates and monitors voluntary and involuntary motor activity.

The incredible expanding brain

Head circumference, which is measured in children up to 3 years, averages 33 to 35.5 cm and should be 2 to 3 cm larger than chest circumference at birth. Fifty percent of brain growth is achieved in the first year of life, 75% by 3 years and 90% by 6 years. The brain comprises 12% of body weight at birth, doubles in weight in the first year and triples by the age of 5 to 6 years.

Separated at birth

Since the skull protects the brain, the anterior and posterior fontanelles are separated at birth to allow for brain growth. The posterior fontanelle normally closes between 4 and 8 weeks, and the anterior fontanelle between 12 and 18 months.

A mass of nerves in a house of bones

Physiologically, the brain is the large, soft mass of nervous tissue housed in the cranium and protected and supported by the meninges and the skull bones. It consists of the:
• cerebrum
• cerebellum
• brain stem.

Other noteworthy figures

Other structures and elements of the brain include the:
• neurones
• meninges
• cerebrospinal fluid (CSF)
• ventricles.

Cerebrum

The cerebrum, the largest portion of the brain, is the nerve centre that controls sensory and motor activities and intelligence.

The outer layer of the cerebrum, the cerebral cortex, consists of neuron cell bodies (grey matter); the inner layers consist of axons (white matter) and basal ganglia, which control motor coordination and steadiness.

Bridging the hemispheres

A longitudinal fissure divides the cerebrum into two hemispheres connected by a wide band of nerve fibres called the corpus callosum. These hemispheres share information through the corpus callosum. Because motor impulses descending

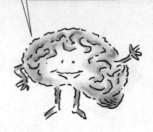

I'm the body's go to organ. When the body needs a stimulus interpreted or a motor activity initiated, I'm the only one for the job.

from the brain cross in the medulla, the right hemisphere controls the left side of the body and the left hemisphere controls the right side of the body.

Not the piercing kind

Several fissures divide the cerebrum into lobes, each of which is associated with specific functions. (See *A look at the lobes*.)

A look at the lobes

Several fissures divide the cerebrum into hemispheres and lobes; each lobe has a specific function.

The great dividers

The *fissure of Sylvius* (lateral sulcus) separates the temporal lobe from the frontal and parietal lobes. The *fissure of Rolando* (central sulcus) separates the frontal lobes from the parietal lobe. The *parieto-occipital fissure* separates the occipital lobe from the two parietal lobes.

Lovely lobes

Each lobe controls specific body functions:

- The *frontal lobe* controls voluntary muscle movements and contains motor areas (including the motor area for speech, or *Broca's area*). It's the centre for personality, behavioural and intellectual functions, such as judgement, memory and problem-solving; for autonomic functions and for cardiac and emotional responses.
- The *temporal lobe* is the centre for taste, hearing and smell. Also, in the brain's dominant hemisphere, it interprets spoken language.
- The *parietal lobe* coordinates and interprets sensory information from the opposite side of the body.
- The *occipital lobe* interprets visual stimuli.

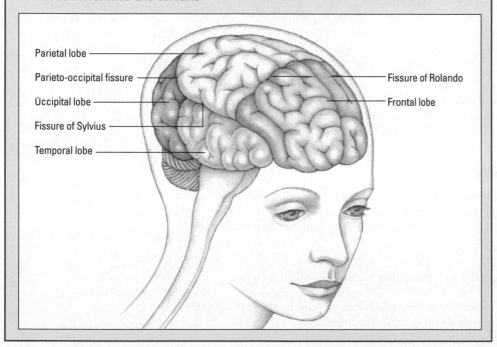

Parietal lobe

Parieto-occipital fissure

Occipital lobe

Fissure of Sylvius

Temporal lobe

Fissure of Rolando

Frontal lobe

Passing the baton

The thalamus, a relay centre below the corpus callosum, further organises cerebral function by transmitting impulses to and from appropriate areas of the cerebrum.

The body's thermostat

The hypothalamus, which lies beneath the thalamus, is an autonomic centre that regulates temperature control, appetite, blood pressure, breathing, sleep patterns and peripheral nerve discharges that occur with behavioural and emotional expression.

Cerebellum

Beneath the cerebrum, at the base of the brain, is the cerebellum. It's responsible for smooth-muscle movements, coordinating sensory impulses with muscle activity and maintaining muscle tone and equilibrium.

Brain stem

The brain stem relays nerve impulses between the spinal cord and other parts of the brain. It houses cell bodies from most of the cranial nerves and includes the:
• midbrain, which is the reflex centre for the third and fourth cranial nerves and mediates pupillary reflexes and eye movements
• pons, which helps regulate respirations and mediate chewing, taste, saliva secretion, hearing and equilibrium
• medulla oblongata, which affects cardiac, respiratory and vasomotor functions
• neurons.

Neurons

The fundamental unit of the nervous system is the neuron, a highly specialised conductor cell that receives and transmits electrochemical nerve impulses. Neurons develop at between 15 and 30 weeks' gestation.

Delicate and impulsive

Its structure contains delicate, threadlike nerve fibres that extend from the central cell body and transmit signals, or axons, which carry impulses away from the cell body, and dendrites, which carry impulses to the cell body.

Meninges

The brain is covered with three thin membranes called meninges:

The outer membrane is the dura mater, or 'hard mother'; it has various folds that separate the brain into compartments.

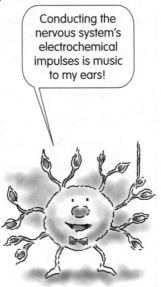

Conducting the nervous system's electrochemical impulses is music to my ears!

The second structure is the arachnoid mater; it has two layers of fibrous and elastic tissue and, between the layers, a spongy, cobweb-like structure containing subarachnoid fluid.

The third structure is the pia mater, or 'tender mother', a very fine membrane that's rich in minute blood plexuses and follows the brain in all its folds. (See *Meningeal layers of the brain*, page 190.)

CSF
The ventricles of the brain and the entire subarachnoid space around the brain and spinal cord contain CSF.

Clear liquid with a protein chaser

CSF is a clear liquid containing water and traces of organic materials (especially protein), glucose and minerals. CSF is formed from blood in capillary networks called choroid plexuses, which are located primarily in the brain's lateral ventricles. The fluid is eventually reabsorbed into the venous blood through the arachnoid villi, located in dural sinuses on the brain's surface.

Better than a bubble bath

The brain floats in, and is bathed by, CSF. It acts as a shock absorber and helps reduce forces that jar or shake the brain. CSF is in contact with the entire brain and spinal cord surface as well as the surfaces of the ventricles.

Ventricles
The four ventricles are large, CSF-filled cavities within the brain. There are two lateral ventricles, one in each cerebral hemisphere. A third ventricle (located directly above the midbrain of the brain stem) communicates with both the lateral ventricles and the fourth ventricle (located in the posterior brain fossa).

> There's nothing like a soothing bath to protect me from the jarring forces of the outside world. Not bad for the ole' noggin either!

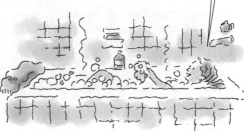

Spinal cord

The spinal cord extends downward from the brain, through the vertebrae, to the level of approximately the second lumbar vertebra. It functions as a conductive pathway to and from the brain. It's also the reflex centre for activities that don't require brain control such as deep tendon reflexes (the jerking reaction elicited by tapping with a reflex hammer).

Can you hear me now?

Within the spinal cord, connections are made between incoming and outgoing nerve fibres. Thirty-one pairs of spinal nerves are connected to the

Meningeal layers of the brain

Three primary membranes, or meninges, help protect the central nervous system: the dura mater, the arachnoid membrane and the pia mater.

Dura mater

The *dura mater* is a fibrous membrane that lines the skull and forms folds (reflections) that descend into the brain's fissures and provide stability. The dural folds include the:

- falx cerebri, which lies in the longitudinal fissure and separates the hemispheres of the cerebrum
- tentorium cerebelli, which separates the cerebrum from the cerebellum
- falx cerebelli, which separates the two cerebellar lobes.

The arachnoid villi (projections of the dura mater into the superior sagittal and transverse sinuses) serve as the exit points for cerebrospinal fluid (CSF) drainage into venous circulation.

Arachnoid membrane

A fragile, fibrous layer with moderate vascularity, the *arachnoid membrane* lies between the dura mater and the pia mater. Injury to its blood vessels during head trauma, lumbar puncture or cisternal puncture may cause haemorrhage.

Pia mater

An extremely thin and highly vascular membrane, the *pia mater* closely covers the brain's surface and extends into its fissures. It contains minute arteries and veins that supply the brain.

Additional layers

Three layers of space further cushion the brain and spinal cord against injury:

- The *epidural space* (a potential space) lies over the dura mater.
- The *subdural space* lies between the dura mater and the arachnoid membrane and is commonly the site of haemorrhage after head trauma.
- The *subarachnoid space*, which is filled with CSF, lies between the arachnoid membrane and the pia mater.

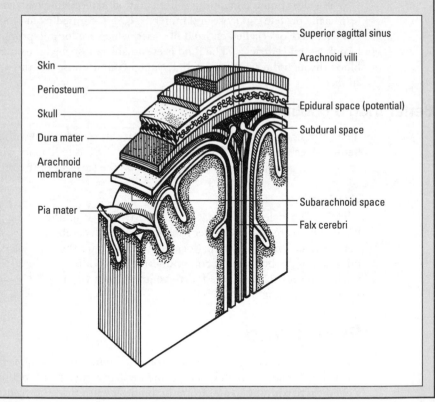

Skin

Periosteum

Skull

Dura mater

Arachnoid membrane

Pia mater

Superior sagittal sinus

Arachnoid villi

Epidural space (potential)

Subdural space

Subarachnoid space

Falx cerebri

cord. The sensory, or ascending, tracts carry sensory impulses up the spinal cord to the brain; the motor, or descending, tracts carry motor impulses down the spinal cord and out to the peripheral nervous system.

Peripheral nervous system

The part of the nervous system outside of the skull and vertebral column is considered the peripheral nervous system. It's composed of 31 spinal nerves and 12 cranial nerves and is divided into two functional systems: the somatic nervous system and the ANS.

Spinal nerves

Messages transmitted through the spinal cord reach outlying areas through 31 pairs of segmentally arranged spinal nerves attached to the spinal cord. Spinal nerves are numbered according to their point of origin in the cord:
- eight cervical nerves–C1 to C8
- twelve thoracic nerves–T1 to T12
- five lumbar nerves–L1 to L5
- one coccygeal nerve.

It's rude to interrupt

After leaving the vertebral column, each spinal nerve separates into rami (branches), distributed peripherally, with extensive but organised overlapping. This overlapping reduces the risk of lost sensory or motor function from interruption of a single spinal nerve.

Cranial nerves

The 12 pairs of cranial nerves transmit motor or sensory messages (or both) primarily between the brain or brain stem and the head and neck. All cranial nerves except the olfactory and optic nerves exit from the midbrain, pons or medulla oblongata of the brain stem. (See *Exit points of the cranial nerves*, page 192.)

Somatic nervous system

The somatic (voluntary) nervous system is activated by will but can function independently. It's responsible for all conscious and higher mental processes as well as subconscious and reflex actions such as shivering.

Autonomic nervous system

The ANS regulates unconscious processes to control involuntary body functions, such as digestion, respiration and cardiovascular function. It's usually divided into two antagonistic systems that balance each other's activities to support homoeostasis under normal conditions:
- The sympathetic nervous system controls energy expenditure, especially in stressful situations, by releasing adrenergic catecholamines.

Exit points of the cranial nerves

As this illustration reveals, 10 of the 12 pairs of cranial nerves (CN) exit from the brain stem. The remaining two pairs – the olfactory and optic nerves – exit from the forebrain.

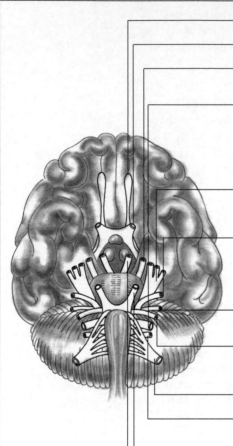

Olfactory (CN I). *Sensory:* smell

Optic (CN II). *Sensory:* visual

Trochlear (CN IV). *Motor:* extraocular eye movement (inferior medial)

Vagus (CN X). *Motor:* movement of palate, swallowing, gag reflex, activity of the thoracic and abdominal viscera, such as heart rate and peristalsis. *Sensory:* sensations of throat, larynx and thoracic and abdominal viscera (heart, lungs, bronchi and GI tract)

Trigeminal (CN V). *Sensory:* transmitting stimuli from face and head, corneal reflex. *Motor:* chewing, biting, and lateral jaw movements

Facial (CN VII). *Sensory:* taste receptors (anterior two-thirds of tongue). *Motor:* facial muscle movement, including muscles of expression (those in the forehead and around the eyes and mouth)

Acoustic (CN VIII). *Sensory:* hearing, sense of balance

Glossopharyngeal (CN IX). *Motor:* swallowing movements. *Sensory:* sensations of throat, taste receptors (posterior one-third of tongue)

Hypoglossal (CN XII). *Motor:* tongue movement

Spinal accessory (CN XI). *Motor:* shoulder movement, head rotation

Abducens (CN VI). *Motor:* extraocular eye movement (lateral)

Oculomotor (CN III). *Motor:* extraocular eye movement (superior, medial, and inferior lateral), pupillary constriction, upper eyelid elevation

- The parasympathetic nervous system helps conserve energy by releasing the cholinergic neurohormone acetylcholine.

Neurological assessment

A complete assessment of the neurological system includes evaluation of:
- mental and emotional status
- cranial nerve function
- sensory function
- motor function
- reflexes.

Knowledge of the child's physical, psychomotor and cognitive developmental milestones is an essential assessment tool for detecting significant deviations.

Mini-assessment

Dependent on the circumstances, the neurological assessment may be a component of advanced paediatric life support and therefore include an assessment on level of consciousness (LOC), pupillary response, motor function, reflexes, sensory functions and vital signs.

Glasgow Coma Scale

The Glasgow Coma Scale (GCS), which assesses eye opening as well as verbal and motor responses, provides a quick, standardised account of neurological status. A paediatric version of the scale considers the pre-verbal child. (See *Paediatric coma scale*, page 194.)

In this test, each response receives a numerical value; the final score is the sum total of the values.
- A score of 15 for all three parts is normal.
- A score of 7 or lower indicates coma.
- A score of 3, the lowest possible score, usually (but not always) indicates brain death.

Motor function

Motor function is also a good indicator of LOC and can point to central or peripheral nervous system damage.

Myelination mastery

The mastery of gross and fine motor skills is related to the myelination of the nervous system and follows the concept of cephalocaudal-proximodistal development. Cephalocaudal development is the sequence in which the greatest growth always occurs at the head and gradually works its way

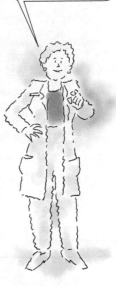

Could you recognise a developmental lag? If you know the milestones, you can tell if a child is falling behind.

Paediatric coma scale

To quickly assess a child's level of consciousness and to uncover baseline changes, use the paediatric coma scale. This assessment tool grades consciousness in relation to eye opening and motor response, and responses to auditory or visual stimuli. A decreased reaction score in one or more categories warns of an impending neurologic crisis. A score of 7 or lower is comatose and probably means severe neurologic damage.

Test	Patient's reaction	Score
Best eye opening response	Open spontaneously	4
	Open to verbal command	3
	Open to pain	2
	No response	1
Best motor response	Obeys verbal command	6
	Localises painful stimuli	5
	Flexion-withdrawal	4
	Flexion-abnormal (decorticate rigidity)	3
	Extension (decerebrate rigidity)	2
	No response	1

Test	Patient's reaction	Score
Best response to auditory and/or visual stimulus	For the child older than age 2 years: Oriented	5
	Confused	4
	Inappropriate words	3
	Incomprehensible sounds	2
	No response	1
	OR For the child younger than age 2 years: Smiles, listens, follows	5
	Cries, consolable	4
	Inappropriate persistent cry	3
	Agitated, restless	2
	No response	1

Total possible score   *3 to 15*

towards the 'tail'. Proximodistal development proceeds from the centre towards the extremities.

Reflex rules

Infant activities are primarily driven by reflex but, with myelination and development, a growing child progressively performs complex tasks requiring coordinated movements.

How strong are you?

To evaluate muscle strength, follow these steps:
• Have the child grip your hands and squeeze.
• Ask them to push against your palm with their foot.
• Compare muscle strength on each side to ensure the results are the same bilaterally.

Pupillary response

Brain damage is indicated by a lack of change in pupil size in response to light. Use a torch to assess pupillary response. While shining the outer edge of the light into the child's eye, observe the initial size of the pupil and the speed of the pupil's response to the light. Compare both eyes to ensure an equal bilateral response.

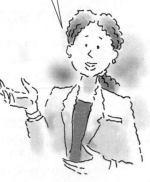

Assess pupillary response at the bedside.

Diagnostic tests

Several invasive and non-invasive tests are used to diagnose neurological disorders.

Minimising emotional trauma

Tests performed to diagnose neurological disorders can be extremely frightening to a child and their parents. Children and parents may have misconceptions related to what will happen and why a test is being performed. Preparing a child helps allay fears and misconceptions and gives them the tools to cope effectively with a frightening experience.

Before a test is performed, follow these steps:
• Tell the child what to expect in age-appropriate terms (what they'll see, hear, and feel) and explain why the test is being performed.
• Be honest about pain or discomfort the child might experience and suggest coping strategies (e.g. 'Count to 5 and the hurting part will be over').
• Always ensure that any analgesics and/or local anaesthetics are prescribed and given before the test allowing them adequate time to work.

I'm really frightened

• Tell the child that it's OK to be afraid, and reassure them that everyone involved is there to help and keep them safe.
• Whenever possible, show the child any equipment (e.g. the scanning machine) before the test.
• Encourage the child to ask questions and express concerns.
• Allow the parents to remain with the child during testing whenever possible; when this isn't possible, tell the child where the parents are and that they are waiting.

A job well done

• Give the child a 'job' to do during the test (e.g. 'Your job is to try and hold very still') to give them a sense of control.
• After the test, praise the child for doing a good job, and encourage them to talk about the test or draw a picture that depicts the experience (to help the child master the experience and put it in perspective).

Specialist to the rescue

Most hospitals have a play specialist who can help prepare the child for the tests and help them make sense of it afterwards.

Brain scan

A brain scan measures gamma rays produced by an IV injection of a radioisotopic material. It's used to identify conditions such as tumour, infarction, intracranial masses and vascular lesions, involving the cortex in patients with headaches, epilepsy and other neurological symptoms.

Nursing considerations

The CYP nurse should explain the procedure to the child and family, and tell the child (in their terms) that the only discomfort is the peripheral venepuncture required for injection of the radioisotope. However, a surface anaesthetic such as Ametop or EMLA should be used to alleviate the discomfort of venepuncture. Assure the child and family that the radioactive material is usually excreted within 6 to 24 hours, and encourage the child to drink fluids after the test to aid in the excretion of the isotope.

CT scan

Computed tomography (CT) scan is indicated when CNS disease is suspected. The X-ray scan produces three-dimensional images that can identify brain tumours, infarction, bleeding and haematomas as well as provide information about the ventricular system of the brain. It is particularly good for imaging bone structures and can be enhanced by the use of contrast dyes.

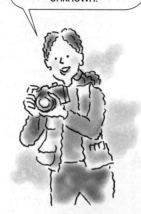

Seeing is believing. Show the child a picture of the imaging machine (or the machine itself) to help allay fear of the unknown.

Nursing considerations

A child who knows what to expect will be less fearful and more cooperative during a CT scan. To help the child know what to expect, consider these steps:
• Explain the procedure to the child. Cooperation is necessary because the child must lie still during the procedure.
• Show the child a picture of the CT machine to help alleviate fears. (It may be necessary to sedate the child.)
• Tell the child that they may hear a clicking noise as the scanner moves around their head but that the machine won't touch them.
• Explain that the child won't be able to eat or drink for 4 hours before the scan (depending on age); contrast dye may cause some nausea.
• Assess the child for any allergy to iodine or shellfish.
• Encourage the child to drink fluids after the scan (because dye is excreted by the kidneys).

EEG

EEG is a graphic recording of the electrical activity of the brain. It's performed to identify and evaluate children having seizures. Pathological conditions involving the brain cortex (such as tumours and infarctions) can also be detected. EEG may also used to confirm brain death.

Nursing considerations

After explaining the procedure to the child and parents:
• reassure the child that they won't feel anything during the test but it may be a little uncomfortable
• make sure the child continues to eat and drink before the test because fasting may cause hypoglycaemia, which could alter the test results
• make sure the child doesn't drink anything with caffeine on the morning of the test because of caffeine's stimulating effect, although coffee is not so good for children anyway!
• tell the child that he needs to remain still during the test; any movement will create interference and alter the EEG recording.

Lumbar puncture

By placing a needle in the subarachnoid space of the spinal column, one can measure the pressure of that space and obtain CSF for examination and diagnosis. The needle is commonly placed between L3 and L4 (or L4 and L5). This examination may assist in the diagnosis of metastatic brain or spinal cord neoplasm, meningitis, cerebral haemorrhage and encephalitis.

Nursing considerations

The procedure should be explained in detail and consent obtained. In addition, follow these steps:
• Local anaesthesia, sedation or general anaesthesia needs to be considered.
• Where possible, instruct the child to empty their bladder and bowels before the procedure.
• Monitor the child's vital signs during and after the procedure because sedation may be used to complete the procedure.
• Explain the importance of remaining still throughout the procedure in the side-lying knee-chest position. (See *Lumbar puncture positioning*, page 198.)
• Gently hold even a cooperative child during the procedure to prevent injury from unexpected or involuntary movement. Relevant guidance including the RCN document 'Restrictive physical intervention and therapeutic holding for children and young people' (RCN, 2010) should be referred to in order to inform practice.

Maintain, encourage, assess

• Keep the child in a reclining position for up to 12 hours after the procedure to avoid the discomfort of potential post-procedure spinal headache.

Advice from the experts

Lumbar puncture positioning

When positioning a child for a lumbar puncture, refer to guidance on restraint and follow these steps:

Have the child lie on their side at the edge of the bed, with chin tucked into the chest and knees drawn up to their abdomen.

Make sure the child's spine is curved and their back is at the edge of the bed (as shown below); this position widens the spaces between the vertebrae, easing insertion of the needle.

To help the child maintain this position, place one of your hands behind their neck; place the other hand behind their knees and pull gently.

Hold the child firmly in this position throughout the procedure to prevent accidental needle displacement. (Typically, the medic inserts the needle between the third and fourth lumbar vertebrae.)

The sitting position may be used for infants. However, because the flexed position may interfere with the infant's breathing, monitor their colour and respiratory status closely during the procedure.

Positioning a young child

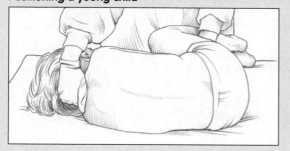

Positioning an infant

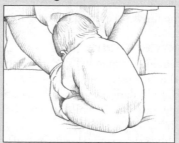

- Encourage the child to drink increased amounts of fluid with a straw to replace the CSF removed during the puncture. (Drinking with a straw allows the child to keep their head flat.)
- Assess the child for numbness, tingling and decreased movement of the extremities; pain at the injection site; drainage of blood or CSF at the injection site and inability to void.

MRI

Magnetic resonance imaging (MRI) is a non-invasive diagnostic procedure that provides valuable information about the body's anatomy in greater detail than a CT scan does. It doesn't require exposure to ionising radiation as it uses magnetic and radio waves to produce an image. MRI is indicated for the evaluation of headache or signs of CNS lesions; it's also used to assess neck and back pain as well as lesions of the bones and joints.

Nursing considerations

Begin by explaining the procedure to the child and family and telling them that there's no exposure to radiation during MRI. In addition, follow these steps:
•   Tell the parents that, because no radiation is used, they may read or talk to their child in the imaging room during the procedure.
•   Inform the parents that young children will need to be sedated because of the need to remain motionless during the procedure.
•   Tell the child that he may eat or drink as usual before and after the procedure. (No food or fluid restrictions are necessary before MRI.)
•   Make sure the child doesn't take their favourite metal toy into the scanner. Magnets and metal don't mix!

PET scan

In positron emission tomography (PET) scanning, radioactive chemicals are administered to the patient. These chemicals are used in the normal metabolic process of the particular organ being studied. Positrons emitted from the radioactive chemicals in the organ are sensed by a series of detectors positioned around the patient.

PET scanning can help detect cerebral dysfunction caused by tumours, seizures and head trauma. It's most commonly used for evaluation of the heart and brain and in many aspects of oncology.

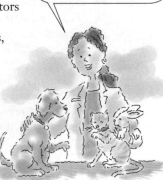

It may not be cute and cuddly, but a PET scan is the best thing going for detecting cerebral dysfunction.

Nursing considerations

Keep in mind that many people haven't heard of PET scanning; the child and parents may be anxious about what they perceive to be a new procedure. To prepare the child and parents for the procedure, follow these steps:
•   Explain the procedure to the child and family.
•   Explain to the child that an IV will be inserted and that this is the only 'hurting part' of the procedure. However, a surface anaesthetic such as Ametop or EMLA should be used to alleviate the discomfort of venepuncture.
•   Explain that food or fluids may need to be restricted for 4 hours prior to the test.
•   Don't sedate the child; they may need to perform certain mental activities during a brain PET scan.
•   After the scan, encourage the child to drink fluids and urinate frequently to aid removal of the radioisotope from the bladder.

Ventricular tap

A ventricular tap is performed if a neonate has unexplained, excessive head growth or a bulging fontanelle caused by increased intracranial pressure (ICP).

An illuminating finding

A ventricular tap is also performed if an infant has a positive transillumination of the skull. In a normal infant, a halo of light can be seen around the rim of the light source. If the infant has hydrocephalus or anencephaly, the halo from the light will be larger or the glow will be visible on the opposite side of the skull.

Going in

When performing a ventricular tap:
• The needle is inserted into the subdural space or the ventricle through the open anterior fontanelles or the coronal suture.
• The fluid is removed slowly to prevent intracranial haemorrhage caused by pressure shifts.

Nursing considerations

Parents are likely to feel anxious when their infant must undergo a procedure that involves pain, discomfort or stress. The nurse should encourage the parents to ask questions and express concerns.
• Explain the procedure to the parents.
• Hold the infant's head securely in the correct position to prevent meningeal laceration.
• Number and label the tubes of fluid in the order in which they're collected.
• Maintain the infant in a semi-erect position (an infant seat may be used) to reduce the possibility of further leakage of fluid from the site of the puncture.
• Assess the pressure dressing for leakage of fluid and bleeding.
• Keep the infant as quiet and comfortable as possible; crying increases ICP.

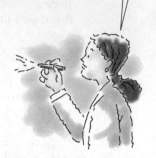

Transillumination is done with a flashlight held closely against the infant's head in a completely dark room.

Procedures and treatments

The care of a child with suspected or diagnosed neurological problems may involve invasive procedures to monitor or treat the child's condition.

ICP monitoring

ICP monitoring allows assessment of the pressure exerted by the blood, brain, CSF and any other space-occupying fluid or mass. In neonates a normal range would be 2–4 mm Hg and in children 5–15 mm Hg with raised ICP defined as pressure sustained at 20 mm Hg or higher.

Look closely ...

Assessment of the child with increased ICP requires close observation because the common signs and symptoms may not appear until ICP is significantly elevated, placing the child in grave danger. The subarachnoid bolt and the intraventricular catheter are the two major instruments used for monitoring ICP in a child:
• The end of the bolt is placed in the subarachnoid space. The top of the bolt is attached to a transducer to conduct a waveform to the monitor.
• The catheter is placed in the lateral ventricle or subarachnoid space. (The catheter provides a method for measuring pressure as well as a conduit to drain off extra fluid into a drainage bag.) The drainage bag and the manometer are part of a sterile closed system. (The manometer is used to measure the ICP within the closed system.)

Less invasive

In an infant, ICP monitoring can be performed without penetrating the scalp. In this external method, a photoelectric transducer with a pressure-sensitive membrane is taped to the infant's anterior fontanelle. The transducer responds to pressure at the site and transmits readings to a bedside monitor and recording system.

Sorry, not for everyone

The external method is restricted to infants because pressure readings can be obtained only at the fontanelles (the incompletely ossified areas of the skull). ICP monitoring from the fontanelles can be inaccurate if the equipment is poorly placed or inconsistently calibrated.

Nursing considerations

Before ICP monitoring is performed, thoroughly explain the procedure to the child (if possible) and the parents. In addition, follow these steps:
• Be thoroughly familiar with the monitoring system being used, and prepare the child and family for what they can expect after placement of the selected monitoring device.
• Explain that the procedure doesn't hurt the child and that they may have bags placed on either side of their head to prevent head movement.
• Assess whether the child has an allergy to iodine preparations.
• Maintain the sterility of the system. Monitor the child closely for signs of infection.
• Monitor the amount of fluid in the drainage bag; assess for signs of infection.
• Constantly monitor the child for signs of increased ICP. Minimise activities that may elevate ICP, such as those that may cause stress, pain or crying; bright lights, noise and other environmental stimuli, and vigorous range-of-motion (ROM) physiotherapy exercises. Remember that suctioning and percussion are contraindicated because they acutely elevate ICP. As

indicated by the paediatric anaesthetist, suctioning may be performed if absolutely necessary by hyperoxygenating the child with 100% oxygen before the procedure. Vibration may be used instead of percussion as it doesn't increase ICP.

VP shunt insertion

A ventriculoperitoneal (VP) shunt is implanted in the child with hydrocephalus to prevent excess accumulation of CSF in the ventricles. The tubing diverts the CSF from the ventricles into the peritoneal cavity, where it's reabsorbed. The procedure is performed under general anaesthesia.

Nursing considerations

Young children may have misconceptions about procedures involving general anaesthesia. When explaining this procedure (and all procedures involving general anaesthesia), make sure the child understands that they will be given 'a special medicine' to make sure they don't feel anything during the procedure.

> Explain that sleeping at night is different from sleeping during general anaesthesia so that the child isn't scared to close their eyes at night or nap time.

A special sleep

Rather than telling a child they'll be asleep (which may make them afraid to go to sleep at night or nap time or cause worry that they won't wake up during the procedure), tell them, 'The medicine gives you a special kind of sleep that isn't like sleeping at night or nap time'.

Monitor and measure

In addition to preparing the child for the procedure, follow these care measures:

Pre-operatively
• Monitor the child for signs of increased ICP.
• Measure head circumference daily at the occipital frontal circumference; place the tape measure just above the top of the ears, around the mid forehead and around the most prominent part of the occiput.
• Gently palpate fontanelles and suture lines for signs of bulging, tenseness and separation, which may indicate increased ICP or increasing ventricular size.

Post-operatively
• Monitor the child for pain, and administer analgesia as prescribed.
• Keep the child positioned flat and on the non-operative side.
• Discuss with medical staff what the child can be allowed to do; the child may be allowed to sit up to reduce ICP.
• Follow the surgeon's instructions and manufacturer's recommendations regarding pumping of the shunt (pressing on it to check for proper function); not all shunt devices require this.

- Observe the child for signs of increased ICP, which may indicate an obstructed shunt.
- Monitor the child for abdominal distension, which may indicate distal catheter placement.
- Be alert for signs of CSF infection (fever, poor feeding, vomiting, decreased LOC, seizures), which is the greatest post-operative risk.
- Administer antibiotics as prescribed.
- Teach the parents how to change dressings and recognise shunt malfunctions.

Neurological disorders

A diagnosis of a neurological disorder, whether acute, chronic or progressive, can be terrifying to a child and his/her parents. They'll look to their nurses to help allay fears and concerns, answer questions and provide ongoing support.

Bacterial meningitis

Meningitis, an inflammation of the meninges, is the most common infectious process of the CNS. It can be bacterial or viral, and can occur as a primary disease or as a result of complications of neurosurgery, trauma, systemic infection or sinus or ear infections.

What causes it

Many organisms can cause meningitis; however, meningococcal meningitis and pneumococcal meningitis are the most common.

Last year's news

Until recently, *Haemophilus influenzae* type B was the most common cause of meningitis in children older than age 1 month, but vaccination with the *H. influenzae* type B vaccine has drastically reduced its incidence.

Still strong but waning

The incidence of *Escherichia coli* and beta-haemolytic streptococcus meningitis is higher during the first 2 years of life, especially during the first month of life. The incidence is expected to decline as more infants and children are immunised with the new pneumococcal 7-valent conjugate vaccine.

How it happens

- Bacteria reach the meninges via the bloodstream from nearby infections (e.g. sinusitis, mastoiditis and otitis media) or by communication of CSF with the exterior (e.g. myelomen-ingocele, penetrating injuries or neurosurgical procedures).

• The organism becomes implanted in CSF and throughout the arachnoid space. Because CSF has relatively low levels of antibodies, complement and white blood cells (WBCs), the infection flourishes.

• As the process continues, increased ICP develops, along with empyaema.

• If the infection spreads to the ventricles, oedema and tissue scarring around the ventricle cause obstruction of the CSF, and subsequent hydrocephalus. Because CSF contains such nutrients as protein and glucose, it's an excellent medium for bacterial growth. Thus, the process of infection, oedema, obstruction and hydrocephalus can occur rapidly.

What to look for

Symptoms of bacterial meningitis are variable and depend on the child's age, pathogen and duration of the illness before diagnosis. Findings in young infants and toddlers (between ages 3 months and 2 years) may include:

• fever
• change in feeding pattern
• vomiting or diarrhoea
• bulging anterior fontanelle
• irritability (becoming more so with rocking and cuddling)
• high-pitched cry.

Bigger kids

In older children, look for:

• fever
• irritability
• lethargy
• confusion
• vomiting
• muscle or joint pain
• headache
• photophobia
• resistance to neck flexion
• hyperextension of the head and neck to relieve discomfort
• seizures
• coma
• positive Kernig's or Brudzinski's sign, or both. (See *Two telltale signs of meningitis*.)

Children with a haemorrhagic rash, first appearing as petaechiae and changing to purpura or large necrotic patches, may have meningococcal meningitis.

What tests tell you

Lumbar puncture is performed to evaluate the CSF for protein and glucose levels and the number of WBCs. The fluid may appear cloudy or milky white. CSF protein levels tend to be high; glucose levels may be low. Polymerase chain reaction techniques are useful when the cultures are negative because of partially treated meningitis.

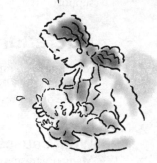

A high-pitched cry is one symptom of bacterial meningitis in infants.

Two telltale signs of meningitis

A positive response to these tests helps to establish a diagnosis of meningitis.

Brudzinski's sign

To test for Brudzinski's sign, place the child in a dorsal recumbent position and put your hands behind their neck and bend it forward. Pain and resistance may indicate meningeal inflammation, neck injury or arthritis. However, if the child also flexes their hips and knees in response to the manipulation, chances are they have meningitis.

Kernig's sign

To test for Kernig's sign, place the child in a supine position. Flex the leg at the hip and knee and then straighten the knee. Pain or resistance points to meningitis.

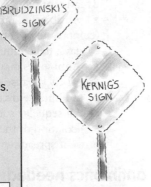

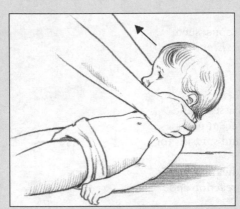

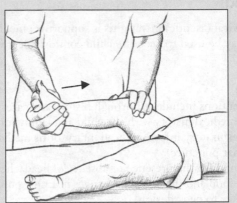

A CT scan can rule out cerebral haematoma, haemorrhage or tumour. Other tests performed to aid in diagnosis include:
* blood cultures
* full blood count (FBC)
* serum electrolytes and osmolality
* clotting factors
* nose and throat cultures.

Complications

The most common neurological complications of meningitis are hearing loss, developmental delay, seizures, visual impairment and behavioural problems. Other complications include cranial nerve dysfunction, brain abscess and syndrome of inappropriate antidiuretic hormone. Death occurs in 10% to 15% of cases (especially neonatal meningitis).

How it's treated

Treatment should begin before the causative organism is identified because it may take up to 3 days to obtain culture results and delays could be fatal. Treatment includes the following:

• Antibiotics, including ampicillin, aminoglycosides, cephalosporins (cefotaxime or ceftriaxone) and penicillin G, may be given IV for 7 to 21 days, depending on the organism and the child's clinical response.

• Antibiotics may be changed when culture and sensitivity results are known, especially because many organisms have resistance to certain antibiotics.

• Adjunctive therapy with dexamethasone may be provided to reduce the risk of sequelae such as hearing loss.

• Isolation of the child is necessary for the first 24 hours of therapy to prevent spreading the infection.

No antibiotics needed

Treatment for viral (aseptic) meningitis is supportive; medications, such as analgesics may be used to keep the child comfortable. (See *Aseptic meningitis*.)

What to do

Nursing interventions include a thorough history and careful assessment:

• Review the medical history with the child and family for recent illnesses, such as upper respiratory infection, head injury, otitis media and sinusitis (or a previous lumbar puncture).

• Assess the child for the presence or absence of headaches, hearing loss, seizure activity, food and fluid intake, changes in LOC, pupil reaction and size and resistance to neck flexion.

• Assess peaks and troughs of antibiotic levels to ensure adequate treatment and prevent ototoxicity.

• Teach the parents about the possible complications of meningitis and about the prescribed medications.

• Question the parents about the child's close contacts because they will need prophylactic treatment. (Close contacts shouldn't wait for signs of meningitis to develop but should seek medical attention promptly because they could be incubating the infection.)

Brain tumours

CNS tumours are the most common solid tumours in children and cause more deaths in children than any other form of malignancy. Most brain tumours in children are supratentorial (above the roofline of the cerebellum); the remaining tumours are infratentorial (below the roofline of the cerebellum).

What causes it

The cause of brain tumours is unknown, but heredity and environment have been associated with their development.

Aseptic meningitis

Aseptic meningitis is a benign syndrome characterised by headache, fever, vomiting and meningeal symptoms. It results from some form of viral infection, including enteroviruses (most common), arboviruses, herpes simplex virus, mumps virus or lymphocytic choriomeningitis virus.

Signs and symptoms

Aseptic meningitis begins suddenly with a fever up to 40° C, alterations in consciousness (drowsiness, confusion, stupor) and neck or spine stiffness, which is slight at first. (The child experiences such stiffness when bending forward.) Other signs and symptoms include headaches, nausea, vomiting, abdominal pain, poorly defined chest pain and sore throat.

Diagnostic tests

A history of recent illness and knowledge of seasonal epidemics are essential in differentiating among the many forms of aseptic meningitis. Negative bacteriologic cultures and cerebrospinal fluid (CSF) analysis showing pleocytosis and increased protein levels suggest the diagnosis. Isolation of the virus from CSF confirms it.

Treatment

Treatment is supportive and includes:

- bed rest
- maintenance of fluid and electrolyte balance
- analgesics for pain
- exercises to combat residual weakness
- careful handling of excretions and good hand-washing technique to prevent spreading the disease (isolation isn't necessary).

How it happens

Brain tumours are generally classified according to the tissue from which they arise: those arising inside the brain substance (such as gliomas and vascular tumours) or those arising outside the brain substance (such as meningiomas and cranial nerve tumours).

Common in kids

The most common brain tumours in children are:
- cerebellar astrocytoma
- medulloblastoma
- ependymoma
- brain stem glioma (See *Locations of brain tumours in children*, page 208.)

What to look for

Signs and symptoms are directly related to the anatomic location and size of the tumour and, to some extent, the age of the child:
- The hallmark symptoms of a brain tumour are headache and early morning vomiting related to the child getting out of bed.
- The child may experience vision changes, such as diplopia, strabismus and nystagmus, which may manifest as difficulties with schoolwork.
- Papilloedema (oedema of the optic disc) may be a late sign; this may be hard to evaluate in children because ophthalmic examinations require the child's cooperation.

Locations of brain tumors in children

Below are the most common types of brain tumour in children, along with their usual location.

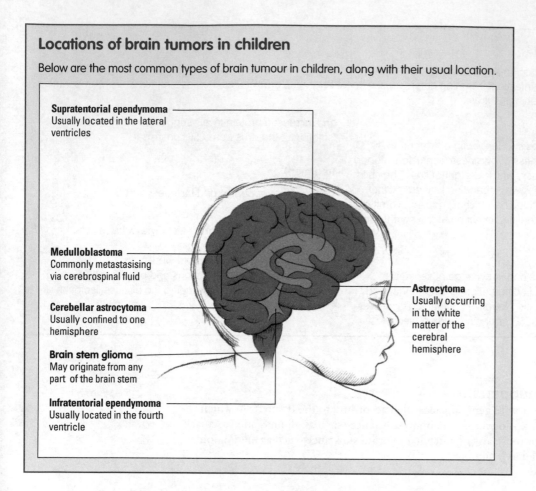

Supratentorial ependymoma
Usually located in the lateral ventricles

Medulloblastoma
Commonly metastasising via cerebrospinal fluid

Cerebellar astrocytoma
Usually confined to one hemisphere

Brain stem glioma
May originate from any part of the brain stem

Infratentorial ependymoma
Usually located in the fourth ventricle

Astrocytoma
Usually occurring in the white matter of the cerebral hemisphere

- Enlargement of the head or bulging fontanelles may be present in children before the closure of cranial sutures (12 to 18 months).
- Personality changes may be most critical and easily observable (such as crying, irritability and not wanting to play).
- Ataxia, or uncoordinated gait, may be mistaken for clumsiness and is the most common sign of cerebellar involvement.

What tests tell you

History, and physical and neurological examinations provide the most important information. Diagnostic studies include:

- MRI (most common), CT scan and PET scan showing the location and extent of the tumour
- lumbar puncture and serology of CSF to assess for the presence of tumour cells (although this isn't performed where there is raised ICP).

Complications

Some children with brain tumours experience some permanent sequelae, especially if they receive radiotherapy. They may have slowed development, lack of coordination, learning disabilities or other effects. In some instances, brain tumours result in death.

How it's treated

Treatment includes:
* removing a resectable tumour
* reducing a non-resectable tumour
* relieving cerebral oedema, increased ICP and other symptoms
* preventing further neurological damage.

The mode of therapy depends on the tumour's histology, radiosensitivity and location; it may include surgery, radiation, chemotherapy or decompression of increased ICP with diuretics, corticosteroids or, possibly, VP shunting of CSF.

Treatment of choice

Surgical excision is usually performed when possible. However, combination therapy (surgery and radiation with or without chemotherapy) has been shown to improve outcomes.

What to do

During your first contact with the child, perform a comprehensive assessment (including a complete neurological evaluation) to provide baseline data and help develop your care plan. In addition, follow these steps:
* Continually assess for signs of increased ICP, including decreasing pulse and respirations, increasing systolic blood pressure and a widening pulse pressure.
* Monitor for changes in the child's LOC. (A change in behaviour is most significant in young children. A change in sleeping and waking patterns may also be significant.)
* Report changes in ocular signs, such as pupil response, shape and size.
* Measure head circumference daily in children younger than age 2 years.

Better safe than sorry

* Observe seizure precautions; seizures are always a possibility in a child with a brain tumour.
* Always keep the bed's side rails up and assist with ambulation because cranial nerve dysfunction may lead to ataxia and weakness.
* Provide emotional support for the child, parents and other family members; referral to a social worker, psychologist or other health care professional may be needed to help the child and family cope with the diagnosis.

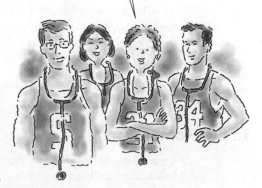

It may take the whole team – a social worker, a psychologist and other health care workers – to help the family cope.

Post-operative care

Children who undergo surgery for a brain tumour require specialised care. Positioning is important and varies with the type of surgery performed, and diligent monitoring of vital signs, neurological status and pain is essential. In addition, follow these steps:

• The child may be kept flat at first; positioning may be limited to a 10 to 20 degree elevation for the first 24 to 48 hours (dependent on local protocols).

• Never place the child in Trendelenburg's position because it increases ICP and the risk of bleeding.

• Assess vital signs, mental status and neurological status frequently because the child is at risk for increased ICP related to cerebral oedema, hydrocephalus or haemorrhage.

High temp, cool blanket

• The child's temperature may be labile (usually elevated) because of oedema of the brain stem; a hypothermia blanket may be used if the child becomes hyperthermic.

• Be careful not to place tension on the suture line when turning the child.

• Assess the child frequently for pain (analgesics should be provided according to prescription).

Hair today, gone tomorrow

• Body image issues (shaven head, oedema or fear of disfigurement) may be a problem for older children; help them to work through these feelings.

• Provide emotional support to the parents; help them to work through their feelings regarding diagnosis, treatment and prognosis (refer them to appropriate agencies and support groups for further assistance).

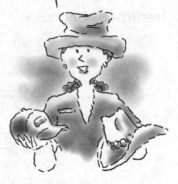

Hair loss from treatment may be more difficult for a child. Suggest using hats, scarves and wigs, and reassure the child that their hair will grow back.

Cerebral palsy

Cerebral palsy (CP) is a non-progressive, neuromuscular disorder of varying degrees resulting from damage or developmental defects in the part of the brain that controls motor function.

Children with CP can't control movements in certain parts of their bodies and may be partially paralysed. They may have completely normal intelligence and may feel as if they're trapped in a body they can't control.

What causes it

Conditions that result in cerebral anoxia, haemorrhage or other damage are probably responsible for CP.

In the womb

Prenatal conditions that may increase the risk of CP include maternal infection (especially rubella), maternal drug ingestion, radiation, anoxia, toxaemia, maternal diabetes, abnormal placental attachment, malnutrition and isoimmunisation.

A shaky start

Perinatal and birth difficulties that increase the risk of CP include forceps delivery, breech presentation, placenta previa, abruptio placentae, metabolic or electrolyte disturbances, abnormal maternal vital signs from general or epidural anaesthetic, prolapsed cord with delay in delivery of the head, premature birth, prolonged or unusually rapid labour and multiple birth (especially infants born last in a multiple birth).

A traumatic legacy

Infection or trauma during infancy that increases the risk of CP includes poisoning, severe kernicterus resulting from erythroblastosis fetalis, brain infection, head trauma, prolonged anoxia, brain tumour, cerebral circulatory anomalies causing blood vessel rupture and systemic disease resulting in cerebral thrombosis or embolism.

How it happens

A perinatal anoxic episode plays the largest role in the pathological state of brain damage. Structural or functional defects occur, impairing motor or cognitive function. Defects may not be distinguishable until several months after birth or when the child fails to meet developmental milestones.

What to look for

There are three distinct types of CP:

spastic

athetoid

ataxic.

Spastic

Spastic CP is the most common type, affecting about 70%. The affected area of the brain is the cortex. Typically, the child with spastic CP walks on his/her toes with a scissor gait, crossing one foot in front of the other. Spastic CP is characterised by:

- increased deep tendon reflexes
- hypertonia
- flexion
- tendency to have contractures
- rapid involuntary muscle contraction and relaxation
- underdevelopment of affected limbs.

Athetoid

In athetoid CP, which affects about 20% of children with CP, involuntary, uncoordinated motion occurs with varying degrees of muscle tension. The area of injury is the basal ganglia. The child exhibits slow, writhing, uncontrolled movements involving all extremities whenever voluntary movement is attempted. Facial grimacing, poor swallowing and drooling make speech difficult.

Ataxic

Ataxic CP accounts for about 10% of those affected. The affected area of the brain is the cerebellum. Its characteristics include poor balance and muscle coordination caused by disturbances in movement and balance. An unsteady, wide-based gait appears as the child begins to learn to walk; overall, the child appears clumsy.

Mixed together

Some children with CP display a combination of these clinical features:
• In most, delayed gross motor development makes eating, especially swallowing, difficult.
• Abnormal motor performance and coordination can manifest early in life as poor sucking and feeding difficulty.
• Spasticity of hip muscles and lower extremities makes putting a nappy on difficult.
• Posture abnormalities occur at rest or when changing position.
• Learning difficulties occur in varying degrees in 18% to 50% of individuals (most children with CP have an IQ that's normal or higher, but they can't demonstrate it on standardised tests).
• Seizures occur in 25% of individuals with CP.
• Many children have sensory deficits related to vision (strabismus), hearing, and speech.

What tests tell you
• Developmental screening reveals delay in achieving milestones.
• EEG may identify the source of seizure activity.
• Neuroimaging studies (CT scan, MRI) determine the site of brain impairment.
• Cytogenic studies (genetic evaluation of the child and other family members) and metabolic studies are performed to rule out other potential causes.

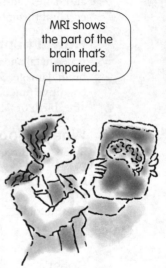

MRI shows the part of the brain that's impaired.

Complications
Children with CP may also have associated disorders, such as impaired intellectual development, seizures, failure to grow and thrive and problems with vision and sense of touch.

How it's treated
CP can't be cured, but proper treatment can help affected children reach their full potential within the limitations set by this disorder. Treatment includes the following:
• A baclofen pump may be inserted to treat spasticity by delivering the skeletal muscle relaxant directly to the intrathecal space around the spinal cord (the pump lasts for 3 to 5 years, after which a new pump must be implanted).
• Oral muscle relaxants may be used or neurosurgery may be required to decrease spasticity.

- Braces or splints and special appliances, such as adapted eating utensils and a low toilet seat with arm rests, can help the child perform activities independently.
- ROM (range of movement) exercises minimise contractures.
- Long-term intensive physiotherapy may improve muscle control.

Correct those contractures

- Orthopaedic surgery may be indicated to correct contractures.
- Phenytoin or another anticonvulsant may be used to control seizures.

What to do

Care of the child with CP involves attention to diet and physical activity:
- Institute a high-calorie diet for the child with increased motor function to help them keep up with increased metabolic demands.
- Assist with locomotion, communication and educational opportunities to enable the child to attain an optimal developmental level.
- Perform ROM exercises to minimise contractures.
- Plan activities that involve gross and fine motor skills (such as holding toys or eating utensils and positioning items to encourage reaching and rolling over).
- Provide a safe environment; have the child use protective headgear or bedsides to prevent injury.

Skilled labour of love

The nurse should also teach the family the skills needed to manage the child's care (such as medication administration, physiotherapy and seizure management). Siblings should be involved in the child's care to prevent feelings of being left out.

Family members need help in setting realistic goals and managing stress. They should be referred, with consent, to child services in order that appropriate support and help is provided. Parents will also be given advice on financial support available to them to manage their child's condition and well-being.

Down's syndrome

Down's syndrome, also known as trisomy 21, is the most common genetic disorder, causing moderate-to-severe learning disabilities.

What causes it

Factors that increase the chances of a child having Down's syndrome include:
- advanced parental age (when the mother is age 35 or older at delivery or the father is age 42 or older)
- cumulative effects of environmental factors, such as radiation or viruses.

How it happens

A spontaneous extra chromosome causes Down's syndrome; the child has 47, rather than 46, chromosomes. The most common chromosome affected is chromosome 21. The child has three copies of chromosome 21 rather than the usual two—hence, the name 'trisomy'.

Down's syndrome may also occur when translocation, an abnormal rearrangement of chromosome material, occurs. There's an unbalanced translocation of chromosome 21, in which the long arm breaks and attaches to another chromosome.

What to look for
The physical signs of Down's syndrome may be apparent at birth, especially hypotonia as well as some dysmorphic facial features and heart defects. The degree of learning disability may not become apparent until the infant grows older.

Facial features
Facial features common in children with Down's syndrome include:
- flat, broad forehead
- flat nasal bridge
- protruding tongue (due to the small oral cavity)
- small head (with slow brain growth)
- Brushfield's spots (speckling of the irises)
- upward slanting eyes
- small, short ears (which may be low-set).

Body features
Body features associated with Down's syndrome include:
- hypotonia
- short stature
- simian crease (a single crease along the palm with an in-curved little finger)
- short, broad hands and neck
- genital abnormalities.

Level of functioning
Intellectual dysfunction associated with Down's syndrome includes mild-to-severe learning disabilities, with intellectual abilities declining with age and the onset of Alzheimer's-type dementia with increasing age.

Level of functioning varies markedly among children (and adults) with Down's syndrome. Some children remain entirely dependent on their parents or caregivers throughout their lives. Other, higher functioning children communicate well, develop relationships outside the home, attend school, and even live independently at some point (although this process takes longer than it does in children without Down's syndrome).

A special gift

Many parents describe their child with Down's syndrome as extraordinarily loving, gentle, affectionate and extremely demonstrative.

What tests tell you

Physical findings at birth, especially hypotonia, may suggest Down's syndrome, but no physical feature is diagnostic by itself. A karyotype showing the specific chromosomal abnormality provides a definitive diagnosis.

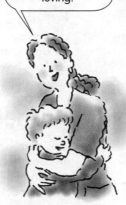

Children with Down syndrome can be extremely engaging, affectionate and loving.

Amnio alert

Amniocentesis allows prenatal diagnosis and is recommended for pregnant women older than age 34, even if the family history is negative. Amniocentesis is also recommended for a pregnant woman of any age when either she or the father carries a translocated chromosome.

Complications

In approximately 60% of children, early death usually results from complications precipitated by associated congenital heart defects; up to 44% die before 1 year. An increased incidence of upper respiratory infections, aspiration, leukaemia and hypothyroidism is common.

How it's treated

Because there's no cure for the disorder, management of Down's syndrome is manifestation-specific and includes surgery to correct cardiac, GI and other congenital problems. Skeletal, immunological, metabolic, biochemical and oncological problems are treated according to the specific problem.

Atlantoaxial instability (a spinal deformity resulting in instability of the upper cervical spine) should be assessed frequently. Growth and development should be monitored using specific growth charts.

What to do

• Offer assistance and support to the parents; give clear explanations to promote understanding and compliance.

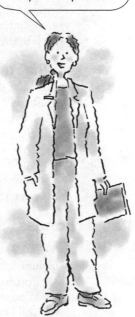

Parents of a child with Down syndrome may need counselling to help them grieve the loss of the healthy child they had hoped for.

Just the way you are

• Assist in identifying positive features and behaviours in the child to alleviate anxiety and promote parental acceptance of the child's disabilities.
• Plan activities based on the child's cognitive and motor abilities, rather than chronological age, to promote a healthy emotional and physical environment.
• Provide activities and toys appropriate for the child to support optimal development.
• Refer the parents to a paediatric dietician for nutritional advice.

Sherlock mom

• Teach parents to recognise symptoms of problems, such as upper respiratory infections and constipation, and to administer thyroid medication if needed.

- Keep the environment as routine as possible; a change in routine commonly results in frustration and decreased coping abilities.
- Refer the parents for genetic counselling to explore the cause of the disorder and to discuss the risk of recurrence in a future pregnancy.

The thrill of success

- Encourage participation in success-oriented activities such as Special Olympics.
- Refer the parents to a community children's or learning disabilities nursing service who can organise appropriate support from the multidisciplinary team; many parents grieve for the 'normal' child they had expected.

Duchenne's muscular dystrophy

Muscular dystrophy is a group of inherited, progressively degenerative diseases that cause muscle fibre degeneration and muscle weakness and atrophy. The most common type of muscular dystrophy is Duchenne's muscular dystrophy (DMD).

What causes it

DMD is a sex-linked recessive disorder and affects mostly males; it occurs in 1 in 3000–4000 male children. Females are usually carriers and pass the defect on to their male offspring.

How it happens

In DMD, there's an absence of the muscle protein dystrophin, which helps support the structure of muscle fibres. This results in degeneration of skeletal or voluntary muscles that control movement. Fat and connective tissue replace the degenerated muscle fibres.

What to look for

Muscular dystrophy affects the upper arms, legs and trunk muscles first. Pelvic muscles begin to weaken between 3 and 5 years. Signs include the following:
- Calves appear large and strong but are weak because of infiltration of the muscles with fat and connective tissue.
- Children have difficulty climbing stairs, running and riding a bicycle.
- The child has a wide stance and a waddling gait.
- Gowers' sign may be displayed when rising from a sitting or supine position. (See *Observing Gowers' sign*.)

Rapid changes

The disease progresses rapidly; by 12 years, the child usually can't walk. Signs include the following:
- Posture changes occur as abdominal and paravertebral muscles weaken.
- Weakened thoracic muscles may cause scapular 'winging' or flaring when the child raises his/her arms.

Observing Gowers' sign

Because Duchenne's muscular dystrophy weakens pelvic and lower extremity muscles, the child must use their upper body to manoeuvre from a prone to an upright position. This manoeuvre is called *Gowers' sign*. Lying on their stomach with arms stretched in front, the child raises their head, backs into a crawling position and then into a half-kneel. Then stopping, braces their legs with hands at the ankles and walks their hands (one after the other) up each leg until pushed upright.

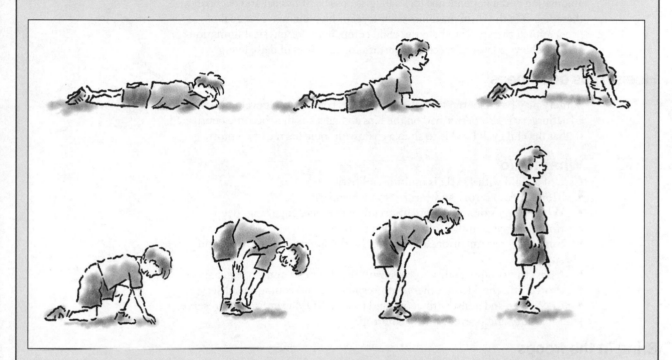

- Bone outlines become prominent as surrounding muscles atrophy.
- In later stages, contractures and pulmonary signs, such as tachycardia and shortness of breath, become noticeable.

What tests tell you
- Muscle biopsy reveals replacement of normal muscle with connective and fatty tissue. It also shows degeneration and necrosis of muscle fibres and a deficiency of the muscle protein dystrophin.
- Electromyography (EMG) shows decreased and weakened electrical impulses in the child with DMD.
- Nerve conduction velocity, in which electrical impulses are sent down the nerves of the arms and legs, reveals abnormal nerve function.
- Creatine kinase levels increase before muscle weakness becomes severe, providing an early indicator of muscular dystrophy.

Complications

Respiratory infections become common as the muscles of the diaphragm weaken. Cardiomyopathy occurs as the heart deteriorates and weakens. Death occurs in the late teens from respiratory failure, heart failure or pneumonia.

How it's treated

Because there's no cure, treatment is supportive and aimed at maintaining ambulation and independence for as long as possible. Physical and occupational therapies help the child maximise their level of functioning. The goal of occupational therapy is to help the child compensate for physical limitations and to achieve a level of success in performing activities of daily living.

Heels, hips and knees

Surgery may be done to release the heel cord as contractures develop in this area. Surgery is also performed on the hips and knees as they become contracted, so that the child will be able to sit in a chair with some degree of comfort.

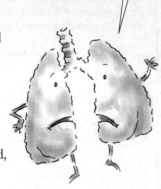

DMD can cause respiratory failure and ultimately death.

What to do

Care of a child with DMD is multidisciplinary:
• Monitor respiratory and cardiac status regularly.
• When respiratory involvement occurs, encourage coughing, deep-breathing exercises and diaphragmatic breathing.
• Ensure proper nutrition, and emphasise the importance of preventing obesity.
• Assess the family's ability to cope with the diagnosis and poor prognosis.
• Protect the child from others with respiratory and contagious diseases.
• Encourage and assist with active and passive ROM exercises to preserve joint mobility and prevent muscular atrophy.

Bring in the troops

• Coordinate other health services that would be beneficial to the child—for example, physiotherapy, occupational therapy and dietetic services.
• As movement becomes more difficult, assist the child with position changes every 2 hours to prevent pressure ulcers.
• Encourage genetic screening and counselling, which are indicated for parents and siblings of children with DMD.
• Refer the parents to agencies that can assist them with the child's needs and provide emotional, physical and financial support.

Guillain–Barré syndrome

Guillain–Barré syndrome is an acute, rapidly progressing, potentially fatal form of polyneuritis. It leads to deteriorating motor function and paralysis that progresses in an ascending pattern. The condition affects the peripheral nervous system, resulting in oedema and inflammation of the affected nerves and a loss of myelin.

What's myelin is your-e-lin

Myelin is the phospholipid protein of the cell membranes that forms the myelin sheath of neurons. It acts as an electrical insulator and increases the velocity of impulse transmission.

What causes it

Guillain–Barré syndrome is caused by an immune response to an infectious organism, usually from a GI or respiratory illness 1 to 3 weeks before onset. It has also been linked to viral immunisations (such as the swine flu vaccine) and cytomegalovirus.

How it happens

The syndrome is commonly preceded by immune system stimulation from a viral illness, trauma, surgery, immunisations, or human immunodeficiency virus. These stimuli are thought to alter the immune system, resulting in sensitisation of lymphocytes to the patient's myelin, and subsequent myelin damage. Demyelination occurs, and the transmission of motor and sensory nerve impulses is stopped or slowed down.

What to look for

Symptoms usually develop 1 to 3 weeks after an upper respiratory or GI infection. Infants have an onset of rapidly progressive and severe hypotonia, possible respiratory distress and feeding difficulties.

Weak from the legs up

Older children have rapidly progressive symmetric weakness and muscle pain with varying degrees of distal paraesthesia and numbness of the legs. The weakness spreads to the upper extremities, trunk, chest, neck, face and head, and there's an ascending loss of deep tendon reflexes with flaccid paralysis. Unexplained autonomic instability may result in hypertension, orthostatic hypotension and sinus tachycardia.

From dysfunction to failure

Other clinical features include urinary and bowel incontinence, cranial nerve dysfunction resulting in Bell's palsy, difficulty swallowing and respiratory failure.

What tests tell you

Diagnosis is based primarily on a patient history revealing a recent febrile illness and typical clinical features. Other tests include the following:
• Lumbar puncture reveals increased protein levels in the CSF.
• EMG and nerve conduction studies are markedly abnormal; an abnormal wave pattern indicates Guillain–Barré syndrome.

Complications

The most serious complication of Guillain–Barré syndrome is respiratory failure, which occurs as paralysis progresses to the nerves that innervate the thoracic area. Most deaths are attributed to respiratory failure. Immobility from the paralysis can cause such problems as paralytic ileus, deep vein thrombosis, thrombophlebitis, pulmonary emboli, muscle atrophy and orthostatic hypotension.

How it's treated

Treatment is primarily supportive with special attention to the respiratory, neurological and cardiovascular systems and with early recognition of deteriorating status. In addition:
- Plasmapheresis, a process that temporarily reduces the number of antibodies in the blood's circulation, is useful during the initial phase but offers no benefit if begun 2 weeks or more after onset.
- High-dose immunoglobulin can be given if plasmapheresis fails or is unavailable.
- The child's nutritional status—including body weight, serum albumin levels, and calorie counts—should be continuously evaluated.
- The child may require mechanical ventilation for respiratory difficulties, and continuous electrocardiogram monitoring for possible cardiac arrhythmias.

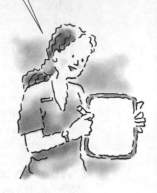

Be prepared when the child with Guillain–Barré syndrome can no longer speak. Age-appropriate tools can help the child communicate.

What to do

Because of the progressive nature of this disorder, it's extremely important to establish a communication system in anticipation of the time when the child can't communicate verbally:
- Perform frequent neurological, cardiovascular and respiratory assessments, and report changes to the doctor.
- Watch for ascending sensory loss, which precedes motor loss.
- Frequently assess respiratory status by monitoring pulse oximeter readings, pulmonary function tests, arterial blood gas values and auscultating breath sounds.
- Perform chest physiotherapy to help prevent complications of immobility.
- To prevent aspiration, test the gag reflex and elevate the head of the bed before giving the child anything to eat.

Survey the signs

- Watch for signs of urine retention and constipation.
- Assess the need for nasogastric tube or gastrostomy feedings, which may become necessary.
- Perform passive ROM exercises to help maintain function and prevent contractures. (See *Care of the immobilised child*.)

Squash the stress

- Help relieve anxiety in the child and his/her parents, and facilitate the child's development with age-appropriate activities.
- Refer the parents to social workers, who can help with financial arrangements and school considerations, and to other health care professionals to help the family cope with the diagnosis.

Advice from the experts

Care of the immobilised child

An immobilised child requires meticulous care to prevent complications. Without constant care, the child is more susceptible to skin breakdown caused by increased pressure on tissues over bony prominences. To care for an immobilised child, follow these steps:

- Change the child's position from side to side every 2 hours.
- Place the child on a sheepskin pad, a convoluted foam mattress, or an alternating–air current mattress.

- Keep the child's body in proper alignment with rolls made of towels or blankets, or with splints.
- Perform passive range-of-motion exercises at least three or four times per day to prevent contractures.
- Emphasise the importance of coughing and deep breathing. Teach the older child to use a spirometer. Younger children can achieve the same effect by blowing bubbles.
- Change soiled or wet nappies frequently to prevent excoriation of the perianal area.

Hydrocephalus

Hydrocephalus is an excessive accumulation of CSF within the ventricles of the brain, resulting from interference with normal circulation or absorption of the fluid.

CSF overload

As excess CSF accumulates in the ventricular system, the ventricles become dilated and the brain is compressed against the skull. This results in enlargement of the skull if the sutures are open, or in signs and symptoms of increased ICP if the sutures are fused.

What causes it

Hydrocephalus that results from an obstruction in CSF flow is called non-communicating hydrocephalus. Causes include faulty foetal development, infection, a tumour, a cerebral aneurysm or a blood clot after intracranial haemorrhage.

Communicating hydrocephalus results from faulty absorption of CSF. Causes of communicating hydrocephalus include a surgical complication, adhesions or meningeal haemorrhage. (See *Hydrocephalus and CSF circulation*, page 222.)

How it happens

In healthy children, CSF circulation is unimpeded:
- CSF is produced from blood in a capillary network (choroid plexus) in the brain's lateral ventricles.

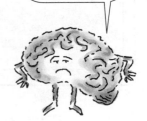

Too much CSF in my ventricles compresses me against my skull.

Hydrocephalus and CSF circulation

In noncommunicating hydrocephalus, the obstruction of cerebrospinal fluid (CSF) circulation occurs most commonly between the third and fourth ventricles, at the aqueduct of Sylvius. However, it can also occur at the outlets of the fourth ventricle (foramina of Luschka and Magendie) or, rarely, at the foramen of Monro.

Absorption distortion
In communicating hydrocephalus, faulty absorption of CSF may result from surgery, adhesions between meninges at the base of the brain or meningeal haemorrhage. Rarely, a tumour in the choroid plexus causes overproduction of CSF, resulting in hydrocephalus.

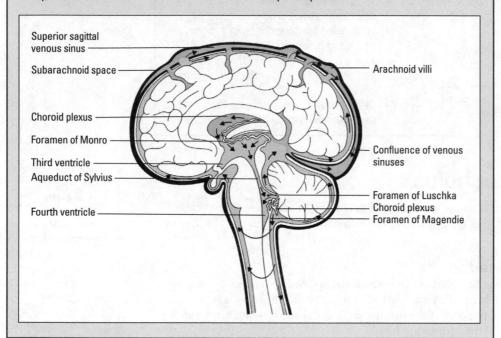

- From the lateral ventricles, CSF flows through the interventricular foramen (foramen of Monro) to the third ventricle.
- From there, it flows through the aqueduct of Sylvius to the fourth ventricle, through the foramina of Luschka and Magendie and to the cisterna of the subarachnoid space.
- The fluid then passes under the base of the brain, upward over the brain's upper surfaces and down around the spinal cord.
- Eventually, CSF reaches the arachnoid villi, where it's reabsorbed into venous blood at the venous sinuses.

What to look for

The signs and symptoms of hydrocephalus vary with the age of the child. In infants, the unmistakable sign of hydrocephalus is rapidly increasing head

circumference that's clearly disproportionate to the infant's growth. Other characteristic changes include:
- widening and bulging of the fontanelles
- distended scalp veins
- thin, shiny, fragile-looking scalp skin
- underdeveloped neck muscles. (See *Signs of hydrocephalus*.)

The setting sun

In severe hydrocephalus, the roof of the orbit is depressed, the eyes are displaced downward and the sclerae are prominent. When the sclera is seen above the iris, it's called the setting-sun sign. Other common signs and symptoms include:
- high-pitched, shrill cry
- abnormal muscle tone of the legs
- irritability
- anorexia
- projectile vomiting.

In older children, indicators of hydrocephalus include decreased LOC, ataxia, incontinence and impaired intellect.

Arnold–Chiari malformation

Arnold–Chiari malformation commonly accompanies hydrocephalus, especially when a myelomeningocele is present. In this condition, an elongated or tongue-like downward projection of the cerebellum and medulla extends through the foramen magnum into the cervical portion of the spinal canal, impairing CSF drainage from the fourth ventricle.

Rigid, noisy and irritable

Infants with this malformation also demonstrate nuchal rigidity, noisy respirations, irritability, vomiting, weak sucking reflex and a preference for hyperextension of the neck.

What tests tell you

Diagnostic tests for hydrocephalus include:
- daily measurement of head circumference, because rapid head enlargement is the first indication of the problem
- skull X-rays, which show thinning of the skull with separation of sutures and widening of the fontanelles
- a CT scan and an MRI, which are used to confirm the diagnosis, assess ventricular dilatation or enlargement, and demonstrate the Arnold–Chiari malformation.

Complications

Potential complications of hydrocephalus include:
- learning difficulties/disabilities
- impaired motor function
- vision loss.

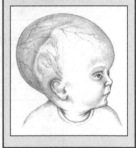

Signs of hydrocephalus

In infants, characteristic changes in hydrocephalus include:

- marked enlargement of the head
- distended scalp veins
- thin, shiny, fragile-looking scalp skin
- weak muscles that can't support the head.

The most serious complication associated with shunt placement is infection. Shunt malfunction is the other major complication and is caused by such mechanical problems as kinking, plugging, migrating and tubing separation.

How it's treated

Treatment involves removal of the obstruction (such as surgical removal of a tumour) or creation of a new CSF pathway to divert excess CSF. The goal of treatment is to bypass the obstruction and drain the fluid from the ventricles to an area where it can be reabsorbed.

It's tubular

This bypass is accomplished with insertion of a VP shunt or tube, which leads from the ventricles, out of the skull, and passes under the skin to the peritoneal cavity. (See *VP shunt*.)

Straight to the heart

An alternative to the VP shunt is the less commonly used ventroatrial shunt, which drains the fluid from the ventricles to the right atrium of the heart.

VP shunt

A ventriculoperitoneal (VP) shunt drains excess cerebrospinal fluid from the brain's lateral ventricle into the peritoneal cavity.

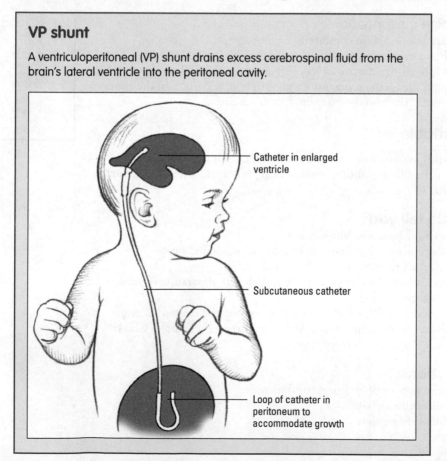

Catheter in enlarged ventricle

Subcutaneous catheter

Loop of catheter in peritoneum to accommodate growth

What to do

Several pre-operative and post-operative nursing interventions are indicated for the child with hydrocephalus.

Pre-operative care

Pre-operative care involves careful monitoring:
- Head circumference should be measured daily, watching for signs of increased ICP.
- Assess respiratory status every 4 hours or more often if necessary.
- Measure intake and output of all fluids.
- Monitor nutritional status and provide small feedings because the child is prone to vomiting. (During feedings, the child's head must be supported carefully and winded frequently.)

Post-operative care

Post-operatively, the child is placed in a flat position on the non-operative side to prevent rapid CSF drainage and pressure on the valves. If CSF is drained too rapidly, the child is at risk for subdural haematoma caused by tears in the vessels secondary to the cerebral cortex pulling away from the dura. Nursing care continues to focus on careful observation of the child's status as well as educating the parents about how to care for the child with the shunt in place:
- Observe for decreased LOC and vomiting.
- Observe the child for signs of shunt infection, such as fever, increased heart and respiratory rates, poor feeding or vomiting, altered mental status, seizures and redness along the shunt tract.
- Observe for abdominal distension or discomfort because shunt placement may cause a paralytic ileus or peritonitis.
- Measure head circumference daily; any increase of more than 0.5 cm is significant and should be reported to medical staff.

Shunt care

- Explain all procedures to the parents.
- Teach the parents signs and symptoms of shunt infection and malfunction, and what to do if they suspect either.
- Teach the parents to foster normal growth and development in their child; the child shouldn't be overprotected but should avoid contact sports.

Neural tube defects

Neural tube defects (NTDs) are serious birth defects that involve the spine or the brain. They result from failure of the neural tube to close at approximately 28 days after conception. The most common forms of NTD are:
- spina bifida (50% of cases)
- anencephaly (40%)
- encephalocele (10%).

Spina bifida

Spina bifida occulta is a visible defect with an external saclike protrusion. It's characterised by incomplete closure of one or more vertebrae without protrusion of the spinal cord or meninges.

What's in the sac?

Spina bifida cystica is a visible defect with an external saclike protrusion. It has two classifications:

• myelomeningocele, in which the external sac contains meninges, CSF and a portion of the spinal cord or nerve roots distal to the conus medullaris
• meningocele, in which the sac contains only meninges and CSF and may produce no neurological symptoms. (See *Forms of spina bifida*.)

Forms of spina bifida

The most common forms of spina bifida are listed below, along with their major characteristics.

Spina bifida occulta
Spina bifida occulta is the least severe of the spinal cord defects. It's characterised by incomplete closure of one or more vertebrae without protrusion of the spinal cord or meninges.

Spina bifida cystica
Spina bifida cystica is a visible defect with an external saclike protrusion. It has two classifications: meningocele and myelomeningocele.

Meningocele
In meningocele, the sac contains only meninges and cerebrospinal fluid (CSF).

Myelomeningocele
In myelomeningocele, the external sac contains meninges, CSF and a portion of the spinal cord or nerve roots distal to the conus medullaris.

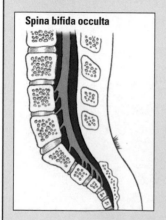

Spina bifida occulta

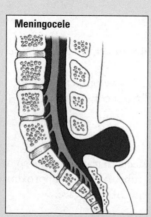

Meningocele

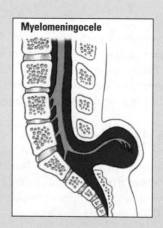

Myelomeningocele

Anencephaly

Anencephaly occurs when both cerebral hemispheres are absent. The closure defect occurs at the cranial end of the neuroaxis and, as a result, part of the entire top of the skull is missing and the brain is severely damaged. It's the most severe NTD and is incompatible with life.

Gone too soon

Many infants with anencephaly are stillborn. If the infant does survive, there's no specific treatment. Because the infant has an intact brain stem, he can maintain vital functions, such as temperature regulation and respiratory and cardiac function. Most live for a few weeks and then die of respiratory failure.

Encephalocele

In encephalocele, a saclike portion of the meninges and brain protrudes through a defective opening in the skull.

What causes it

NTDs may be isolated birth defects, may result from exposure to a teratogen (factor that increases risk of congenital disorder in an embryo) or may be part of a multiple malformation syndrome. It's believed that isolated NTDs (those not due to a specific teratogen or associated with other malformations) are caused by a combination of genetic and environmental factors. Although most of the specific environmental triggers are unknown, recent research has identified a lack of folic acid in the mother's diet as one of the risk factors.

How it happens

During the fourth week of gestation, ventral induction of the neural tube fails to occur. The degree of impairment depends on the size and level of the defect and whether it involves the spinal cord and nerves. Associated malformations include hydrocephalus and Arnold–Chiari malformation.

What to look for

The signs and symptoms of NTDs vary widely according to the type of the defect.

Search the sacrum

In spina bifida occulta, a depression or dimple, a small tuft of hair, a haemangioma or a port wine naevi in the lower lumbar or sacral area usually accompanies the defect. Because there's no herniation of the spinal cord or meninges, spina bifida occulta usually doesn't cause neurological dysfunction, but it's occasionally associated with foot weakness or bowel and bladder disturbances.

Sac on the back

In myelomeningocele and meningocele, a saclike structure protrudes over the spine. Meningocele seldom causes neurological symptoms. Myelomeningocele is associated with permanent neurological symptoms, such as flaccid or spastic paralysis, bowel and bladder incontinence, clubfoot, knee contractures, hydrocephalus and, possibly, learning disabilities, Arnold–Chiari malformation and curvature of the spine.

Poor prognosis

Clinical effects of encephalocele include paralysis, hydrocephalus and severe cognitive developmental delay or retardation. Anencephaly is invariably fatal.

What tests tell you

Diagnostic tests include the following:
• Alpha-fetoprotein (AFP) screening to measure AFP levels in the blood at 16 to 18 weeks' gestation. AFP is a foetal-specific gamma-1 globulin in the amniotic fluid that indicates the presence of myelomeningocele. If the AFP screen is abnormal, amniocentesis and foetal ultrasound are performed.
• Amniocentesis may reveal the presence of AFP in the amniotic fluid.
• Ultrasound may be used to detect open NTDs or ventral wall defects.
• Transillumination of a protruding spinal sac can sometimes distinguish between myelomeningocele (in which the sac transilluminates) and meningocele (in which the sac doesn't transilluminate).
• Skull X-rays and CT scans identify the defects.

Complications

Complications of NTDs include decreased motor activity below the defect, paralysis, multiple musculoskeletal handicaps, neurogenic bladder and bowel, CNS infections, hydrocephalus and death.

Latex liability

Children with spina bifida are at high risk for developing latex allergies, possibly because of frequent exposure to latex during catheterisations and multiple surgical procedures. Allergic reactions can range from mild signs and symptoms to anaphylactic shock.

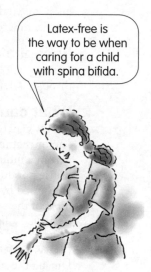

Latex-free is the way to be when caring for a child with spina bifida.

How it's treated

Immediate surgical closure (within 48 hours) is the most common choice of treatment, although spina bifida occulta usually requires no surgery. The rationale for early surgical closure is to decrease the risk of infection, morbidity, and mortality, and to prevent further spinal cord and spinal nerve damage. Surgery doesn't reverse neurological deficits.

Scheduled for surgery

A shunt may also be needed to relieve related hydrocephalus. Treatment of encephalocele includes surgery during infancy to place protruding tissues back in the skull, excise the sac and correct associated craniofacial abnormalities.

What to do

Nursing interventions begin prenatally and, after the child is born, continue with pre-operative and post-operative care.

Prenatal care

Prenatally, care focuses on educating and supporting the parents:
- Refer the prospective parents to a genetic counsellor who can provide information and support the couple's decision on how to manage the pregnancy.
- Inform women of childbearing age to take a folic acid supplement until menopause or the end of childbearing potential. Research has indicated that the risk of an open NTD may be reduced 50% to 100% in pregnant women who take folic acid.
- Provide psychological support to help the parents accept the diagnosis and prognosis.

Pre-operative care

Before surgery, many nursing interventions focus on preventing complications associated with the sac:
- Prevent the sac from drying by covering it with warmed saline-soaked sterile dressings.
- Check for leakage from the sac, monitor for redness and infection around the sac and assess for signs and symptoms of CNS infection.
- Assess for sensory and motor activity below the sac, including bowel and bladder function.

No pressure, please

- Prevent trauma by keeping pressure off the sac; keep the child on his/her side with knees flexed, or on his/her abdomen.
- Institute measures to keep the sac free from infection; avoid contamination from urine and stool. (A 'mud flap' can be made using a strip of plastic with adhesive backing on the top portion; this is placed directly below the defect, and will prevent contamination from stool.)
- Measure head circumference to establish baseline data.
- Be aware of the increased incidence of latex allergies in these children, and take appropriate precautions.

Teach and support

- Provide emotional support to the parents. Be aware that surgery is usually performed 24 to 48 hours after birth.
- Teach parents and other family members about measures to prevent contractures, pressure ulcers, urinary tract infections and other complications.

Post-operative care

After surgery, provide routine post-operative care, including monitoring vital signs, positioning and observation of the operative site. In addition, follow these steps:
- Provide thorough skin care if paralysis is present (to prevent complications such as pressure ulcers).
- Assess motor activity and bowel and bladder function to compare with the pre-operative condition.

- Measure head circumference daily, and perform ROM exercises.
- Teach clean intermittent catheterisation to parents.
- Maintain splints, braces and casts; use wheelchairs, walkers and other assistive devices as needed.

Reye's syndrome

Reye's syndrome is an acute childhood illness that causes fatty infiltration of the liver with concurrent hyperammonaemia, encephalopathy and increased ICP. Fatty infiltration of the kidneys, brain and myocardium may occur.

Equal opportunity syndrome

Reye's syndrome affects children from infancy to adolescence and occurs equally in boys and girls.

What causes it

Reye's syndrome typically begins within 1 to 3 days of an acute viral infection, such as an upper respiratory tract infection, type B influenza or varicella.

Nada to ASA

Use of aspirin in children younger than age 15 isn't recommended because of its link to Reye's syndrome. Fortunately, Reye's syndrome has become rare because professionals and parents now give children paracetamol instead of aspirin for a range of issues.

How it happens

In Reye's syndrome, damaged hepatic mitochondria disrupt the urea cycle, which normally changes ammonia to urea for its excretion from the body. This disruption results in hyperammonaemia, hypoglycaemia and an increase in serum short-chain fatty acids, leading to encephalopathy. Fatty infiltration occurs simultaneously in renal tubular cells, neuronal tissue and muscle tissue (including the heart).

> To prevent Reye's syndrome, never give aspirin to a child younger than age 15. Use paracetamol or NSAIDs instead.

What to look for

The severity of the child's signs and symptoms varies with the degree of encephalopathy and cerebral oedema. In all cases, Reye's syndrome develops in five stages:

The first stage is the initial viral infection.

A brief recovery period follows, when the child doesn't seem seriously ill.

A few days later the child develops intractable vomiting, lethargy, rapidly changing mental status (mild-to-severe agitation, confusion, irritability and delirium), rising blood pressure and respiratory and pulse rate and hyperactive reflexes.

The syndrome commonly progresses to coma.

As coma deepens, seizures develop, followed by decreased tendon reflexes and, usually, respiratory failure.

What tests tell you

Diagnosis of Reye's syndrome is based on the abrupt change in the child's LOC and on findings from diagnostic tests. At the time of diagnosis, the child usually has already progressed to stage III—coma and decorticate posturing:
• Blood studies reveal liver enzyme levels (aspartate aminotransferase or alanine aminotransferase) elevated to twice their normal levels as well as elevated ammonia levels, below normal blood glucose levels and prolonged prothrombin time.
• Liver biopsy, which is usually performed to confirm the diagnosis, reveals small fat deposits.

Complications

Developmental and neurological deficits may occur and are more severe in children younger than 2 years. Cerebral oedema is the major factor contributing to morbidity and mortality. Other complications may include respiratory failure and death.

How it's treated

The goal of medical management is to provide supportive treatment to prevent the secondary effects of cerebral oedema and metabolic injury; it includes assisted ventilation for the comatose child, monitoring for signs of increased ICP (caused by cerebral oedema) and IV glucose for hypoglycaemia. Close monitoring of electrolytes, blood chemistry and blood pH is also done.

What to do

In stage I, follow these steps:
• Assess hydration status.
• Monitor skin turgor, mucous membranes, intake and output and urine-specific gravity.
• Maintain a patent IV line for hydration.

Respiratory inventory

In stages II through V, follow these steps:
• Assess respiratory status, noting changes in rate and pattern, presence of cyanosis, restlessness or agitation.
• Assess circulatory status by taking vital signs frequently.
• Note skin colour, temperature and the presence of abnormal heart sounds or neck vein dissention.

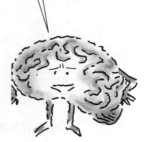

Respiratory failure and cerebral oedema can cause death in children with Reye's syndrome.

Know your neuro

In all stages, follow these steps:
• Assess neurological status.
• Immediately report to medical staff signs of coma that require invasive, supportive therapy such as intubation.
• Monitor LOC, pupil response, motor coordination, extremity movement, orientation, posturing and seizure activity.
• Support the child and family. Explain treatments and procedures, incorporating family members in treatments as appropriate.
• Provide additional parental and community education to ensure early recognition and treatment.

Seizure disorders

A seizure is a sudden, episodic, involuntary alteration in consciousness, motor activity, behaviour, sensation or autonomic function caused by abnormal electrical discharges by the neurons in the brain. Seizures can accompany a variety of disorders, or they may occur spontaneously without apparent cause. Epilepsy is a condition in which a person has spontaneously recurring seizures.

What causes it

The most common causes of seizure during the first 6 months of life are:
• severe birth injury
• congenital defects involving the CNS
• infections
• inborn errors of metabolism.
   Other causes include birth trauma (inadequate oxygen supply to the brain, blood incompatibility or haemorrhage), infectious diseases (meningitis, encephalopathy or brain abscess), ingestion of toxins, head trauma, metabolic disorders (hypoglycaemia, hypocalcaemia, hyponatraemia, hypernatraemia or hyperbilirubinaemia) and high fever.

How it happens

In recurring seizures (epilepsy), a group of abnormal neurons seem to undergo spontaneous firing.

Consciously electric

Electrical discharges come from central areas in the brain that affect consciousness. The discharges may be localised in one area of the brain and cause responses specific to the anatomic focus controlled by that area. They may be initiated in a localised area of the brain and then spread to other areas, resulting in a generalised response.

Cellular excitement

Hyperexcitable cells, called the epileptogenic focus, spontaneously release the discharges. These discharges can be triggered by either environmental or physiological stimuli, such as emotional stress, anxiety, fatigue, infection or metabolic disturbances.

What to look for

Seizures can take various forms, depending on their origin and whether they're localised to one area of the brain (as in partial seizures) or occur in both hemispheres (as in generalised seizures). If a partial seizure generalises, it's still classified as a partial seizure. (See *Classifying seizures*.)

Classifying seizures

This chart lists and describes each type of seizure, along with signs and symptoms.

Type	Description	Signs and symptoms
Partial		
Simple partial	Seizure activity begins in one hemisphere or focal area. There's no change in level of consciousness.	May have motor (change in posture), sensory (hallucinations) or autonomic (flushing, tachycardia) symptoms; no loss of consciousness
Complex partial	Seizure activity begins in one hemisphere or focal area. There's an alteration in consciousness.	Loss of consciousness, aura of visual disturbances; postictal seizures
Generalised		
Absence (petit mal)	Sudden onset; lasts 5 to 10 seconds; can have 100 daily; precipitated by stress, hyperventilation, hypoglycemia, fatigue; differentiated from daydreaming	Loss of responsiveness but continued ability to maintain posture control and not fall; twitching eyelids; lip smacking; no postictal symptoms
Myoclonic	Sudden, short contractures of a muscle or muscle group	No loss of consciousness; sudden, brief shocklike involuntary contraction of one muscle group
Clonic	Opposing muscles contract and relax alternately in rhythmic pattern; may occur in one limb more than others	Mucous production
Tonic	Muscles are maintained in continuous contracted state (rigid posture)	Variable loss of consciousness; pupils dilate; eyes roll up; glottis closes; possible incontinence; may foam at mouth
Tonic-clonic (grand mal, major motor)	Violent, total-body seizure	Aura first (20 to 40 seconds); clonic next; postictal symptoms
Atonic	Drop-and-fall attack; needs to wear protective helmet	Loss of posture tone
Akinetic	Sudden brief loss of muscle tone or posture	Temporary loss of consciousness
Febrile	Seizure threshold lowered by elevated temperature; only one seizure per fever; common in 4% of population under age 5; occurs when temperature is rapidly rising	Lasts less than 5 minutes; generalised, transient and nonprogressive; doesn't generally result in brain damage; EEG is normal after 2 weeks
Status epilepticus	Prolonged or frequent repetition of seizures without interruption; may result in anoxia and cardiac and respiratory arrest	Consciousness not regained between seizures; lasts more than 30 minutes

What tests tell you

A complete history, physical and neurological examination—including birth and development history, significant illnesses and injuries, family history, history of febrile seizures and a comprehensive neurological assessment—should be performed. Laboratory and other tests include:

• FBC and blood chemistry to detect electrolyte imbalances
• blood glucose levels to detect hypoglycaemic episodes
• lumbar puncture to rule out meningitis as a cause of the seizures
• EEG to help differentiate epileptic from non-epileptic seizures (each seizure has a characteristic EEG tracing).

CT, MRI—both can help identify

If the child is taking anticonvulsants, blood levels should be monitored. Lead levels, toxicology screening and radiological tests, such as CT scanning or MRI, may be performed to identify structural lesions.

Complications

Complications from seizures include physical injury during the seizure, brain damage and respiratory insufficiency or arrest.

How it's treated

Most children are treated with anticonvulsants, preferably a single medication to minimise adverse effects. Children who continue to have seizures with the single medication are treated with multiple anticonvulsants. Medication dosage adjustments are usually needed as the child grows. Serum drug levels are monitored to achieve therapeutic levels or when toxicity is possible. Surgery may be necessary to remove a tumour, lesion or portion of the brain that has been identified as causing the seizure.

Kudos for ketogenic

A ketogenic diet may occasionally be used for children younger than age 8 years with myoclonic or absence seizures. A ketogenic diet is a high-fat, low-carbohydrate, low-protein diet that causes ketosis as the body uses fat for metabolism. Ketosis is believed to slow the electrical impulses that cause seizures. It is increasing in usage but researchers are still exploring the most effective form of the diet as well as to how it might work!

Keep it cool

Children with febrile seizures are usually treated by lowering the fever through the administration of antipyretics such as paracetamol and ibuprofen (NIHCE guidelines on Feverish Illness in Children, 2007). In some situations, the child may be treated with an anticonvulsant such as diazepam throughout the presenting febrile illness; long-term anticonvulsants aren't generally used.

What to do

The nurse caring for a child who has seizures should focus on maintaining airway patency, ensuring safety, administering medications, observing and treating the seizure, educating the child and parents and providing psychosocial intervention. In addition, he/she should:
- stay with the child during a seizure
- move the child to a flat surface, out of danger; if standing, gently assist to the floor
- provide a patent airway and place the child on one side to allow saliva to drain out
- avoid trying to interrupt the seizure (Instead, gently support the child's head and keep their hands from inflicting self-harm, but do not restrain)
- pad the cot or bed rails to prevent physical injury.

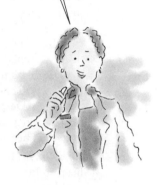

Never try to interrupt a seizure. Instead, stay with the child and take appropriate measures to keep them safe.

Out with the noise, in with the calm

- reduce external stimuli and environmental noise
- avoid using tongue blades because they add stimuli
- administer anticonvulsants as prescribed
- record seizure activity, and assess neurological status and vital signs after the seizure subsides
- monitor serum levels of anticonvulsants to ensure therapeutic levels and prevent toxicity.

A helping hand

Having a seizure can be extremely frightening to a child; it can also be embarrassing, especially when a seizure occurs in the presence of peers. To the child's parents, and others who witness a seizure, the experience can be terrifying. The child and parents need a great deal of education and emotional support:
- Instruct the parents (and the child, if old enough) in all aspects of seizure control measures such as how to control fever if the child has febrile seizures.
- Stress to the parents the need to treat the child as normally as possible.
- Encourage the parents and the child to express their fears and anxieties; answer their questions honestly.

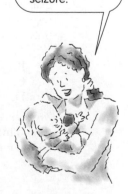

Always make sure that all of a child's potential caregivers know what to do – and what not to do – in the event of a seizure.

It takes a village

- Instruct the parents to make sure that the child's teachers, nursery providers, babysitters and other caregivers know what to do in the event of a seizure.
- If the child has had a seizure at school, suggest that the parents discuss this with the School Health Nurse who may talk to the child's classmates, obviously with consent.
- Refer the family to organisations that will provide them with more information and support such as Epilepsy Action (http://www.epilepsy.org.uk/).

• Remind the parents that their child should wear some form of medical identification such as a medical identification bracelet.

Quick quiz

1.   A child who had bacterial meningitis is scheduled to have a hearing test before discharge. The mother asks the nurse why the test is necessary. The most appropriate nursing response is:
    A.   'It's necessary to make sure your child is developing appropriately'.
    B.   'The test will identify attention deficit problems related to your child's illness'.
    C.   'It's necessary to make sure the steroid therapy your child had in the hospital didn't affect their hearing'.
    D.   'Despite treatment, some children with bacterial meningitis suffer neurological damage, especially to the nerve responsible for hearing'.

Answer: D. The most common neurological complications of meningitis are hearing loss, mental retardation, seizures, visual impairment and behavioural problems.

2.   A nurse is caring for a 2-year-old child with a VP shunt. Assessment indicates the child is afebrile but irritable and less responsive than previously. The most appropriate nursing action is to:
    A.   lower the head of the bed and position the child on his/her stomach.
    B.   increase the oxygen to 100%.
    C.   increase the fluids the child is receiving.
    D.   notify the medical staff.

Answer: D. The nurse should notify the medical staff of indications of increased ICP, including irritability and lethargy.

3.   An 18-month-old is admitted to the emergency department with a diagnosis of seizure. Upon assessment, vital signs are temperature of 40°C, respirations at 26 breaths/minute, pulse at 120 beats/minute and blood pressure of 90/69 mm Hg. The nurse should:
    A.   reduce the child's temperature.
    B.   tepid sponge the child.
    C.   do a blood glucose measurement.
    D.   place a fan in the room directed toward the child.

Answer: A. An elevated temperature could lead to a febrile seizure. The nurse should intervene to lower the core body temperature by offering oral fluids, and administering prescribed antipyretics.

4. A 9-year-old is admitted with weakness in their legs and a history of the flu. A diagnosis of Guillain–Barré syndrome is made. The nurse must notify the medical staff immediately if what symptom is observed?
    A. Tingling in the hands
    B. Increasing hoarseness
    C. Weak muscle tone in the arms
    D. Weak muscle tone in the feet

Answer: B. The most serious complication of Guillain–Barré syndrome is respiratory failure, which occurs as paralysis progresses to the nerves that innervate the thoracic area. Increasing hoarseness may be a sign of impending respiratory distress.

Scoring

☆☆☆ If you answered all four items correctly, fantastic! There's no deficit in your understanding of neurological problems.

☆☆ If you answered three items correctly, great work! Your brain is in tip-top condition.

☆ If you answered fewer than three items correctly, don't despair! Just scan the chapter again (no MRI needed).

Cardiovascular 8 problems

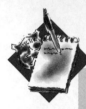

Just the facts

In this chapter, you'll learn:
♦ anatomy and physiology of the cardiovascular system
♦ diagnostic testing for cardiovascular problems
♦ treatments and procedures for cardiovascular problems
♦ cardiovascular system disorders that occur in children
♦ nursing care for the child with cardiovascular problems.

Anatomy and physiology

Understanding cardiovascular problems in children requires a sound, working knowledge of normal cardiac structure and function.

Structures of the heart

The heart is a muscular organ located behind the sternum in the chest and covered by a sac called the pericardium. Its main purpose is to pump blood throughout the body by continuous rhythmic contractions. The heart is composed of four chambers (two atria and two ventricles) and four valves.

Heart chambers
The four chambers of the heart are the right and left atria and the right and left ventricles.

Atria
The atria serve as reservoirs during ventricular contraction (systole) and as pumps during ventricular relaxation (diastole). The right atrium and left atrium are separated by an atrial septum.

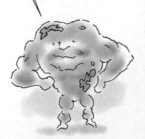

It isn't bragging to say I'm muscular. After all, it's my impressive physique that allows me to pump blood throughout the entire body.

A look inside the heart

Within the heart lie four chambers (two atria and two ventricles) and four valves (two atrioventricular and two semilunar valves). A system of blood vessels carries blood to and from the heart.

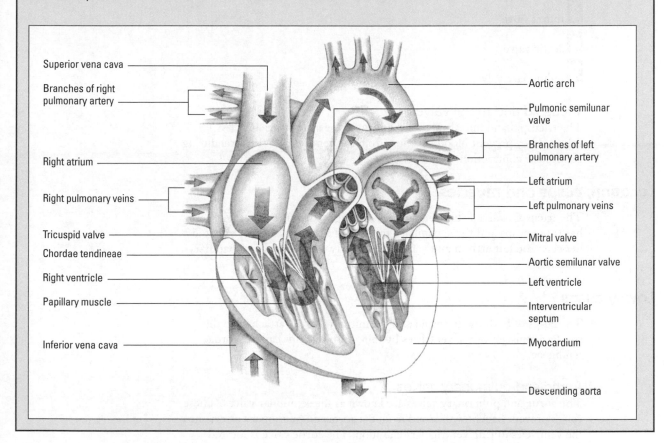

Superior vena cava

Branches of right pulmonary artery

Right atrium

Right pulmonary veins

Tricuspid valve

Chordae tendineae

Right ventricle

Papillary muscle

Inferior vena cava

Aortic arch

Pulmonic semilunar valve

Branches of left pulmonary artery

Left atrium

Left pulmonary veins

Mitral valve

Aortic semilunar valve

Left ventricle

Interventricular septum

Myocardium

Descending aorta

Ventricles

The left ventricle propels blood through the aorta to the rest of the body. The right ventricle sends blood through the pulmonary artery to the lungs. The ventricles are separated by an interventricular septum.

Equal at birth

At birth, the ventricles are relatively equal in size because of low-resistance placental circulation. When the left ventricle begins functioning against systemic resistance that increases after birth, however, it becomes thicker than the right ventricle. (See *A look inside the heart*.)

Heart valves

The heart has four valves:

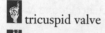 tricuspid valve

mitral valve

aortic valve

pulmonary valve.

Tricuspid and mitral valves

The tricuspid and mitral valves are known as the atrioventricular (AV) valves. They prevent blood backflow from the ventricles to the atria during ventricular contraction.

Location, cusps and muscles

The tricuspid valve is located between the right atrium and ventricle. It has three cusps and three papillary muscles. The mitral valve is situated between the left atrium and ventricle. It has two cusps and two papillary muscles.

Lovely cusps

The cusps of both the tricuspid and the mitral valve are attached to the papillary muscles of the ventricles by thin, fibrous bands called chordae tendineae.

Aortic and pulmonary valves

The aortic and pulmonary valves are known as the semilunar valves. These valves prevent backflow of blood from the aorta and pulmonary artery into the ventricles during ventricular relaxation. The aortic valve is located between the left ventricle and the aorta. The pulmonary valve is located between the right ventricle and the pulmonary artery.

Circulation

Blood is returned to the heart via the veins. Veins are small, thin-walled blood vessels that carry deoxygenated blood from the capillaries to the heart.

A long day's journey

Blood enters the right atrium from the inferior and superior vena cave and then goes into the right ventricle. From there, it's pumped into the pulmonary artery to the lungs, where it gains oxygen and loses carbon dioxide.

Return to sender

The pulmonary veins bring the oxygenated blood from the lungs to the left atrium. The oxygenated blood then passes into the left ventricle, is pumped into the aorta and is delivered to the rest of the body via the arteries. Arteries are large, thick-walled blood vessels that distribute oxygenated blood to the capillaries.

Pulmonary role reversal

The pulmonary artery is the only artery in the body that carries deoxygenated blood. The pulmonary veins are the only veins in the body that carry oxygenated blood.

Conduction system

The heart's conduction system is an electrical system that initiates myocardial contractions to move blood through the heart and maintain its rhythmic pumping action. This system is composed of several specialised cells:
• The sinoatrial node (also called the pacemaker of the heart) is located within the right atrial wall near the opening of the superior vena cava. It initiates electrical impulses and sends them throughout the atria.
• The AV node is located within the right atrium near the lower end of the septum. It transmits impulses from the atria to the ventricle.

Bundles and branches

• The AV bundle (bundle of His) extends from the AV node to each side of the interventricular septum and divides into right and left bundle branches. It facilitates rapid conduction of the impulses through the ventricles.
• The Purkinje fibres extend from the AV bundle into the walls of the ventricles and rapidly conduct impulses through the heart muscle.

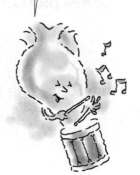

I've got rhythm, I've got pumping. Blood moves through me. Who could ask for anything more?

Cardiac physiology

The heart's primary purpose is to pump the blood that delivers oxygen and nutrients to tissues throughout the body and to remove waste products such as carbon dioxide. To do this, the heart must maintain an adequate cardiac output.

Cardiac output is the amount of blood ejected by the heart in 1 minute. Cardiac output can be determined by multiplying the heart rate in 1 minute by the stroke volume. Stroke volume is the amount of blood ejected by the heart at each heartbeat (or contraction).

Stroke volume is affected by three factors:

Preload, or the stretch of the myocardial fibres, is simply the circulating blood volume.

Afterload is the resistance against which the ventricle must pump during its contraction, which can be affected by blood pressure. (Hypertension will increase afterload, as the heart must pump harder to force blood into circulation.)

Contractility is the force of left ventricular ejection.

Chillin' with homeostasis

To maintain homeostasis, the body will make many adjustments to the factors that contribute to cardiac output.

Cardiac adaptations at birth

During foetal circulation, blood is oxygenated and waste products are removed in the placenta. Blood is shunted away from those organs that aren't yet fully functional, such as the lungs and the liver.

Perfusion only – no exchange

In the foetus, the lungs are filled with fluid and aren't yet the site of gas exchange. The amount of blood that passes through the lungs is just enough to perfuse lung tissue.

Farewell placenta, hello lungs!

At birth, however, the neonate moves from a reliance on the placenta to a reliance on lungs for oxygenation. This change is normally accomplished within the first few breaths after birth.

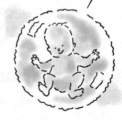

Right now I get all the oxygen I need from the placenta. But as soon as I get out of here, my lungs will take over.

Many keys, one lock

Key structures that maintain foetal circulation include:
• umbilical vein, which carries oxygenated blood from the placenta to the foetus
• umbilical arteries, which carry deoxygenated blood from the foetus to the placenta
• foramen ovale, which serves as the septal opening between the atria of the foetal heart
• ductus arteriosus, which connects the pulmonary artery to the aorta, allowing blood to bypass the foetal lungs
• ductus venosus, which carries oxygenated blood from the umbilical vein to the inferior vena cava, bypassing the liver.

Out with fluid, in with air

Cardiac adaptations at birth occur gradually, resulting from structural and pressure changes in the lungs, heart and major vessels. With the first few breaths after birth, the fluid in the neonate's lungs is absorbed and replaced with air. Inspired oxygen dilates the pulmonary vessels, resulting in decreased pulmonary vascular resistance and increased pulmonary blood flow. More blood will now travel to the lungs.

The drama unfolds

The pressure in the right atrium, right ventricle and pulmonary artery decreases. Simultaneously, a gradual increase in systemic vascular resistance occurs when the umbilical cord is clamped and the low-resistance placental circulation is removed. At that point, left atrial pressure increases more than right atrial pressure. The foramen ovale closes as a result of this unequal pressure. The ductus arteriosus begins to close because of increased pulmonary blood flow and the dramatic reduction in pulmonary vascular resistance.

Out of a job

Function of the foramen ovale ceases immediately or soon after birth. Ductus arteriosus functioning ceases after the infant is 4 days old. Anatomic closure, however, takes considerably longer. If the foramen ovale or ductus arteriosus fails to close, persistent shunting of foetal blood away from lungs will result. (See *From foetal to neonatal circulation*.)

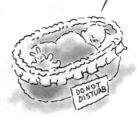

After only a few breaths, I'm breathing oxygen, dilating my pulmonary vessels and sending more blood to my lungs. How about me!

From foetal to neonatal circulation

These illustrations show the changes in circulation that occur at birth, allowing all neonatal blood to pass through the lungs.

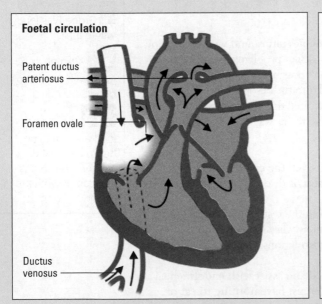

Foetal circulation

Patent ductus arteriosus

Foramen ovale

Ductus venosus

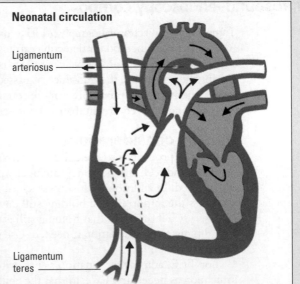

Neonatal circulation

Ligamentum arteriosus

Ligamentum teres

Murmurs

Murmurs are produced by vibrations within the chambers of the heart or major arteries from the back-and-forth flowing of blood through these structures. In children, murmurs may be called:
• innocent, which means there's no anatomical or physiological cause
• functional, when there's a physiological cause, such as anaemia, but no anatomical abnormality
• organic, when there's some anatomical defect in the heart, with or without the existence of a physiological abnormality.

Diagnostic tests

Diagnostic tests of the cardiovascular system in children include:
• echocardiography
• electrocardiography (ECG)
• magnetic resonance imaging (MRI).

Echocardiography

Echocardiography is used to evaluate cardiac structures and functions using echoes from pulsed, high-frequency sound waves. An ultrasound transducer is placed on the chest, and the sound waves produce an image of the heart. The test is non-invasive and painless and is one of the most commonly used tests to detect cardiac problems in children.

Ultrasound–endoscopy combo

Transesophageal echocardiography (TEE) combines ultrasound with endoscopy. It's an alternative method for detecting cardiovascular problems in children and is used when the transthoracic approach isn't possible or would be difficult. During the procedure, the transducer is passed into the oesophagus to an area behind the atria. The procedure is more complicated than the transthoracic approach and may require intubation to preserve the airway in young children.

Nursing considerations

Explain the procedure to the child and parents; tell the child what they'll see, hear, and feel, and be honest about any pain or discomfort that might be experienced. In addition, follow these steps:
• Stress the importance of holding still during the test, and assist as necessary. (Tell the child that holding still is their 'very important job'.)
• Administer mild sedation if needed. Use distractions such as a DVD to help calm the child.
• For TEE, administer sedation as prescribed and assist with endotracheal intubation as necessary. Explain that the child must have nothing to eat or drink before the procedure.

Grading murmurs

Use the system outlined here to describe the intensity of a murmur. When recording findings, use roman numerals as part of a fraction, always with 'VI' as the denominator. For example, a grade III murmur would be recorded as 'grade III/VI'.

Grade I is a barely audible murmur.

Grade II is audible but quiet and soft.

Grade III is moderately loud, without a thrust or thrill.

Grade IV is loud, with a thrill.

Grade V is very loud, with a thrust or a thrill.

Grade VI is loud enough to be heard before the stethoscope comes into contact with the chest.

Electrocardiography

ECG provides a graphic representation of the heart's electrical activity. It's used to detect the presence of ischaemia, injury, necrosis, bundle-branch block, fascicular blocks, conduction delay, chamber enlargement and arrhythmias.

Nursing considerations

Explain the test to the child and parents, stressing that there's no pain involved. In addition:
• describe the equipment that will be used for the test; show the child a picture or, if possible, the actual equipment
• explain that the child may have to lie on their left side, inhale and exhale slowly, or hold their breath at intervals during the test
• encourage the child to be still during the test; they may sit on the parent's lap if necessary.

Magnetic resonance imaging

MRI uses magnetic fields and radio frequencies to show a cross-sectional view of the heart and its structures. It's useful in identifying some congenital heart defects. MRI is generally a non-invasive test; however, contrast media may be used.

Nursing considerations

When explaining the test to the child, show a picture of the scanner or, whenever possible, let the child see the actual scanner. Tell the child that no pain is involved; prepare appropriately if contrast media must be used. In addition:
• tell the child that their parents may stay in the room during the scan
• prepare the child for the movements and the loud, clicking noises made by the scanner; reassure that the machine won't actually touch them
• because no metal can go in the scanner, assist the child in removing hair clips, jewellery and other metal items as necessary – remember, no metal toys!
• if necessary, provide sedation to ensure that the child remains still during the test
• assess for a history of iodine or other allergies before the procedure if a contrast medium is to be used.

Treatments and procedures

Treatments and procedures used for cardiac problems in childhood include:
• valve replacement
• cardiac catheterisation
• cardiac surgery
• cardiac transplantation.

Teach expectations

Many of the treatments and procedures done for children with cardiac problems involve surgery. When a child knows what to expect before a surgical procedure, they may be less frightened, more cooperative and more trusting of the nurses who provide care. (See *Preparing children for surgery*.)

Valve replacement

Valve replacement with a prosthetic valve is indicated for heart valve narrowing (stenosis) and heart valve leaking (insufficiency). Valvular problems are commonly caused by rheumatic fever and congenital heart defects. They may also be caused by heart failure and infective endocarditis.

Nursing considerations

Nursing interventions focus on monitoring and educating the child and parents.
• After surgery, monitor for hypotension, arrhythmias and thrombus formation.
• Monitor vital signs arterial blood gas (ABG) values, intake, output, daily weight, blood chemistries, chest X-rays and pulmonary artery catheter readings.

Heed the signs

• Because lifelong anticoagulant therapy will be necessary, teach the parents (and the child, if old enough) to recognise the signs and symptoms of bleeding, including black, tarry stools (from GI bleeding), oral bleeding (a small, soft bristle toothbrush should be used to prevent this) and excessive bleeding from minor cuts and scrapes.
• Stress to the child and parents the importance of antibiotic therapy before dental treatment and other invasive procedures to prevent infective endocarditis. Children who undergo valve replacement will always need this type of prophylactic antibiotic therapy.
• Teach the child and parents the importance of good oral hygiene to reduce the risk of oral infection, which may lead to bacteraemia.
• Inform the child and parents that clicking of the mechanical heart valve may be heard outside of the chest. Reinforce that this sound is normal.
• Help them to ensure a medical alert bracelet or card is carried with/by the child at all times.

Cardiac catheterisation

Cardiac catheterisation is performed with a radiopaque catheter that's passed through the femoral artery directly into the heart and lungs. It may also be performed in conjunction with angiography, in which a radiopaque contrast medium is injected through the catheter into the circulation, allowing visualisation of blood circulation through the heart chambers.

Preparing children for surgery

Many of the interventions performed for cardiac problems involve major surgery. What a child imagines about surgery is likely much more frightening than the reality. A child who knows what to expect ahead of time may be less fearful and more co-operative and will learn to trust caregivers. A child who's well prepared for medical procedures is much less likely to experience emotional trauma, which can have long-lasting effects.

Developmental concerns

Many of the concerns that children may have about hospitalisation and surgery relate to their particular stage of development.

Infants, toddlers and preschoolers

- Infants and toddlers are most concerned about separation from their parents. Stranger anxiety may make a necessary separation (during surgery) especially difficult.
- Because toddlers think concretely, showing is a necessary adjunct to telling when preparing a toddler for surgery.
- Preschoolers may view medical procedures, including surgery, as punishment for some type of perceived bad behaviour.
- Preschoolers are also likely to have many misconceptions about what will happen during surgery.

School-age children

- School-age children have concerns about fitting in with peers, and may view surgery as something that sets them apart from their friends.
- A desire to appear 'grown up' may make the school-age child reluctant to express fears.

- Despite a reluctance to express fear, because this age is a time when children are especially curious and interested in learning, school-age children are very receptive to pre-operative teaching and will likely ask many important questions (although they may need to be given the 'permission' to do so).

Young people

- Young people struggle with the conflict between wanting to assert their independence and needing their parents (and other adults) to take care of them during illness and treatment.
- Young people may want to discuss their illness and treatment without a parent present.
- In addition, young people may have a hard time admitting that they're afraid or experiencing pain or discomfort.

Before surgery

Whenever the situation permits, arrange for the child to visit the hospital before admission. Ideally, the formal preparation for surgery is done during the pre-admission visit.

Explanations should be honest and age-appropriate and should involve the parents (unless the young person would rather be prepared alone). The explanation should focus on what the child will see, hear and feel; where their parents will be waiting and when they'll be reunited.

If a child will initially be cared for in an intensive care setting, allow them to visit the area ahead of time and to meet some of the nurses who will be providing care. Prepare the young person for the equipment and the other young people he/she may see.

Principles of preparation

Here are some principles to keep in mind when preparing a child for surgery:
- Begin by asking the child to tell you what they think are going to happen during surgery.
- Ask the child about worries or fears. Chances are, they'll be worried about something that isn't going to happen at all.
- Provide an age-appropriate explanation of why the surgery is being performed; encourage the child to ask questions.
- Reassure the child that they won't wake up during the surgery, but that the doctor knows how and when to wake them up afterwards.
- Show the child an induction mask (if it will be used) and allow them to 'practice' by placing it on their face (or yours).
- Prepare the child for equipment (monitors, drains, and IVs, for example) that they'll wake up with.
- Tell the child about the sights and sounds of the operating room.
- Tell the child that their doctor and nurse will be in the operating room with them. Reassure them that they'll talk to and tell him/her what's happening.
- If possible, show the child where they will be waking up in the recovery room and where their parents will be waiting.
- Tell the child it's perfectly fine to be afraid and to cry.
- After the surgery, encourage the child to talk about the experience; they may also express their feelings through art or play.

Measure for measure

Cardiac catheterisation is used to evaluate ventricular function and measure heart chamber pressures and oxygen saturation in the blood. It also serves as a method for obtaining cardiac muscle biopsy specimens and for performing electrophysiological studies.

Complications

Complications of cardiac catheterisation include acute haemorrhage, transient arrhythmias, temporary diminished circulation to the catheterised extremity because of clot or haematoma formation, allergic reaction to the contrast medium and nausea and vomiting.

Nursing considerations

Nursing interventions for cardiac catheterisation begin when the procedure is scheduled and continues throughout the recovery period. In most cases, the procedure is performed under a general anaesthetic (GA), although older children may just be sedated. Providing recovery is not compromised, the child should be able to go home some hours after the procedure.

Before the procedure

Before catheterisation, nursing interventions focus on preparing the child physically and emotionally for both the anaesthetic/sedation and the procedure. The following will depend on whether a GA or sedation is used.
• Explain the procedure for the GA.
• Describe to the child and parents the procedure room as well as the equipment that will be used during the procedure. Show the child where on their body the catheter will be inserted, using doll play to prepare them, as necessary.
• Tell the child that the lights in the room will be dimmed after the catheter is placed.
• Reassure them that you'll be right there and will talk to them throughout the procedure.
• Tell the child that they may feel warm after the contrast medium is injected.
• Weigh the child and record their baseline observations.
• Assess the child's colour, temperature of their extremities and pedal pulses. Mark the dorsalis pedis and posterior tibial pulses with indelible ink before the procedure, allowing for easy assessment after the procedure.

After the procedure

After catheterisation, nursing care focuses on ensuring recovery from the GA or sedation, preventing complications, monitoring the catheterised extremity and ensuring adequate fluid intake.
• Keep the affected extremity immobile to prevent haemorrhage, usually for 4 to 6 hours after the procedure.
• Keep the catheter site clean and dry; monitor for bleeding and haematoma formation.

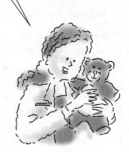

'Performing' a procedure on a 'friend' gives the child a sense of control, and helps them learn what to expect – in a non-threatening way.

• Compare post-catheterisation assessment data to pre-catheterisation baseline data, paying special attention to pulses and neurovascular status in the catheterised extremity.
• Ensure adequate fluid intake (IV and oral) to compensate for blood loss during the procedure and the diuretic action of some contrast media used. Doing so will also aid in flushing the contrast medium from the circulation.
• Provide thorough post-procedure teaching for the parents. (See *Instructions after cardiac catheterisation*.)

Cardiac surgery

Treatment of almost all congenital heart defects is achieved through cardiac surgery. The specific procedure performed will depend on the defect. Also the time spent in hospital will differ but fast-track cardiac procedures allows the child to be discharged within a few days. Even so, certain methods are used no matter which procedure is performed.

Heart–lung vacation

Cardiopulmonary bypass machines are typically used to oxygenate body tissues because surgery may necessitate stopping the heart. During the procedure, the child is placed in a hypothermic state to minimise blood loss (which enhances recovery) and to reduce the body's need for oxygen. An incision into the chest (thoracotomy) is commonly performed and chest tubes are inserted.

Complications
Complications of cardiac surgery may include arrhythmias, acid–base and electrolyte imbalances, hypoxia and trauma to the conduction pathways of the heart.

Nursing considerations
Prepare the child (and his parents) for what they'll see, hear and feel after surgery. When a child and the parents know ahead of time that certain events are 'normal', those events may be less stressful and frightening when they occur.
• Monitor the child's heart rate closely. (It will normally increase after surgery.) Changes in regularity and rhythm should be reported to the medical staff immediately.
• Auscultate the lungs every hour, assessing for diminished or absent breath sounds, which may require further medical evaluation.

Keep the heat

• Keep the child warm to prevent heat loss. (Infants may be placed under radiant heat warmers).
• Monitor body temperature closely. It may rise to about 37.8°C in the first 48 hours after surgery due to the inflammatory process initiated by tissue

It's all relative

Instructions after cardiac catheterisation

Cardiac catheterisations can be performed on an outpatient basis. Provide parents with these clear instructions about caring for their child at home:

• Remove the pressure dressing the day after the procedure.
• Keep the site covered with an adhesive bandage for several days after the procedure.
• Keep the insertion site clean and dry; give only sponge baths until the site is healed.
• Observe the site for redness, swelling, drainage and bleeding.
• Monitor the child's temperature, and report fever promptly.
• Have the child avoid strenuous exercise.
• Provide a regular diet for the child.
• Administer paracetamol or ibuprofen as needed for discomfort or pain.
• Keep follow-up appointments.

trauma. (Further temperature elevation may indicate an infection, requiring immediate action to determine the cause.)

• Maintain mechanical ventilation of the child in the immediate post-operative period. Extubation may occur in the operating room or in the early post-operative period.

• After extubation, an oxygen mask, head box (if below 8 months) or nasal cannula is used to deliver humidified oxygen.

Turn and breathe

• Implement turning and deep breathing hourly, using adjunct analgesics and splinting of the incision to prevent discomfort and pain. Firm stuffed animals can be used effectively for incisional support during deep-breathing and spirometry exercises.

• Prepare the child for chest tube removal (typically between the first and third post-operative day), which can be a painful and frightening procedure for a child. Topical anesthetics or analgesics are commonly administered before removal. (Creams, such as EMLA, must be applied 3 hours in advance.) (See *Chest tube removal*.)

Rx:TLC

• Provide emotional support and comfort because surgery can be frightening as well as painful to the child. (Encourage parental involvement in the child's care to foster feelings of comfort and security.)

• Provide detailed discharge teaching. (*See Teaching about cardiac surgery*.)

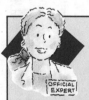

Advice from the experts

Chest tube removal

Follow these guidelines to prepare the child for chest tube removal and to reduce complications:

• Tell the child they'll experience momentary sharp pain as the chest tube is removed.
• Administer anaesthetics or analgesics as prescribed.
• Instruct the child to take a deep breath. (The tube should be removed at the end of inspiration.)

• Cover the wound with sterile petroleum gauze.
• Cover the wound with a clear, occlusive film dressing, such as Tegaderm, making sure all sides are securely attached to the skin for an airtight seal.
• Monitor the site for drainage, bleeding and infection. Change the dressing according to your hospital's policy.

Cardiac transplantation

For infants and children with worsening heart failure and limited life expectancy, heart transplantation has become an option. Indications for transplantation in children include cardiomyopathy and end-stage congenital heart disease.

One of two

There are two surgical options for cardiac transplantation:
• orthotopic procedure, in which the diseased heart is removed in its entirety and a new, healthy heart from a donor (who has been declared brain dead) is implanted
• heterotopic procedure (rarely performed in children), in which the child's own heart is kept in place and a 'piggyback' heart is implanted to serve as an additional pumping organ to assist the diseased heart.

Who knows NHSODR?

The process begins by placing the child on the NHS Organ Donation Register to match a donor with the recipient.

Whilst waiting

For some children, their hearts are not strong enough to maintain circulation and oxygenate tissues so a Berlin heart device may be used to allow time for a transplant donor to be found or in some rare cases for recovery to occur. The Berlin heart is a ventricular assist device that supports the child's heart and assists with pumping blood around the body.

Crucial 6 months

Complications are most common during the first 6 months to 1 year after transplantation. During this period, the family must adjust to a totally new lifestyle that will require lifelong management. The leading cause of demise after heart transplantation is organ rejection. Because lifelong immunosuppressive therapy is required, infection is always a risk.

Nursing considerations

The child and parents must be prepared thoroughly for this major procedure. Preparation should include a visit to the children's cardiac intensive care unit (CICU) and, if possible, the family and child should be introduced to the nurses who will be providing care. Parents should be made aware of the arrangements in the hospital to allow them spend as much time with their child as possible.

During this time, the family will probably have lots of questions and so constant support and information is important. There are many sources of information but a great one for both children and adults is Transplant Kids (http://www.transplantkids.co.uk/index.html)

It's all relative

Teaching about cardiac surgery

Be sure to include these points in your teaching plan for the parents of a child who has undergone cardiac surgery:

• dietary restrictions, if any
• fluid requirements and restrictions
• activity and exercise restrictions
• operative site care and inspection
• medication regimen
• follow-up tests and out-patient visits
• home care needs
• importance of encouraging the child to talk and express their feelings about the surgery and hospitalisation.

The hard part is over

Post-operative care involves:
• monitoring the child closely for signs of rejection, infection and adverse reactions from immunosuppressive therapy
• restricting fluids as ordered to prevent hypervolaemia and heart strain
• providing adequate rest periods with gradual activity increases to further decrease the workload of the heart
• encouraging compliance with the complex drug therapy is required, especially for older children
• providing emotional support to the child and family and offering resources for additional support such as Contact a Family
• helping the parents (and the child, if age appropriate) come to terms with the reality that someone had to die for a heart to become available. (This concept is too confusing and upsetting for most young children; parents should be encouraged to provide age-appropriate explanations when the child begins to ask where this new heart came from).

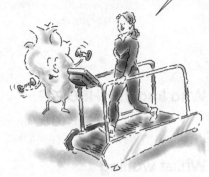

Activity is important after heart transplantation. Teach children to go slowly, and intersperse gradual activity increases with lots of rest.

Congenital heart defects that increase pulmonary blood flow

Congenital heart defects that increase pulmonary blood flow include atrial septal defect (ASD), patent ductus arteriosus (PDA) and ventricular septal defect (VSD).

Atrial septal defect

In a child with ASD, an opening between the left and right atria allows blood to flow from the left side of the hear to the right side, resulting in ineffective pumping of the heart, thus increasing the risk of heart failure. (See *Looking at ASD*.)

ASDs come in threes

The three types of ASDs are:

ostium secundum defect, the most common type, which occurs in the region of the fossa ovalis at the centre of the atrial septum and, occasionally, extends inferiorly, close to the vena cava

sinus venosus defect, which occurs in the superior–posterior portion of the atrial septum, sometimes extends into the vena cava, and is almost always associated with abnormal drainage of pulmonary veins into the right atrium

ostium primum defect, which occurs in the inferior portion of the septum primum and is usually associated with AV valve abnormalities (cleft mitral valve) and conduction defects.

Benign when small

ASD accounts for about 10% of congenital heart defects and is almost twice as common in females as in males, with a strong familial tendency. Although an ASD is usually a benign defect during infancy and childhood, delayed development of symptoms and complications makes it one of the most common congenital heart defects diagnosed in adults.

The prognosis is excellent for asymptomatic children and for those with uncomplicated surgical repair. The prognosis is poor, however, in children with cyanosis caused by large, untreated defects.

What causes it

The cause of ASD is unknown. Ostium primum defects commonly occur in children with Down's syndrome.

How it happens

In ASD, blood shunts from the left atrium to the right atrium because the left atrial pressure is normally slightly higher than the right atrial pressure. The difference in pressure forces large amounts of blood through the defect. This shunt results in right heart volume overload, affecting the right atrium, right ventricle and pulmonary arteries.

Enlarge and dilate

Eventually, the right atrium enlarges, and the right ventricle dilates to accommodate the increased blood volume. If pulmonary artery hypertension develops, increased pulmonary vascular resistance and right ventricular hypertrophy follow.

What to look for

Signs and symptoms of ASD include:
- fatigue after exertion
- early to midsystolic murmur at the second or third left intercostal space
- low-pitched diastolic murmur at the lower left sternal border (more pronounced on inspiration)
- fixed, widely split S2 due to delayed closure of the pulmonary valve
- systolic click or late systolic murmur at the apex
- clubbing and cyanosis if a right-to-left shunt develops. (See *Cyanosis and crying*, page 254.)

What tests tell you

A history of increasing fatigue and characteristic physical features suggest ASD. These tests confirm the diagnosis:

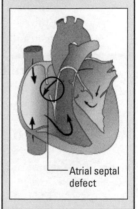

Looking at ASD

An atrial septal defect (ASD) is an opening between the left and right atria that allows blood to flow from the left side of the heart to the right side, as shown here.

Atrial septal defect

- Chest X-ray shows an enlarged right atrium and right ventricle, a prominent pulmonary artery and increased pulmonary vascular markings.
- ECG results may be normal but commonly show right-axis deviation, prolonged PR interval, varying degrees of right bundle-branch block, right ventricular hypertrophy, atrial fibrillation and, in ostium primum defect, left-axis deviation.
- Echocardiography measures right ventricular enlargement, may locate the defect and shows volume overload in the right side of the heart. (It may also reveal right ventricular and pulmonary artery dilation.)
- Two-dimensional echocardiography with colour Doppler flow and contrast echocardiography has supplanted cardiac catheterisation as the confirming tests for ASD. (Cardiac catheterisation is used if inconsistencies exist in the clinical data or if significant pulmonary hypertension is suspected.)

Complications

Complications of ASD may include physical underdevelopment, respiratory infections, heart failure, atrial arrhythmias and mitral valve prolapse.

How it's treated

Operative repair is advised for uncomplicated ASD with evidence of significant left-to-right shunting. Ideally, this is performed when the child is between ages 2 and 4. An operative repair shouldn't be performed on a child with a small defect and trivial left-to-right shunt.

Procrastination preferred

Because ASD seldom produces complications in an infant or toddler, surgery can be delayed until preschool or early school age. In some cases, the ASD closes over time so regular monitoring is all that is needed. A large defect may need immediate surgical closure with sutures or a patch graft. Alternatively, placement of an atrial occluder during cardiac catheterisation is becoming a more common intervention than open-heart surgery and means the child will only be in hospital for a few days.

What to do

Before cardiac catheterisation, explain pre-test and post-test procedures to the child and parents. Whenever possible, use drawings or other visual aids to enhance the explanation.

- As needed, teach the parents (and child) about antibiotic prophylaxis to prevent infective endocarditis.
- If surgery is scheduled, prepare the child and parents for what they'll experience in the intensive care unit and introduce them to the staff. Show the parents where they can wait during the operation, and explain post-operative procedures, tubes, dressings and monitoring equipment.
- After surgery, closely monitor the child's vital signs, central venous and intra-arterial pressures and intake and output. (Watch for atrial arrhythmias, which may remain uncorrected.)

Cyanosis and crying

An infant may be cyanotic because they have a cardiac or pulmonary disorder. Cyanosis that worsens with crying is most likely associated with cardiac causes because crying increases pulmonary resistance to blood flow, resulting in an increased right-to-left shunt. Cyanosis that improves with crying is most likely due to pulmonary causes because deep breathing improves tidal volume.

It's a bird, it's a plane, it's ... antibiotics! For the child with ASD, we're the first line of defence against the evil endocarditis!

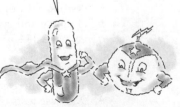

Persistent ductus arteriosus

The ductus arteriosus is a foetal blood vessel that connects the pulmonary artery to the descending aorta, just distal to the left subclavian artery. Normally, the ductus closes within days after birth. In PDA, the lumen of the ductus remains open after birth. This defect creates a left-to-right shunt of blood from the aorta to the pulmonary artery and results in recirculation of blood through the lungs.

Postdated PDA

Initially, PDA may not produce clinical effects. Over time, however, it can precipitate pulmonary vascular disease, causing symptoms to appear by age 40. PDA affects twice as many females as males. (See *Looking at PDA*.)

Smaller is better

In PDA, prognosis is good if the shunt is small or surgical repair is effective. Otherwise, PDA may advance to intractable heart failure, which may be fatal.

What causes it

PDA is associated with:
* premature birth, probably as a result of abnormalities in oxygenation or the relaxant action of prostaglandin E, which prevents ductal spasm and contracture necessary for closure
* rubella syndrome
* coarctation of the aorta
* VSD
* pulmonary and aortic stenosis
* living at high altitudes.

How it happens

The ductus arteriosus normally closes as prostaglandin levels from the placenta fall and oxygen levels rise. This process should begin as soon as the neonate takes his first breath, but may take as long as 3 months in some children.

Back to the aorta

In PDA, relative resistance in pulmonary and systemic vasculature and the size of the ductus determine the quantity of blood that's shunted from left to right. Because of increased aortic pressure, oxygenated blood is shunted from the aorta through the ductus arteriosus to the pulmonary artery and the lungs. The blood returns to the left side of the heart and is pumped out to the aorta once more.

The left atrium and left ventricle must accommodate the increased pulmonary venous return by increasing filling pressure and workload on the left side of the heart. This compensation causes left-sided hypertrophy and, possibly, heart failure.

Looking at PDA

In patent ductus arteriosus (PDA), the lumen of the ductus arteriosus stays open after birth, causing a left-to-right shunt of blood from the aorta to the pulmonary artery, resulting in recirculation of arterial blood through the lungs.

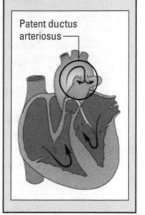

Patent ductus arteriosus

Reverse to cyanosis

In the final stages of untreated PDA, the left-to-right shunt leads to chronic pulmonary artery hypertension that becomes fixed and unreactive. This condition causes the shunt to reverse so that deoxygenated blood enters the systemic circulation, causing cyanosis.

What to look for

Signs and symptoms of PDA may include:
• respiratory distress with signs of heart failure in infants, especially those who are premature
• classic machinery murmur (Gibson murmur), a continuous murmur heard throughout systole and diastole
• thrill palpated at the left sternal border
• prominent left ventricular impulse
• bounding peripheral pulses
• widened pulse pressure
• slow motor development
• faltering growth
• fatigue and dyspnoea on exertion, which may develop in adults with undetected PDA.

What tests tell you

These tests help diagnose PDA:
• Chest X-rays may show increased pulmonary vascular markings, prominent pulmonary arteries and enlargement of the left ventricle and aorta.
• ECG may be normal or may indicate left atrial or ventricular hypertrophy and, in pulmonary vascular disease, biventricular hypertrophy.
• Echocardiography detects and estimates the size of a PDA. It also reveals an enlarged left atrium and left ventricle or right ventricular hypertrophy from pulmonary vascular disease.

Complications

Possible complications of PDA may include infective endocarditis, heart failure and recurrent pneumonia.

How it's treated

Correction of PDA may involve:
• indometacin a prostaglandin inhibitor, to induce ductus spasm and closure in premature infants
• left thoracotomy to ligate the ductus if medical management can't control heart failure (Asymptomatic infants with PDA don't require immediate treatment; if symptoms are mild, surgical ligation of the PDA is usually delayed until the child is 1 year old.)
• visual assisted thoracoscopic surgery (VATS) to ligate the ductus as an alternative to surgery with a thoracotomy (VATS may be done at the bedside or in a procedure room and involves three small incisions in the left chest through which a clip is placed on the ductus.)

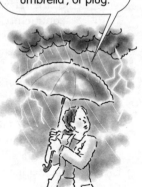

Plug up the ductus! In a child with a PDA, shunting can sometimes be stopped by inserting an 'umbrella', or plug.

- prophylactic antibiotics to protect against infective endocarditis
- treatment of heart failure with fluid restriction, diuretics and digoxin
- other therapy, including cardiac catheterisation, to deposit a plug (or 'umbrella') or coils in the ductus to stop shunting.

What to do

PDA necessitates careful monitoring, child and family teaching and emotional support.
- Watch carefully for signs of PDA in all premature neonates.
- Be alert for respiratory distress symptoms resulting from heart failure, which may develop rapidly in a premature neonate. Frequently assess vital signs, ECG, electrolyte levels and intake and output, and document the child's response to diuretics and other therapy.
- If the infant receives indometacin for ductus closure, watch for possible adverse effects, such as diarrhoea, jaundice, bleeding and renal dysfunction.

Explain, prepare, meet and greet

- Before surgery, carefully explain all treatments and tests to the parents.
- Arrange for the parents to meet the intensive care unit staff. Tell the parents about expected IV lines, monitoring equipment and post-operative procedures.
- Immediately after surgery, the child may have a central venous pressure catheter and an arterial line in place. Carefully assess vital signs, intake and output and arterial and venous pressures. Provide pain relief as needed.

Tell one, tell all

- Stress the need for regular medical follow-up examinations, and advise the parents to inform any health professional who treats their child about the history of surgery for PDA – even if the child is being treated for an unrelated medical problem.
- Before discharge, review instructions to the parents about activity restrictions based on the child's tolerance and energy levels. (Advise the parents how to avoid becoming overprotective as their child's tolerance for physical activity increases.)

Ventricular septal defect

In the child with VSD, an opening in the septum between the ventricles allows blood to shunt between the left and right ventricles. This opening results in ineffective pumping of the heart and increases the risk of heart failure. (See *Looking at VSD*.)

VSDs account for up to 30% of all congenital heart defects. The prognosis is good for defects that close spontaneously or are correctable surgically. Prognosis is poor, however, for untreated defects, which are sometimes fatal in children by the age of 1 year, usually from secondary complications.

Looking at VSD

In a ventricular septal defect (VSD), an opening in the interventricular septum allows blood to shunt between the left and right ventricles.

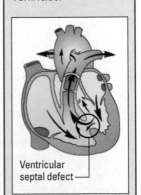

Ventricular septal defect

What causes it
VSD may be associated with:
- foetal alcohol syndrome
- Down syndrome and other autosomal trisomies
- renal anomalies
- PDA and coarctation of the aorta
- prematurity.

How it happens
In infants with VSD, the ventricular septum fails to close completely by eight-week gestation. VSDs are located in the membranous or muscular portion of the ventricular septum and vary in size. Some defects close spontaneously; in other defects, the septum is entirely absent, creating a single ventricle. Small VSDs are likely to close spontaneously. Large VSDs should be surgically repaired before pulmonary vascular disease occurs or while it's still reversible.

Undercover VSD

VSD isn't readily apparent at birth because right and left pressures are approximately equal and pulmonary artery resistance is elevated. Alveoli aren't yet completely opened, so blood doesn't shunt through the defect. As the pulmonary vasculature gradually relaxes between 4 and 8 weeks after birth, right ventricular pressure decreases, allowing blood to shunt from the left to the right ventricle.

Leading with the left

Initially, large VSD shunts cause left atrial and left ventricular hypertrophy. Later, an uncorrected VSD causes right ventricular hypertrophy due to increasing pulmonary resistance. Eventually, right- and left-sided heart failure and cyanosis (from reversal of the shunt direction) occur. Fixed pulmonary hypertension may occur much later in life with right-to-left shunting, causing cyanosis and clubbing of the nail beds.

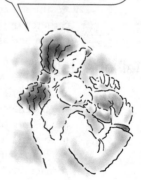

Because it isn't readily apparent at birth, VSD can sometimes go undiagnosed until an infant is 8 weeks old.

What to look for
Signs and symptoms of VSD may include:
- thin, small infant who gains weight slowly (when a large VSD is present)
- loud, harsh, widely transmitted systolic murmur heard best along the left sternal border at the third or fourth intercostal space
- palpable thrill
- loud, widely split pulmonary component of S2
- point of maximal impulse displacement to the left
- prominent anterior chest
- liver, heart and spleen enlargement
- feeding difficulties
- sweating, tachycardia, and rapid, grunting respirations
- cyanosis and clubbing if right-to-left shunting occurs later in life.

What tests tell you

These tests help diagnose VSD:
- Chest X-rays appear normal in children with small defects. In children with large defects, X-rays may show cardiomegaly, left atrial and left ventricular enlargement and prominent vascular markings.
- ECG may be normal with small VSDs, whereas in large VSDs it may show left and right ventricular hypertrophy, suggesting pulmonary hypertension.
- Echocardiography can detect a VSD in the septum, estimate the size of the left-to-right shunt, suggest pulmonary hypertension and identify associated lesions and complications.
- Cardiac catheterisation determines the size and exact location of the VSD and the extent of pulmonary hypertension, detects associated defects and calculates the degree of shunting by comparing the blood oxygen saturation in each ventricle. (The oxygen saturation of the right ventricle is greater than normal because oxygenated blood is shunted from the left to the right ventricle.)

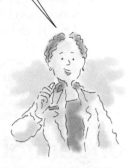

Small VSDs might not be detected by chest X-rays or ECG.

Complications

Complications of VSD may include pulmonary hypertension, infective endocarditis, pneumonia and heart failure.

How it's treated

Many VSDs (20% to 60%) may close spontaneously during the first year of life, especially small VSDs. Correction of VSD may involve:
- early surgical correction for a large VSD, usually performed using a patch graft, before heart failure and irreversible pulmonary vascular disease develop
- placement of a permanent pacemaker, which may be necessary after VSD repair if complete heart block develops from interference with the bundle of His during surgery
- surgical closure of small defects using sutures (such defects may not be surgically repaired if the child has normal pulmonary artery pressure and a small shunt)
- pulmonary artery banding to normalise pressures and flow distal to the band and to prevent pulmonary vascular disease if the child has other defects and will benefit from delaying surgery
- digoxin, sodium restriction and diuretics before surgery to prevent heart failure
- prophylactic antibiotics before and after surgery to prevent infective endocarditis.

What to do

Although the parents of an infant with VSD commonly suspect something is wrong with their child before diagnosis, they may need psychological support to help them accept the reality of a serious cardiac disorder. Also, because surgery may take place months after diagnosis, parent teaching is vital to

prevent complications until the child is ready for surgery or the defect closes. Thorough explanations of all tests are also essential. In addition, follow these steps:
• Instruct the parents to watch for signs of heart failure, such as poor feeding, sweating and heavy breathing.
• If the child is receiving digoxin or other medication, tell the parents how to give it and how to recognise adverse effects. (Caution them to keep medication out of the reach of all children.)
• Teach the parents how to recognise and report early signs of infection and to avoid exposing the child to people with obvious infections.
• Encourage the parents to let the child engage in normal activities.
• Stress the importance of prophylactic antibiotics before and after surgical procedures.

Congenital obstructive defects

Defects that obstruct the flow of blood out of the heart include coarctation of the aorta, aortic stenosis and pulmonary stenosis.

Coarctation of the aorta

Coarctation is a narrowing of the aorta, usually just below the left subclavian artery, near the site where the ligamentum arteriosum (the remnant of the ductus arteriosus) joins the pulmonary artery to the aorta.

Coarctation may occur with aortic valve stenosis (usually of a bicuspid aortic valve) and with severe cases of hypoplasia of the aortic arch, PDA and VSD. The obstruction to blood flow results in ineffective pumping of the heart and increases the risk of heart failure. (See *Looking at coarctation of the aorta*). The impact may be worsened if the child has other cardiac conditions.

What causes it
Although the cause of this defect is unknown, it may be associated with Turner syndrome. Turner syndrome is a chromosome abnormality affecting only females, caused by the complete or partial deletion of the X chromosome.

How it happens
Coarctation of the aorta may develop as a result of spasm and constriction of the smooth muscle in the ductus arteriosus as it closes. This contractile tissue may extend into the aortic wall, causing narrowing. The obstructive process causes hypertension in the aortic branches above the constriction (arteries that supply the arms, neck and head) and diminished pressure in the vessel below the constriction (that supplies the trunk and lower extremities).

Looking at coarctation of the aorta

In coarctation of the aorta, a narrowing of the aorta occurs, usually near the site of insertion of the ductus arteriosus.

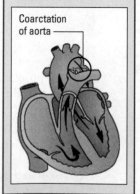
Coarctation of aorta

Under pressure

Restricted blood flow through the narrowed aorta increases the pressure load on the left ventricle and causes dilation of the proximal aorta and ventricular hypertrophy.

A leggy problem

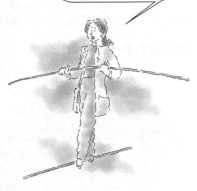

Walking can be difficult and painful for a child with coarctation of the aorta.

As oxygenated blood leaves the left ventricle, a portion travels through the arteries that branch off the aorta proximal to the coarctation. If PDA is present, the rest of the blood travels through the coarctation, mixes with deoxygenated blood from the PDA and travels to the legs. If the PDA is closed, the legs and lower portion of the body must rely solely on the blood that gets through the coarctation.

Untreated, this condition may lead to left-sided heart failure. If coarctation remains asymptomatic in infancy, it usually remains so throughout adolescence as collateral circulation develops to bypass the narrowed segment.

What to look for

Signs and symptoms of coarctation of the aorta may include:
• tachypnoea, dyspnoea, pulmonary oedema, pallor, tachycardia, failure to thrive, cardiomegaly and hepatomegaly during an infant's first year of life
• claudication
• hypertension in the upper body
• headache, vertigo and epistaxis
• pink upper extremities and cyanotic lower extremities
• bounding pulses in the arms and absent or diminished femoral pulses
• in most cases, normal heart sounds unless a coexisting cardiac defect is present
• more developed chest and arms than legs
• upper extremity blood pressure greater than lower extremity blood pressure.

What tests tell you

Physical examination reveals the cardinal signs of coarctation of the aorta, including resting systolic hypertension in the upper body, absent or diminished femoral pulses and a wide pulse pressure. In addition, these tests may indicate the condition:
• Chest X-rays may demonstrate left ventricular hypertrophy, heart failure, a wide ascending and descending aorta and notching of the undersurfaces of the ribs due to erosion by collateral circulation.
• ECG may reveal left ventricular hypertrophy.
• Echocardiography may show increased left ventricular muscle thickness, coexisting aortic valve abnormalities and the coarctation site.

Complications

Possible complications may include heart failure, severe hypertension, cerebral aneurysms and haemorrhage, rupture of the aorta, aortic aneurysm and infective endocarditis.

How it's treated

Correction of coarctation of the aorta may involve:
- digoxin, diuretics, oxygen and sedatives in infants with heart failure
- prostaglandin infusion to keep the ductus open
- antibiotic prophylaxis against infective endocarditis before and after surgery
- antihypertensive therapy for children with previous undetected coarctation until surgery is performed.

Resect, patch, ligate

Surgery may be performed early for infants with heart failure or hypertension, or it may be delayed until the preschool years. Options include:
- end-to-end anastomosis, in which the area of coarctation is resected and the distal and proximal aorta are anastomosed end-to-end
- patch aortoplasty, in which the area of coarctation is incised and an elliptical Dacron patch is sutured in place to widen the diameter
- subclavian flap aortoplasty, in which the distal subclavian artery is divided and the flap of the proximal portion of this vessel is used to expand the coarcted area.

The ductus arteriosus is always ligated with each of these surgical techniques.
- balloon angioplasty may be performed for older children or if re-coarctation occurs.

What to do

When providing care to an infant:
- if coarctation requires rapid digitalisation, monitor vital signs closely and watch for digoxin toxicity (poor feeding and vomiting)
- monitor intake and output carefully, especially if the infant is receiving diuretics with fluid restriction.

Bigger and bigger

For an older child:
- regularly assess blood pressure in the extremities, explain exercise restrictions, stress the need to take medication properly and to watch for adverse effects and teach about tests and other procedures.

Post-op checklist

After corrective surgery, follow these steps:
- Monitor blood pressure closely using an intra-arterial line. Take blood pressure in all extremities.
- Monitor intake and output.
- If the child develops hypertension and requires nitroprusside administer it as prescribed by continuous IV infusion using an infusion pump. Watch for severe hypotension and regulate the dosage carefully.
- Provide pain relief and encourage a gradual increase in activity.
- Stress the importance of continued endocarditis prophylaxis.

Aortic Stenosis

In aortic stenosis, narrowing or fusion of the aortic valve interferes with left ventricular outflow to the aorta. This defect, which is most common in males, causes left ventricular hypertrophy, causing pulmonary venous and arterial hypertension. (See *Looking at aortic stenosis*.)

What causes it
Aortic stenosis may result from congenital aortic bicuspid valves, congenital stenosis of valve cusps or rheumatic fever.

How it happens
Increased left ventricular pressure attempts to overcome the resistance of the narrowed valvular opening. The added workload increases the demand for oxygen, and diminished cardiac output causes poor coronary artery perfusion, ischemia of the left ventricle and left-sided heart failure. If left-sided heart failure develops, increased pressure in the left atrium with resulting increased pressure in the pulmonary veins can cause pulmonary oedema.

What to look for
Signs and symptoms of aortic stenosis may include:
• rough, systolic murmur heard loudest at the second intercostal space
• diminished carotid pulses
• systolic thrill
• syncope
• hypotension
• poor feeding
• angina-like chest pain on activity and exercise intolerance.

What tests tell you
Tests used to diagnose aortic stenosis and determine its severity include:
• chest X-ray, which shows left ventricular hypertrophy and prominent pulmonary vasculature
• ECG, which shows left ventricular hypertrophy
• echocardiography, which shows a thickened aortic valve and left ventricular wall
• cardiac catheterisation, which demonstrates the degree of stenosis.

Complications
Complications of aortic stenosis may include infective endocarditis, pulmonary oedema, heart failure and sudden death due to myocardial ischemia.

How it's treated
Digoxin and diuretics are given for signs of heart failure. Anticoagulant therapy is used to prevent thrombus formation around the stenotic or replaced valve. Prophylactic antibiotics are given to prevent infective endocarditis.

Looking at aortic stenosis

In aortic stenosis, narrowing or fusion of the aortic valve causes left ventricular hypertrophy and interferes with ventricular outflow to the aorta.

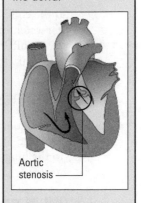

Aortic stenosis

Surgery may involve aortic valvulotomy or prosthetic valve replacement, and balloon angioplasty may be used to dilate the stenotic valve.

What to do

When caring for a child with aortic stenosis:
• watch closely for signs of heart failure or pulmonary oedema and for adverse effects of drug therapy
• teach the child and parents about the importance of medications and consistent follow-up care.

Post-surgical steps

If the child has had surgery:
• watch for hypotension, arrhythmias and thrombus formation
• monitor vital signs, ABG values, intake and output, daily weight, blood chemistry, chest X-rays and pulmonary artery catheter readings.

Pulmonary stenosis

In pulmonary stenosis, a narrowing or fusing of pulmonary valve cusps at the entrance of the pulmonary artery interferes with right ventricular outflow to the lungs, decreasing blood flow to the lungs. (See *Looking at pulmonary stenosis*.)

What causes it

Pulmonary stenosis results from congenital stenosis of the valve cusp or rheumatic heart disease. It's also associated with tetralogy of Fallot.

How it happens

Obstructed right ventricular outflow causes right ventricular hypertrophy, eventually resulting in right-sided heart failure.

What to look for

Children with pulmonary stenosis may be asymptomatic, or they may show:
• cyanosis
• signs of heart failure
• systolic murmur heard loudest at the upper left sternal border and a split S2.

What tests tell you

Evidence of right ventricular hypertrophy may be seen on chest X-ray, ECG and echocardiography. Cardiac catheterisation demonstrates the degree of the stenosis.

Complications

Complications of pulmonary stenosis may include infective endocarditis and heart failure.

Looking at pulmonic stenosis

In pulmonic stenosis, a narrowing or fusing of the pulmonic valve interferes with right ventricular outflow to the lungs.

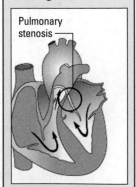

Pulmonary stenosis

How it's treated

Digoxin and diuretics are given for signs of heart failure and anticoagulant therapy is used to prevent thrombus formation around the stenotic or replaced valve. Prophylactic antibiotics are given to prevent infective endocarditis. Balloon angioplasty during cardiac catheterisation is widely used to relieve pulmonary stenosis. Valvulotomy may be necessary.

What to do

The child and parents should be taught about the importance of medication and consistent follow-up care. The child must be watched closely for signs of heart failure or pulmonary oedema and for adverse effects of drug therapy.

If the child has had surgery:
- watch for hypotension, arrhythmias and thrombus formation
- monitor vital signs, ABG values, intake and output, daily weight, blood chemistry, chest X-rays and pulmonary artery catheter readings.

Mixed congenital heart defects

In defects that cause mixed blood flow, oxygenated and deoxygenated blood mix in the heart or great vessels. Such defects include hypoplastic left heart syndrome (HLHS) and transposition of the great arteries.

Hypoplastic left heart syndrome

HLHS refers to underdevelopment of the left side of the heart. The defects of this syndrome include:
- aortic valve atresia or stenosis
- mitral valve atresia or stenosis
- diminutive or absent left ventricle
- severe hypoplasia of the ascending aorta and aortic arch. (See *Looking at hypoplastic left heart syndrome*, page 266.)

What causes it

The cause of HLHS is unknown.

How it happens

Blood from the left atrium travels through a patent foramen ovale to the right ventricle and pulmonary artery, entering the systemic circulation via the ductus arteriosus. Patency of the ductus arteriosus, which allows blood flow to the systemic circulation, is necessary to sustain life.

What to look for

Signs and symptoms may include:
- cyanosis
- weak or absent pulses
- signs of heart failure, such as tachycardia, sweating, cardiomegaly, tachypnoea, cyanosis and peripheral oedema.

Looking at hypoplastic left heart syndrome

Hypoplastic left heart syndrome consists of these defects:

- aortic valve atresia or stenosis
- mitral valve atresia or stenosis
- diminutive or absent left ventricle
- severe hypoplasia of the ascending aorta and aortic arch.

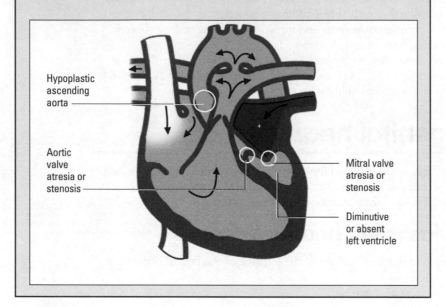

Hypoplastic ascending aorta

Aortic valve atresia or stenosis

Mitral valve atresia or stenosis

Diminutive or absent left ventricle

Close call

If the ductus arteriosus closes, the infant will progressively deteriorate with worsening cyanosis, decreased cardiac output and eventual cardiovascular collapse.

What tests tell you

Echocardiography provides visualisation of the defect.

Complications

HLHS is very difficult to treat and in many cases only supportive palliative care can be offered. Many children die from this condition.

How it's treated

Prostaglandin E is used to maintain patency of the ductus arteriosus. Digoxin and diuretics are administered to control heart failure.

Certain surgery

Without surgery, death will occur in early infancy. Surgical procedures include heart transplantation in the neonatal period (although not common because of the shortage of neonatal organs, risk of rejection and need for chronic immunosuppression) or the more commonly performed staged reconstruction, which is a series of surgeries to restructure the heart to be as efficient as possible without an adequately functioning left ventricle. Typically, three procedures are performed:
- Norwood procedure (performed soon after birth)
- bidirectional Glenn operation (performed at 4 to 6 months)
- modified Fontan procedure (the final stage performed at 2 to 3 years).

What to do

Explain the heart defect to the parents, prepare the child for surgery and answer any questions. In addition, follow these steps:
- Monitor vital signs, pulse oximetry and intake and output to assess renal function and detect changes.
- Assess cardiovascular and respiratory status to detect early signs of decompensation.
- Take the child's apical pulse for 1 minute before giving digoxin, and withhold the drug to prevent toxicity if the heart rate is below 90 to 110 beats/minute in infants and young children (below 70 beats/minute in older children).
- Monitor fluid status, enforcing fluid restrictions as appropriate to prevent fluid overload. Weigh the child daily and record.
- Organise nursing care activities around long periods of uninterrupted rest to decrease the child's oxygen demands.

Transposition of the great arteries

In transposition of the great arteries, the aorta rises from the right ventricle and the pulmonary artery rises from the left ventricle. This defect produces two non-communicating circulatory systems. (See *Looking at transposition of the great arteries*.)

What causes it

The cause of transposition of the great arteries is unknown.

How it happens

The transposed pulmonary artery carries oxygenated blood back to the lungs, rather than to the left side of the heart. The transposed aorta returns deoxygenated blood to the systemic circulation rather than to the lungs.

Communication between the pulmonary and systemic circulation is necessary for survival; the presence of other congenital defects, such as PDA, ASD and VSD, allows for such communication. These defects cause holes in the heart that allow blood to get from one side of the heart to the other so that oxygenated and deoxygenated blood can mix and flow to the rest of the body, which is necessary to sustain life.

Looking at transposition of the great arteries

In transposition of the great arteries, the aorta rises from the right ventricle, and the pulmonary artery from the left ventricle, producing two noncommunicating circulatory systems.

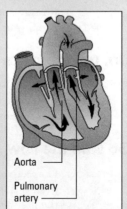

Aorta

Pulmonary artery

What to look for

Signs and symptoms of transposition of the great arteries include:
- cyanosis from birth and tachypnoea (worsening with crying)
- gallop rhythm
- tachycardia
- dyspnoea
- cardiomegaly
- hepatomegaly
- murmurs of ASD, VSD or PDA, and loud S2
- diminished exercise tolerance
- fatigue
- clubbing.

What tests tell you

Chest X-rays may show increased pulmonary vascular markings; right atrial and ventricular enlargements give the heart a characteristic oblong appearance. In addition:
- ECG may indicate right axis deviation and right ventricular hypertrophy
- echocardiography demonstrates the reversed position of the aorta and pulmonary artery and may detect other cardiac defects
- cardiac catheterisation shows decreased oxygen saturation in left ventricular blood and aortic blood; increased right atrial, right ventricular and pulmonary artery oxygen saturation and right ventricular systolic pressure equal to systemic pressure. (Dye injection reveals transposed vessels and the presence of any other cardiac defects.)

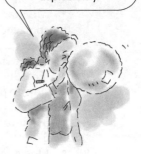

In a child with transposition of the great arteries, the patent foramen ovale is sometimes enlarged with atrial balloon septostomy.

Complications

Complications of transposition of the great arteries may include infective endocarditis and death.

How it's treated

Prostaglandin E is given to maintain patency of the ductus arteriosus. Prophylactic antibiotics will be needed to prevent infective endocarditis.

Up, up and away

Atrial balloon septostomy may be performed during cardiac catheterisation to enlarge the patent foramen ovale, which improves oxygenation by allowing greater mixing of the pulmonary and systemic circulations.

Go with the flow

Corrective surgery may be performed to redirect blood flow by switching the positions of the major blood vessels. This procedure is typically performed in the first few weeks of life, although for some children the 'switch' cannot be performed and alternative surgical procedures may be needed.

What to do

Nursing care begins with child education. Teach the parents about the defect and answer any questions they may have. The child should be prepared for surgery and other invasive procedures.

- Monitor vital signs, pulse oximetry and intake and output to assess renal function and detect changes.
- Assess cardiovascular and respiratory status to detect early signs of decompensation.
- Monitor fluid status, enforcing fluid restrictions as appropriate to prevent fluid overload. Weigh the child daily.
- Offer the child high-calorie foods that are easy to ingest and digest.
- Encourage parents to help their child assume new activity levels and independence.

Congenital heart defects that decrease pulmonary blood flow

Defects that decrease pulmonary blood flow include tetralogy of Fallot and tricuspid atresia.

Tetralogy of Fallot

Tetralogy of Fallot is a combination of four cardiac defects:
- VSD
- right ventricular outflow obstruction (pulmonary stenosis)
- right ventricular hypertrophy
- overriding aorta (aorta positioned above the VSD).

Blood shunts from right to left through the VSD, allowing deoxygenated blood to mix with oxygenated blood, which results in cyanosis. This heart defect accounts for about 10% of all congenital defects and occurs equally in males and females. (See *Looking at tetralogy of Fallot*, page 270.)

What causes it

The cause of tetralogy of Fallot is unknown; however, it may be associated with foetal alcohol syndrome. In the past, it has been associated with thalidomide use during pregnancy.

How it happens

In tetralogy of Fallot, deoxygenated venous blood returning to the right side of the heart may pass through the VSD to the left ventricle, bypassing the lungs or it may enter the pulmonary artery, depending on the extent of the pulmonary stenosis. Rather than originating from the left ventricle, the aorta overrides both ventricles.

Looking at tetralogy of Fallot

Tetralogy of Fallot is a combination of four defects:

- ventricular septal defect (VSD)
- right ventricular outflow obstruction (pulmonic stenosis)
- right ventricular hypertrophy
- overriding aorta (aorta positioned over the VSD).

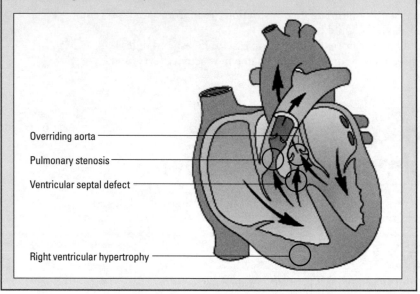

Overriding aorta

Pulmonary stenosis

Ventricular septal defect

Right ventricular hypertrophy

VSD usually lies in the outflow tract of the right ventricle. Severe obstruction of right ventricular outflow produces a right-to-left shunt, causing decreased systemic arterial oxygen saturation, cyanosis, reduced pulmonary blood flow and hypoplasia of the entire pulmonary vasculature. Right ventricular hypertrophy develops in response to the extra force needed to push blood into the stenotic pulmonary artery. Milder forms of pulmonary stenosis result in a left-to-right shunt or no shunt at all.

What to look for

Cyanosis is the hallmark of tetralogy of Fallot. Children may have cyanotic or 'blue' spells ('tet' spells), characterised by dyspnoea; deep, sighing respirations; bradycardia; fainting; seizures and loss of consciousness after exercise, crying, straining, infection or fever.

Other signs and symptoms include:
- clubbing, diminished exercise tolerance, increasing dyspnoea on exertion, growth retardation and eating difficulties in older children
- squatting with shortness of breath

- loud systolic murmur best heard along the left sternal border, which may diminish or obscure the pulmonary component of S2
- continuous murmur of the ductus in a child with a large PDA
- thrill at the left sternal border
- obvious right ventricular impulse and prominent inferior sternum associated with right ventricular hypertrophy.

What tests tell you

Findings from chest X-rays, ECG and echocardiography demonstrate the defects:
- Chest X-ray demonstrates a boot-shaped cardiac silhouette and decreased pulmonary vascular markings.
- ECG shows right ventricular hypertrophy, right axis deviation and, possibly, right atrial hypertrophy.
- Echocardiography and cardiac catheterisation provide visualisation of the defects.

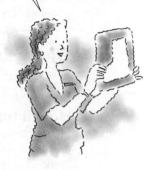

Tetralogy of Fallot gives the heart 'the boot'. Actually, the cardiac silhouette is boot-shaped on X-ray.

Complications

Complications of tetralogy of Fallot may include hypercyanotic 'tet' spells, right ventricular dysfunction, infective endocarditis, polycythaemia and death.

How it's treated

Tetralogy of Fallot may be managed by:
- knee-chest position and administration of oxygen and morphine to improve oxygenation
- propranolol to prevent 'tet' spells and prophylactic antibiotics to prevent infective endocarditis
- palliative surgery to reduce hypoxia during 'tet' spells (involving the Blalock–Taussig procedure, which joins the subclavian artery to the pulmonary artery)
- complete surgical closure to relieve pulmonary stenosis and close the VSD, directing left ventricular outflow to the aorta (Brock procedure).

What to do

Educating the parents (and the child, if old enough) is a major part of nursing care:
- Explain tetralogy of Fallot to the parents; explain that their child will set their own exercise limits and will know when to rest.
- Teach the parents how to recognise 'tet' spells, which can cause dramatically increased cyanosis; deep, sighing respirations and loss of consciousness (tell them to place the child in the knee-chest position and to report such spells immediately; emergency treatment may be necessary).
- During hospitalisation, alert the staff to the child's condition.
- Because of the right-to-left shunt through the VSD, treat IV lines like arterial lines, and remember that a clot dislodged from a catheter tip in a vein can cross the VSD and cause cerebral embolism (which can also happen if air enters the venous lines).

• If the child requires medical attention for an unrelated problem, advise the parents to inform the health professionals immediately of the child's history of tetralogy of Fallot; any treatment must take this serious heart defect into consideration.

Tricuspid atresia

Tricuspid atresia is failure of the tricuspid valve to develop. This defect prevents blood from entering the right ventricle from the right atrium. (See *Looking at tricuspid atresia*.)

What causes it

The cause of tricuspid atresia is unknown, but it may be associated with pulmonary stenosis or transposition of the great arteries.

How it happens

Deoxygenated blood shunts from the right atrium through an ASD or a patent foramen ovale to the left atrium, where it mixes with oxygenated blood. This mixed blood then passes to the left ventricle and through a VSD to the right ventricle, pulmonary artery and lungs, or mixed blood from the aorta refluxes back through the PDA to the lungs.

What to look for

Signs and symptoms may include cyanosis, tachycardia, dyspnea and a heart murmur.

What tests tell you

In a child with tricuspid atresia:
• chest X-ray shows an enlarged right atrium and decreased pulmonary blood flow
• ECG indicates left-axis deviation and absent right ventricular forces
• echocardiography provides visualisation of the defect and shunting.

Complications

Complications of tricuspid atresia include infective endocarditis, brain abscess and stroke.

How it's treated

Prostaglandin E is administered to maintain ductal patency until surgery. Surgical repair may involve a subclavian-to-pulmonary artery shunt to improve blood flow to the lungs, or the modified Fontan procedure, which connects the right atrium directly to the pulmonary artery.

What to do

Explain the heart defect to the parents, prepare the child for surgery and answer any questions. In addition, follow these steps:
• Monitor vital signs, pulse oximetry and intake and output to assess renal function and detect changes.

Looking at tricuspid atresia

In tricuspid atresia, the tricuspid valve fails to develop, preventing blood from entering the right ventricle from the right atrium.

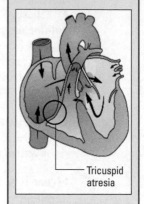

Tricuspid atresia

- Assess cardiovascular and respiratory status to detect early signs of decompensation.
- Monitor fluid status, enforcing fluid restrictions as appropriate to prevent fluid overload.
- Weigh the child daily.
- Organise nursing care around periods of uninterrupted rest to reduce the child's oxygen demands.

Other cardiovascular disorders

Other cardiovascular disorders affecting children and adolescents include endocarditis, heart failure and less commonly Kawasaki disease (KD).

Endocarditis

Endocarditis (also known as infective or bacterial endocarditis) is an infection of the endocardium, heart valves or cardiac prosthesis resulting from bacterial or fungal invasion.

Untreated endocarditis is usually fatal but, with proper treatment, 70% of children recover. The prognosis is worst when endocarditis causes severe valvular damage, leading to insufficiency and heart failure, or when it involves a prosthetic valve.

What causes it

Most cases of endocarditis in children occur in children with:
- abnormal heart valves
- prosthetic heart valves
- congenital heart defects (especially VSD, PDA and tetralogy of Fallot)
- rheumatic heart disease.

Other predisposing conditions include Marfan syndrome, degenerative heart disease, IV drug use and, rarely, a syphilitic aortic valve.

The root of the problem

Some children with endocarditis have no underlying heart disease. Infecting organisms differ among these groups. In children with native valve endocarditis, causative organisms usually include (in order of frequency) streptococci (especially *Streptococcus viridans*), staphylococci and enterococci. Although other bacteria occasionally cause the disorder, fungal causes are rare in this group. The mitral valve is involved most commonly, followed by the aortic valve.

In older children who may be IV drug abusers, *Staphylococcus aureus* is the most common infecting organism. Less commonly, streptococci, enterococci, gram-negative bacilli or fungi cause the disorder. The tricuspid valve is involved most commonly, followed by the aortic valve, and then the mitral valve.

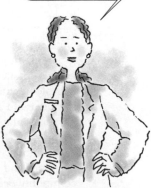

Bacteremia from something as simple as a dental extraction may be enough to cause endocarditis.

Post-prosthesis predicament

In children with prosthetic valve endocarditis, early cases (those that develop within 60 days of valve insertion) are usually due to staphylococcal infection. However, gram-negative aerobic organisms, fungi, streptococci, enterococci or diphtheroids may also cause the disorder.

The course is usually fulminant and is associated with a high mortality rate. In late cases (occurring after 60 days), children show signs and symptoms similar to those of native valve endocarditis.

How it happens

In endocarditis, bacteraemia even transient bacteraemia following dental or urogenital procedures introduces the pathogen into the bloodstream. This infection causes fibrin and platelets to aggregate on the valve tissue and engulf circulating bacteria or fungi that flourish and form friable wartlike vegetative growths on the heart valves, the endocardial lining of a heart chamber or the epithelium of a blood vessel. (See *Degenerative changes in endocarditis*.)

It's a cover up

Such growths may cover the valve surfaces, causing ulceration and necrosis, or extend to the chordae tendineae, leading to rupture and subsequent valvular insufficiency. Ultimately, they may embolise to the spleen, kidneys, central nervous system and lungs.

What to look for

Early clinical features of endocarditis are usually non-specific and include malaise, weakness, fatigue, weight loss, anorexia, arthralgia, night sweats, chills, valvular insufficiency and, in 90% of children, an intermittent fever that may recur for weeks. A more acute onset is associated with organisms of high pathogenicity such as *S. aureus*.

Murmur by megaphone

Endocarditis commonly causes a loud, regurgitant murmur typical of the underlying heart lesion. A sudden change in the murmur or the discovery of a new murmur in the presence of fever is a classic physical sign of endocarditis.

In about 30% of children, embolisation from growing lesions or diseased valvular tissue may produce:
• splenic infarction – pain in the left upper quadrant, radiating to the left shoulder and abdominal rigidity
• renal infarction – haematuria, pyuria, flank pain and decreased urine output
• pulmonary infarction – cough, pleuritic pain, pleural friction rub, dyspnoea and haemoptysis (most common in right-sided endocarditis, which commonly occurs among IV drug abusers and after cardiac surgery)

Degenerative changes in endocarditis

This illustration shows typical growths on the endocardium produced by fibrin and platelet deposits on infection sites.

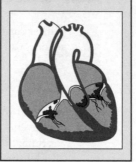

- cerebral infarction – haemiparesis, aphasia or other neurological deficits
- peripheral vascular occlusion – numbness and tingling in an arm, leg, finger or toe, or signs of impending peripheral gangrene.

Pinpoint spots

Other signs of endocarditis may include splenomegaly; petechiae of the skin (especially common on the upper anterior trunk) or buccal, pharyngeal or conjunctival mucosa and splinter haemorrhages under the nails.

Osler, Roth and Janeway

Rarely, endocarditis produces Osler's nodes (tender, raised, subcutaneous lesions on the fingers or toes), Roth's spots (hemorrhagic areas with white centres on the retina) and Janeway lesions (purplish macules on the palms or soles).

What tests tell you

Three or more blood cultures in a 24- to 48-hour period (each from a separate venepuncture) identify the causative organism in up to 90% of children. Blood cultures should be drawn from three different sites, with 1 hour between each venepuncture.

The remaining 10% of children may have negative blood cultures, possibly suggesting fungal infection or infections that are difficult to diagnose such as *Haemophilus parainfluenzae*.

Other abnormal but non-specific laboratory test results may include:
- normal or elevated white blood cell (WBC) count
- abnormal histiocytes (macrophages)
- elevated erythrocyte sedimentation rate (ESR)
- normocytic, normochromic anaemia (in 70% to 90% of children)
- proteinuria and microscopic haematuria (in about 50% of children)
- positive serum rheumatoid factor (in about 50% of all children after endocarditis is present for 3 to 6 weeks)
- valvular damage, identified by echocardiography, particularly TEE
- atrial fibrillation and other arrhythmias that accompany valvular disease, identified by ECG.

Complications

Complications of endocarditis may include heart failure, death, aortic root abscesses, myocardial abscesses, pericarditis, cardiac arrhythmia, meningitis, cerebral emboli, brain abscesses, septic pulmonary infarcts, arthritis, glomerulonephritis and acute renal failure.

How it's treated

The goal of treatment is to eradicate the infecting organism. First-line therapy is usually a combination of penicillin and an aminoglycoside, usually gentamicin. Antimicrobial therapy should start promptly and continue over 4 to 6 weeks.

The right fit

Selection of an antibiotic is based on identification of the infecting organism and on sensitivity studies. While awaiting results, or if blood cultures are negative, empiric antimicrobial therapy is based on the likely infecting organism.

Supportive treatment includes rest, paracetamol for fever and aches, and sufficient fluid intake. Severe valvular damage, especially aortic or mitral insufficiency, may require corrective surgery if refractory heart failure develops or in cases requiring that an infected prosthetic valve be replaced.

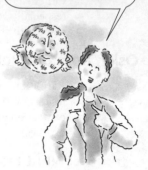

Watch the clock! Giving antibiotics at their prescribed times will keep blood levels consistent in a child with endocarditis.

What to do

Provide reassurance by teaching the child and family about this disease and the need for prolonged treatment. In addition, follow these steps:
• Before giving antibiotics, obtain the child's history of allergies. Administer antibiotics on time to maintain consistent antibiotic blood levels.

Monitoring marathon

• Observe for signs of infiltration or inflammation at the venepuncture site, possible complications of long-term IV drug administration; to reduce the risk of these complications, rotate venous access sites.
• Watch for signs of embolisation (haematuria, pleuritic chest pain, left upper quadrant pain or paresis), a common occurrence during the first 3 months of treatment (tell the parents – and the child, if old enough – to watch for and report these signs, which may indicate impending peripheral vascular occlusion or splenic, renal, cerebral or pulmonary infarction.
• Monitor the child's renal status (blood urea nitrogen [BUN] levels, creatinine clearance and urine output) to check for signs of renal emboli or evidence of drug toxicity.
• Observe for signs of heart failure, such as dyspnoea, tachypnoea, tachycardia, crackles, jugular vein distension, oedema and weight gain.
• Teach the child about antibiotic prophylaxis against endocarditis.

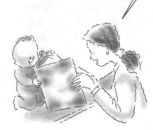

A book, song or board game is a good choice for a child who needs some diversion but can't handle physical exertion.

The education edge

• Instruct the parents to watch closely for fever, anorexia and other signs of relapse about 2 weeks after treatment stops. Suggest quiet diversionary activities to prevent excessive physical exertion.
• Prophylactic antibiotics prior to specific procedures such as dental care are no longer recommended; however, the health professional must assess the needs of the child.
• Teach the child how to recognise symptoms of endocarditis, and tell parents immediately.

Heart failure

Heart failure occurs when the heart can't pump enough blood to meet the body's metabolic needs. It results in intravascular and interstitial volume overload and poor tissue perfusion.

What causes it

Heart failure most commonly occurs in children secondary to structural defects (such as congenital heart defects), resulting in increased blood volume and pressure within the heart itself. Other causes include:
• ventricular impairment from myocardial infarction (MI)
• cardiomyopathy
• arrhythmias
• lung disease
• severe electrolyte imbalances
• sepsis or severe anaemia, which can place excessive demands on the normal heart muscle.

How it happens

Right-sided heart failure results from ineffective right ventricular contractile function; blood isn't pumped effectively through the right ventricle to the lungs, causing it to back up into the right atrium and the peripheral circulation. The child gains weight and develops peripheral oedema and engorgement of the liver, kidneys and other organs.

Left-sided heart failure occurs as a result of ineffective left ventricular contractile function. As the pumping ability of the left ventricle fails, cardiac output falls. Blood is no longer effectively pumped out into the body; it backs up into the left atrium and then into the lungs, causing pulmonary congestion, dyspnoea and activity intolerance. If the condition persists, pulmonary oedema and right-sided heart failure may result.

Reverse, reverse!

The body will attempt to compensate for heart failure by increasing cardiac output through such mechanisms as increased sympathetic activity, ventricular dilation and ventricular hypertrophy.

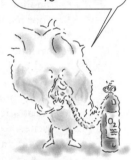

Increased ventricular muscle mass improves my output, but it also increases my oxygen needs.

Increased sympathetic activity

Increased sympathetic activity – a response to decreased cardiac output and blood pressure – enhances peripheral vascular resistance, contractility, heart rate and venous return. Signs such as cool extremities and clamminess may indicate impending heart failure.

Ventricular dilation

In ventricular dilation, an increase in end-diastolic ventricular volume (preload) causes increased stroke work and stroke volume during contraction, stretching cardiac muscle fibres so that the ventricle can accept the increased intravascular volume. Eventually, the muscle becomes stretched beyond optimum limits and contractility declines.

Ventricular hypertrophy

In ventricular hypertrophy, an increase in ventricular muscle mass allows the heart to pump against increased resistance to the outflow of blood, improving cardiac output. This increased muscle mass, however, also increases myocardial oxygen requirements. An increase in the ventricular diastolic pressure necessary to fill the enlarged ventricle may compromise diastolic coronary blood flow, limiting the oxygen supply to the ventricle and causing ischemia and impaired muscle contractility.

What to look for

In children, total adequate heart functioning depends on both the right and left sides of the heart because they work together to pump blood. Because a failure of one chamber causes reciprocal change in the opposite chamber, children don't show separate right- or left-sided signs and symptoms, as observed in adults. Typically, a combination of symptoms is seen because right- and left-sided heart failure occurs simultaneously in children.

Gallops, wheezes and weight

Signs and symptoms of heart failure in children may include:
* tachycardia (one of the earliest signs)
* gallop heart rhythm
* diaphoresis
* poor feeding
* failure to thrive
* peripheral oedema
* tachypnoea, dyspnoea and orthopnoea
* retractions and flaring nares in the infant
* rales, rhonchi and wheezes
* hepatomegaly
* ascites
* weight gain.

What tests tell you

A chest X-ray may reveal cardiomegaly with pulmonary vascular markings resulting from increased pulmonary blood flow. ECG may identify ventricular hypertrophy, and echocardiography may reveal the cause of heart failure such as a congenital heart defect.

Complications

Acute complications of heart failure include pulmonary oedema, acute renal failure and arrhythmias. Chronic complications include activity intolerance, renal impairment, metabolic impairment and thromboembolism.

How it's treated

Because heart failure in children occurs mainly as a result of congenital heart defects, treatment guidelines are directed towards the specific defect involved. Other therapies for heart failure in children may include:
* digoxin to increase myocardial contractility, improve cardiac output, reduce the volume of the ventricle and decrease ventricular stretch

- angiotensin-converting enzyme (ACE) inhibitors to reduce the production of angiotensin II, resulting in preload and afterload reduction (in children, most commonly captopril)
- diuretics to reduce fluid volume overload and venous return
- sodium-restricted diet to reduce accumulated sodium (less common in children)
- oxygen administration to improve tissue oxygenation, especially in those with pulmonary oedema and increased pulmonary vascular resistance.

Give the heart a break!

To reduce the workload on the heart, minimise metabolic demands by:
- maintaining a normothermic state in a neutral thermal environment
- providing treatment of infection, if present
- decreasing respiratory effort (providing oxygen and keeping the child in a semi-Fowler's position if their age allows)
- providing sedation or analgesics as needed for pain or discomfort
- decreasing stimuli to promote a quiet, restful environment.

What to do

Children with heart failure tend to require close monitoring. Because congenital heart defects are the main cause of heart failure in children, be alert for signs and symptoms of heart failure when caring for a child with a congenital heart defect.
- Prepare the child for the intensive care environment and various equipment that may be in use. Also, make sure parents are aware of visiting policies.

Oxygen as ordered

- Place the child in semi-Fowler's position and provide supplemental oxygen as ordered to help him/her breathe more easily.
- Weigh the child daily, and check for peripheral oedema.
- Carefully monitor vital signs and IV intake and output. Auscultate the heart for murmur or gallop rhythm and the lungs for crackles or rhonchi. Report changes at once.

Shhhhhh … they're sleeping

- Group nursing care measures to allow for periods of uninterrupted sleep.
- Frequently monitor BUN, creatinine, serum potassium, sodium, chloride and magnesium levels.

Feed the heart well

- Increase calorific intake to meet the body's increased metabolic needs as the heart is working harder.
- Monitor the child's apical pulse for 1 full minute before administering a digoxin dose. Although the drug may be given to adults with apical rates above 60 beats/minute, digoxin should be withheld in infants and young children

if the apical rate is below 90 to 110 beats/minute (below 70 beats/minute in older children).
• Stress the importance of taking digoxin exactly as prescribed, and tell parents to watch for and immediately report signs of toxicity, such as anorexia, nausea, vomiting and bradycardia.

Kawasaki disease

A child with heart failure has higher metabolic needs, so bring on the healthy high-calorie treats!

Kawasaki disease (KD), also known as mucocutaneous lymph node syndrome, is an acute, systemic vasculitis. It has become a leading cause of acquired heart disease in children in the UK. The majority of cases occur in children younger than age 5, with 1½ times the incidence in boys than in girls.

Although KD is a self-limiting disorder, cardiac sequelae may develop in about 20% of children who aren't treated. These sequelae may include damage to the coronary arteries and myocardium.

What causes it

The cause of KD is unknown. It has geographic or seasonal outbreaks in late winter or early spring, suggesting an infectious process. However, it isn't spread person to person.

How it happens

In KD, inflammation of the small-to-medium blood vessels occurs throughout the body. However, the coronary arteries and, subsequently, the myocardium are most vulnerable to damage. Later progression of the vasculitis may damage the walls of medium-sized vessels, possibly leading to coronary artery aneurysms. Systemic vasculitis usually begins to subside in 6 to 8 weeks.

What to look for

The three phases of KD are acute, subacute and convalescent.

Acute phase

The acute phase of KD involves abrupt onset of high fever that doesn't respond to antipyretics and antibiotic therapy. Signs and symptoms during this phase include:
• fever
• irritability (possibly inconsolable)
• cervical lymphadenopathy
• congested conjunctivae and dry eyes
• erythema of the oral cavity, lips and tongue, leading to the characteristic 'strawberry tongue'
• desquamation of the palms of the hands and soles of the feet
• myocarditis
• intermittent signs of heart failure
• transient arthritis of the small joints. (See *Clinical criteria for KD.*)

Subacute phase

The subacute phase begins as fever subsides and continues until all clinical signs have resolved. Because the damaged coronary arteries will stretch to their maximum diameter during this phase, the child is at risk for coronary thrombosis and aneurysms. Signs and symptoms that may occur during this phase include:

- irritability
- periungual desquamation (peeling that occurs around the nails of the fingers and toes)
- arthritis of larger, weight-bearing joints.

Convalescent phase

By the convalescent phase, all of the clinical signs of KD have resolved. Laboratory results may, however, still be abnormal, and this phase will end when those results are normal. This phase usually occurs 6 to 8 weeks after the onset of fever, and the child usually seems to be 'back to normal' by the end of the convalescent phase.

What tests tell you

Along with the clinical findings, diagnostic tests may show:

- elevated platelet count
- elevated ESR and C-reactive protein
- tissue biopsy showing initial proliferation of the adventitia and intima of vessels and thickening of vessel walls
- echocardiogram showing changes to the myocardium or coronary arteries.

Complications

Thrombosis formation in the coronary arteries may cause MI or ischemia. Less than 1% may die from the disease.

How it's treated

High-dose IV immune globulin (IVIG) may reduce the duration of fever as well as coronary artery involvement (if given in the first 10 days of the disease course). Salicylate therapy is used to reduce fever and inflammation – this is one of the few times aspirin can be used in children under 16 years. For the occurrence of giant aneurysms, anticoagulation therapy in the form of aspirin may be instituted.

Most children recover completely following treatment, but cardiovascular involvement may lead to serious morbidity, usually due to coronary thrombosis.

What to do

Monitor cardiovascular status and intake and output carefully, including daily weights. Observe the child for fluid volume overload due to myocarditis, and assess him frequently for signs of heart failure. In addition, follow these steps:

- Administer IVIG as you would a blood product, obtaining vital signs during and immediately following the infusion and being alert for signs of allergic reaction (the single infusion is usually given over 10 to 12 hours).

Clinical criteria for KD

To be diagnosed with Kawasaki disease (KD), a child must have a fever that's unresponsive to antibiotics for more than 5 days and show four of the following five signs and symptoms:

- bilateral conjunctivitis without discharge
- strawberry tongue and mucous membrane dryness with possible fissures
- erythema of the palms or soles with peeling (usually at week 2 or 3) and peripheral edema
- polymorphous rash
- cervical lymph node swelling (one node greater then 1.5 cm).

Soft and soothing

- Decrease skin inflammation with cool compresses, unscented lotions and the use of soft clothing.
- Provide gentle mouth care during the acute phase of the illness along with a diet of clear liquids and soft foods.
- Maintain a quiet environment to promote rest and reduce irritability. Teach parents that irritability is a hallmark symptom of KD (because parents are at times surprised by their child's uncharacteristic behaviour).

Hush little baby, don't you cry

- Support the parents' efforts to console their crying child, and reassure them that irritability usually subsides during the convalescent phase.
- Because antibody development may be suppressed, don't administer live immunisations, such as the measles-mumps-rubella or varicella vaccines, until 11 months after IVIG administration.

Come on in – the water's fine

- Because arthritis symptoms may persist for several weeks in weight-bearing joints, provide warm baths and passive exercises to maintain joint function and reduce stiffness.
- Teach the parents signs and symptoms of MI in children, such as abdominal pain, vomiting, restlessness, inconsolable crying and pallor (possibly chest pain in older children). Instruct the parents how to perform basic life support.

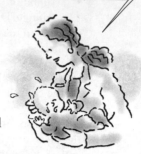

The inconsolable crying of a child with Kawasaki disease is as hard on the parents as it is on the child.

Quick quiz

1. Which sign best indicates the presence of coarctation of the aorta?
    A. Clubbing of fingers and toes
    B. Generalised cyanosis, especially with crying
    C. Rapid and irregular apical heartbeat
    D. Bounding brachial pulses with weak femoral pulses

Answer: D. The child with coarctation of the aorta has bounding pulses in the upper extremities and weak pulses in the lower extremities because the narrowed aorta causes higher blood pressure in the upper extremities.

2. Which nursing intervention is most important to perform before administering digoxin to a child?
    A. Checking apical pulse for 1 full minute
    B. Positioning the child with the head slightly elevated
    C. Counting the child's respiratory rate for 1 full minute
    D. Calculating the child's urine output

Answer: A. The child's apical heart rate should be counted for 1 full minute before digoxin administration. If the heart rate is below the rate specified in the order (typically, 90 to 110 beats/minute for infants and young children or below 70 beats/minute in older children), the dose should be withheld and the doctor notified.

Muscles affected by Duchenne's muscular dystrophy

Duchenne's muscular dystrophy, also known as *pseudohypertrophic dystrophy*, is a congenital disorder characterised by progressive wasting of skeletal muscles (without neural or sensory deficits) that strikes during childhood and is typically fatal during the second decade of life. It has an insidious onset and initially affects the legs, pelvis and shoulders. Children with Duchenne's muscular dystrophy have difficulty climbing stairs, fall frequently and exhibit Gower's sign when standing from a sitting position. They also toe-walk and have a waddling gait and lumbar lordosis.

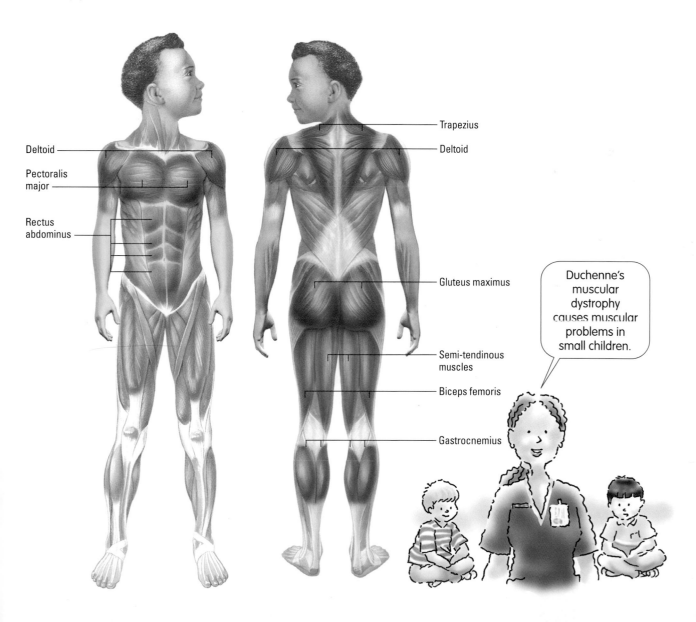

Classifications and complications of otitis media

Otitis media is one of the most common disorders of childhood. It occurs most commonly in children aged 6 months to 2 years and primarily results from eustachian tube dysfunction. Otitis media can be classified as acute otitis media or otitis media with effusion. Complications may include atelectasis, perforation or cholesteatoma.

Classifications

Acute otitis media

In acute otitis media, there's infected fluid in the middle ear and rapid onset of symptoms such as pain; symptoms, however, have a short duration.

Otoscopic view

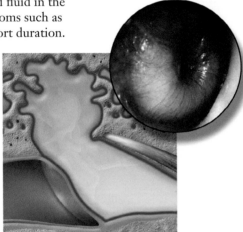

Otitis media with effusion

In otitis media with effusion, there's usually asymptomatic fluid in the middle ear. It may be acute, subacute or chronic in nature.

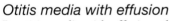

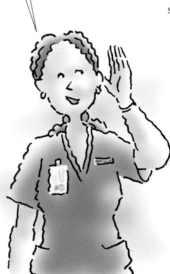

Listen up! Complications of otitis media can cause permanent ear damage.

Complications

Atelectasis

Atelectasis occurs as the tympanic membrane becomes thin and can potentially collapse.

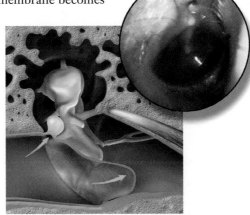

Perforation

A hole in the tympanic membrane signals perforation. It's caused by chronic negative pressure in the middle ear, inflammation or trauma.

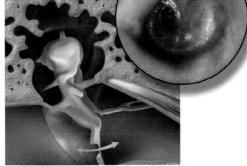

Cholesteatoma

Cholesteatoma is a mass of entrapped skin in the middle ear or temporal lobe.

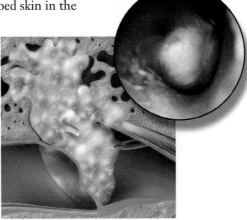

Hydrocephalus

Hydrocephalus is an excessive accumulation of cerebrospinal fluid within the ventricle spaces of the brain. In infants, hydrocephalus causes the head to grow at an abnormal rate. In infants and children, it may cause signs of increased intracranial pressure, such as a tense and bulging anterior fontanel, irritability and lethargy.

Normal brain – Lateral view

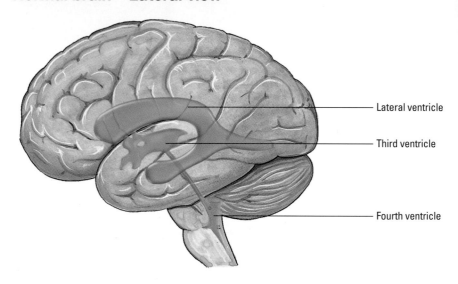

Lateral ventricle

Third ventricle

Fourth ventricle

Ventricular enlargement in hydrocephalus

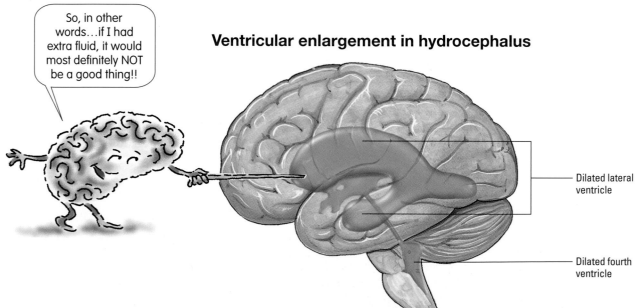

So, in other words…if I had extra fluid, it would most definitely NOT be a good thing!!

Dilated lateral ventricle

Dilated fourth ventricle

3. An infant is diagnosed with PDA. Which drug may be administered to achieve pharmacological closure of the defect?
    A. digoxin.
    B. prednisone.
    C. furosemide.
    D. indometacin.

Answer: D. Indometacin is administered to an infant with PDA in an effort to close the defect.

4. Which cardiac defect is associated with VSD, right ventricular hypertrophy, right ventricular outflow obstruction and an overriding aorta?
    A. Tricuspid atresia
    B. Hypoplastic left heart syndrome
    C. PDA
    D. Tetralogy of Fallot

Answer: D. Tetralogy of Fallot has four cardiac defects: VSD, right ventricular outflow obstruction, right ventricular hypertrophy and an overriding aorta.

Scoring

☆☆☆ If you answered all four items correctly, fabulous! You've gone straight to the heart of cardiac problems.

☆☆ If you answered three items correctly, good work! Your knowledge of cardiac problems is heart-felt.

☆ If you answered fewer than three items correctly, don't take it to heart! A quick review will get your knowledge pumping.

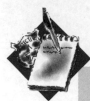

Just the facts

In this chapter, you'll learn:

♦ respiratory anatomy and physiology

♦ tests used to diagnose respiratory disorders in children

♦ treatments and procedures used for children with respiratory problems

♦ respiratory disorders that affect children and nursing interventions for each.

Anatomy and physiology

The structures of the respiratory system are responsible for oxygen distribution and gas exchange. A child's respiratory tract is constantly growing and changing for the first 12 years of life. It differs anatomically from an adult's respiratory system in ways that predispose the child to respiratory difficulties, making respiratory problems common during childhood. (See *Structures of the respiratory system*.)

Chest and lungs

The lungs are the main component of the respiratory system. They inspire air, extract oxygen and exhale the waste product carbon dioxide.

Totally lobular

The right lung has three lobes; the left has two. The mediastinum is the space between the two lungs. The lungs are surrounded by a framework of ribs, vertebrae (posteriorly) and the sternum (anteriorly), creating the chest.

In with the oxygen, out with the carbon dioxide. Breathe easy – we're on the job!

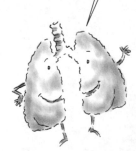

Structures of the respiratory system

This illustration shows the structures of the respiratory system.

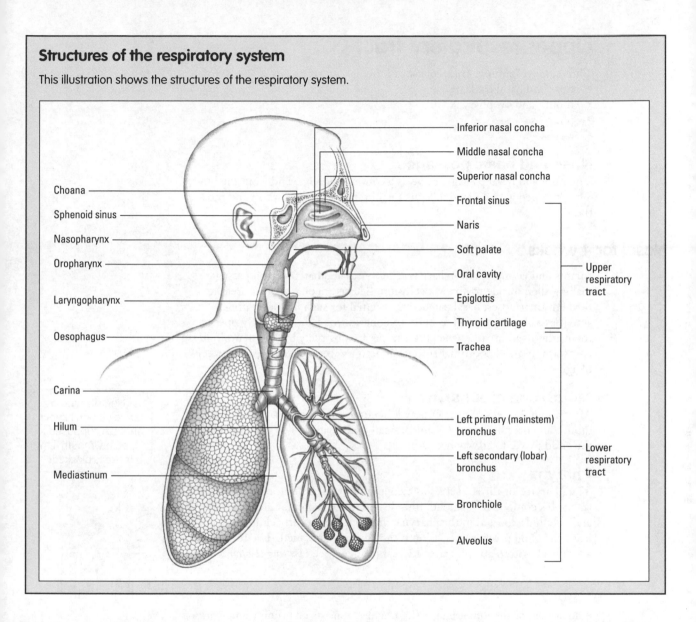

Choana

Sphenoid sinus

Nasopharynx

Oropharynx

Laryngopharynx

Oesophagus

Carina

Hilum

Mediastinum

Inferior nasal concha

Middle nasal concha

Superior nasal concha

Frontal sinus

Naris

Soft palate

Oral cavity

Epiglottis

Thyroid cartilage

Trachea

Left primary (mainstem) bronchus

Left secondary (lobar) bronchus

Bronchiole

Alveolus

Upper respiratory tract

Lower respiratory tract

Roll out the barrel

At birth, the chest is relatively round-shaped. It will gradually develop into a flattened shape across the front and back as the child grows. However, certain respiratory diseases can alter the shape of the chest. For example, obstructive diseases like asthma and cystic fibrosis can produce a barrel-shaped chest when they become severe.

Upper respiratory tract

The upper respiratory tract consists of the:
- nose and nasal passages
- mouth and oropharynx
- pharynx
- larynx.

Nose and nasal passages

The nose and nasal passages serve as a conduit for air to and from the lungs. They're lined with ciliated mucous membranes that filter, warm and moisten the air.

Nasal for 4 weeks

Infants and young children have smaller nares and narrow nasal passages, making them prone to airway occlusion. Because neonates must breathe through their noses, nasal patency is essential for such life-sustaining activities as breathing and feeding. (Neonates won't automatically open their mouths to breathe when their noses are obstructed.) The neurological pathways that will coordinate mouth breathing won't develop until 4 weeks of age.

Mouth and oropharynx

After about 4 weeks of age, air may also enter the respiratory system via the mouth and oropharynx. The child's small oral cavity and large tongue leave the child prone to airway occlusion.

Pharynx

The pharynx, or throat, serves as a conduit for the respiratory and digestive tracts. It's composed of smooth muscle and mucous membranes. The tonsils and adenoids, located in the pharynx, grow rapidly in early childhood and can leave the child prone to occlusion if they become inflamed. The tonsils and adenoids begin to atrophy after 12 years of age. (See *Locating the tonsils and adenoids*.)

Larynx

The larynx, or the upper end of the trachea, consists of a rigid framework of cartilage. It contains the epiglottis, a flap-like structure that overhangs the entrance to the trachea and the glottis, the opening to the trachea.

No solids or fluids beyond this point

The epiglottis and glottis prevent solids and fluids from entering the air passages during swallowing. The glottis contains the vocal cords, which produce vocal sounds when they vibrate. The child's long, floppy epiglottis is vulnerable to swelling that may lead to obstruction.

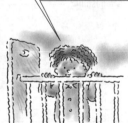

Hey, give me a break. I don't know that I'm supposed to open my mouth if my nose is blocked!

Locating the tonsils and adenoids

These illustrations show the locations of the tonsils and adenoids. Because of their locations, inflammation of these structures can cause airway occlusion.

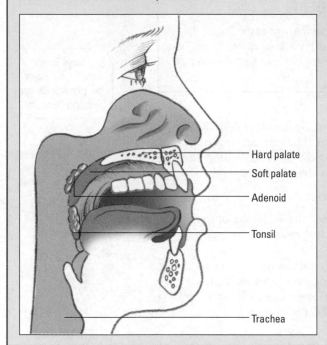

- Hard palate
- Soft palate
- Adenoid
- Tonsil
- Trachea

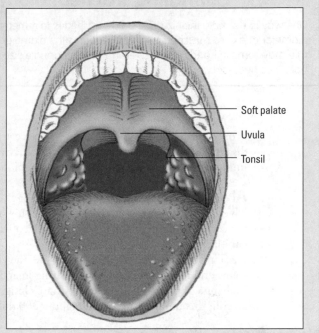

- Soft palate
- Uvula
- Tonsil

Lower respiratory tract

The lower respiratory tract is comprised of the:
- trachea
- bronchi
- alveoli.

Trachea

The trachea acts as a passageway for air into the lungs. It's made up of C-shaped rings of cartilage and is supported by smooth muscle. In infants, the cartilage is soft, making the airway more easily collapsible when the neck is flexed. A child's trachea is higher than an adult's and gives rise to two major bronchi: the right and the left. The right bronchus is shorter, wider and situated more vertically than the left. (See *Estimating tracheal diameter*, page 288.)

Bronchi

The bronchi, the larger air passages of the lungs, are composed of the same cartilaginous rings and smooth muscle as the trachea. The bronchi divide into progressively smaller passages called bronchioles.

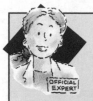

Advice from the experts

Estimating tracheal diameter

One way to estimate the size of a child's trachea is to remember the 'rule of the finger'. The diameter of a child's trachea is roughly equal to the diameter of his little (or pinky) finger. This rule may come in handy when selecting the appropriate size endotracheal tube if intubation becomes necessary.

As a child grows taller in stature, there's increased branching of the bronchioles, leading to greater lung surface area. The cartilaginous rings disappear as the bronchioles get smaller, leaving the smallest divisions with a lining of a single layer of cells. The bronchioles terminate in alveoli.

Alveoli

Alveoli are the small, saclike structures in which the exchange of oxygen for carbon dioxide takes place. Each alveolus is surrounded by many capillaries.

Throughout the first 12 years of life, the alveoli change in size and shape and increase in number, resulting in an increased area available for gas exchange as the child grows. A neonate's lung tissue contains about 25 million alveoli; this number increases to about 300 million by 8 years.

No confusion – it's diffusion

The alveoli promote gas exchange by diffusion (the passage of gas molecules through the respiratory membranes). By diffusion, oxygen from the alveoli passes to the blood, and carbon dioxide, a by-product of cellular metabolism, passes out of the blood into the alveoli, where it's channelled away during exhalation.

Airway resistance

Airway resistance (the effort or force required to move air into the lungs) is greater in children than in adults because children's airways are narrower than those of adults. In infants, airway resistance is about 15 times that of an adult. When there's oedema or swelling in the airway due to an irritant or infectious process, the airway is further narrowed, increasing the airway resistance even more.

Child labour

Increased airway resistance makes the child work harder to breathe. This is indicated by:
• increased respiratory rate

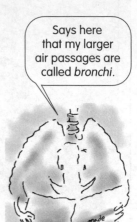

Says here that my larger air passages are called *bronchi*.

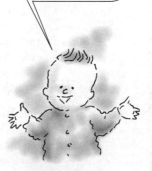

Being a child isn't all fun and games. My airway is narrower than my mom's, so I have to work harder to breathe than she does.

- recession
- nasal flaring.

Pulmonary circulation

In pulmonary circulation, blood passes through the lungs to obtain oxygen to distribute to the cells and tissues of the body in a four-step process:

Deoxygenated blood enters the lungs from the pulmonary artery that arises from the heart's right ventricle.

Blood then flows through the main pulmonary arteries into the smaller vessels of the main bronchi, through the arterioles and, eventually, into the capillary networks that surround the alveoli.

There oxygen diffuses into the capillaries from the alveoli, and the oxygenated blood flows through progressively larger vessels, enters the main pulmonary vein, and flows into the left atrium.

From there, the oxygenated blood passes into the left ventricle and exits the heart through the aorta for distribution throughout the body.

Inspiration and expiration

An infant's ribs are primarily cartilage and are very flexible, making them inefficient in ventilating. Infants primarily engage in diaphragm breathing, also known as abdominal breathing. As the diaphragm moves downward during inspiration, a negative pressure is created, allowing the lungs to expand to draw air in.

Muscles to stabilise, muscles to breathe

The intercostal muscles of the chest are used for stabilisation. However, after 6 years, a child will begin to use the intercostal muscles for breathing. Then, contraction and relaxation of these respiratory muscles moves air into and out of the lungs. Normally, expiration is passive. (See *Normal paediatric respiratory rates*.)

Retractions reveal distress

When an infant or child is having difficulty breathing, retractions of the respiratory muscles will occur. The depth and location of the retractions will indicate the severity of the respiratory distress:
- In mild distress, there are isolated intercostal retractions.
- In moderate distress, there are subcostal, suprasternal and supraclavicular retractions.
- In severe distress, there are all of the retractions mentioned above along with accessory muscle use. (See *Looking for retractions*, page 290.)

Normal paediatric respiratory rates

This chart shows the normal respiratory rates from birth to 18 years.

Age	Breaths per minute
Birth to 6 months	30 to 60
6 months to 2 years	20 to 30
3 to 10 years	20 to 28
10 to 18 years	12 to 20

Looking for retractions

This illustration shows you where to look for retractions. The types of retractions you see in a child can indicate the severity of his/her respiratory distress.

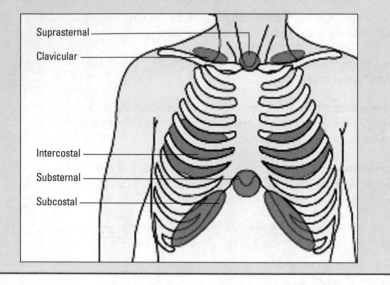

Suprasternal
Clavicular
Intercostal
Substernal
Subcostal

Adventitious breath sounds

Adventitious breath sounds are sounds not normally heard on auscultation of the lungs. Because of the thinness of the chest wall, breath sounds seem louder and harsher in infants and young children, and adventitious breath sounds may transmit over larger areas.

Ventriloquist lungs

Sounds may seem to originate in the lungs when they're actually referred from the upper airway, such as when there's mucus in the nose or throat. Auscultating in the axillae of infants and small children is a good way to hear adventitious breath sounds if they're present. (See *Types of adventitious breath sounds*.)

Blown away

When assessing breath sounds:
• encourage small children to breathe deeply by asking them to pretend they're blowing out candles or have them blow away a tissue
• listen with the bell of the stethoscope for low-pitched sounds
• listen with the diaphragm for higher-pitched sounds.

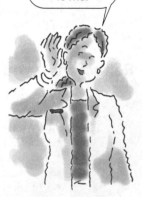

Hmmm. Sounds like adventitious breath sounds to me.

Types of adventitious breath sounds

This chart describes the types of adventitious breath sounds you might hear in a child.

Breath sound	Characteristics	Causes
Wheezing	• Continuous, musical, high-pitched sounds heard in mid-to-late expiration (may be audible without a stethoscope)	• Indicative of oedema and obstruction in small airways
Crackles	• Intermittent, medium- to high-pitched popping sounds heard during inspiration (may clear with coughing)	• Caused by fluid in the alveoli, bronchioles or bronchi
Rhonchi	• Continuous, snoring, low-pitched sounds heard throughout respiration (may clear with coughing)	• Due to oedema and obstruction in large bronchi and the trachea
Stridor	• High-pitched crowing sound heard on inspiration	• Caused by upper airway obstruction at or above the vocal cords
Pleural friction rub	• Grating, rubbing, loud, high-pitched sound heard during inspiration and expiration	• Due to inflamed pleural surfaces

Diagnostic tests and monitoring techniques

Children with suspected or diagnosed respiratory problems may need to undergo invasive or non-invasive diagnostic tests as well as monitoring procedures.

Arterial blood gas

An arterial blood gas (ABG) analysis assesses gas exchange. It also assesses the respiratory control system, determines the blood's acid–base balance and monitors the effectiveness of respiratory therapy. The respiratory and metabolic systems work together to keep the body's acid–base balance within normal limits. (See *Understanding acid–base disorders*, page 292.)

ABG analysis is done on a blood sample taken from a peripheral arterial puncture or an arterial catheter, such as an umbilical arterial catheter, arterial line or central catheter. The normal paediatric values are similar to those for adults.

Nursing considerations

If the sample is to be drawn from an arterial catheter, reassure the child that they won't feel any pain. If the sample is to be taken via an arterial puncture, keep in mind that this is more painful than a venous puncture. Help minimise the trauma from a peripheral arterial puncture:

Understanding acid–base disorders

Acid–base disorders may have several causes and signs and symptoms, as outlined in the chart below along with arterial blood gas (ABG) analysis findings for each disorder.

Disorder and ABG findings	Possible causes	Signs and symptoms
Respiratory acidosis (excess carbon dioxide retention) pH < 7.35 HCO_3^- > 26 mEq/L (if compensating) $PaCO_2$ > 5.98 kPa	• Central nervous system depression from drugs, injury or disease • Asphyxia • Hypoventilation from pulmonary, cardiac, musculoskeletal or neuromuscular disease	Diaphoresis, headache, tachycardia, confusion, restlessness, apprehension, flushed face
Respiratory alkalosis (excess carbon dioxide excretion) pH > 7.45 HCO_3^- < 22 mEq/L (if compensating) $PaCO_2$ < 4.65 kPa	• Hyperventilation from anxiety, pain or improper ventilator settings • Respiratory stimulation from drugs, disease, hypoxia, fever or high room temperature • Gram-negative bacteremia	Rapid, deep respirations; paresthesia; light-headedness; twitching; anxiety; fear
Metabolic acidosis (bicarbonate loss, acid retention) pH < 7.35 HCO_3^- < 22 mEq/L $PaCO_2$ < 4.65 kPa (if compensating)	• Bicarbonate depletion from diarrhea • Excessive production of organic acids from hepatic disease, endocrine disorders, shock or drug intoxication • Inadequate excretion of acids from renal disease	Rapid, deep breathing; fruity breath; fatigue; headache; lethargy; drowsiness; nausea; vomiting; coma (if severe); abdominal pain
Metabolic alkalosis (bicarbonate retention, acid loss) pH > 7.45 HCO_3^- > 26 mEq/L $PaCO_2$ > 5.98 kPa (if compensating)	• Loss of hydrochloric acid from prolonged vomiting or gastric suctioning • Loss of potassium from increased renal excretion (as in diuretic therapy) or steroids • Excessive alkali ingestion	Slow, shallow breathing; hypertonic muscles; restlessness; twitching; confusion; irritability; apathy; tetany; seizures; coma (if severe)

• Be honest about the painful part of the procedure. (For example, say, 'This is going to hurt for a few seconds. It's OK to be scared, but you're going to do a great job and it's going to be over very quickly.')
• Where possible use a surface anaesthetic and ensure that this is left for the optimal time to maximise its effectiveness

Blood borrowing

• Explain that only a small amount of blood will be taken, and that the child's body will quickly make new blood to replace it. (Young children think they have a finite amount of blood and may have many misconceptions about what happens to them when some of that blood is removed.)
• Allow the parent to comfort the child during the blood taking. A parent's presence reassures the child that nothing terrible will happen to him.

Count and squeeze

• Give the child coping mechanisms. (For example, say, 'Count to 5 and the hurting part will be over', or, 'Squeeze your mother's hand if it hurts'.)

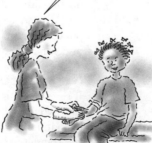

- Praise the child for doing a good job regardless of how they react.
- Comfort the child and apply a bandage as soon as the sample has been drawn; covering the site reassures the child that the hurting part is truly over.

Obtaining the sample

If a peripheral arterial puncture is performed, check arterial circulation to the area (e.g. with the Allen test) before the puncture is made. After the puncture, apply firm pressure to the arterial site to stop the bleeding; then frequently assess the site for bleeding or haematoma formation.

To obtain the sample, follow these steps:
- Draw the blood sample into a heparinised syringe because unclotted blood is required.
- Remove air bubbles from the sample to avoid altering the gas concentration.
- Keep the blood sample on ice and transport it immediately to the blood gas analyser or the laboratory.

Chest X-ray

A chest X-ray is used to visualise internal structures on film. On a chest X-ray, soft tissues, such as organs and muscles, appear as grey forms.

Dem bones, dem bones

Dense tissue such as bone appears white and clearly defined. The chest X-ray is used to rule out foreign body aspiration, determine infectious process and gain information on cardiac size and contour, vessel and cardiac chamber size and status of pulmonary blood flow.

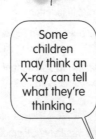

> You'd be surprised what a child can aspirate! On a chest X-ray, an aspirated foreign body will appear white.

Inspiration, expiration, front and back

Inspiratory and forced expiratory films are best to rule out foreign body aspiration. Anterior-posterior and lateral films are best to view internal structures for diagnosis of disease processes in the chest.

Nursing considerations

Explain the procedure to the child, assuring them that there are no 'hurting parts' to the test. If possible, show the child an actual X-ray film (if available as most units now use digital radiography and so do not produce a film) to illustrate what the X-ray can and can't show. (Young children may think an X-ray machine will be able to tell what he's thinking and feeling.)
- Protect the child (and parent if present) from radiation exposure by covering the gonads and thyroid gland with lead shields during the test.
- Make sure the child stays still during the test and tell them that doing so is their special job. (You may need to assist the child to do so.)

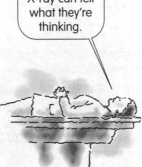

> Some children may think an X-ray can tell what they're thinking.

Pulmonary function tests

Pulmonary function tests (PFTs) are a series of measurements used to evaluate respiratory function. They aid in the assessment of lung function in children with acute or chronic respiratory disorders. (See *Understanding PFT results*.)

Serial testing

Normal values can change dramatically with growth. For this reason, serial determination of pulmonary function is more informative than a single PFT,

---

Understanding PFT results

You may need to interpret pulmonary function test (PFT) results in your assessment of a patient's respiratory status. Use this chart as a guide to common PFTs.

Restrictive and obstructive

The chart mentions restrictive and obstructive defects.

- A restrictive defect is one in which a person can't inhale a normal amount of air; it may occur with chest-wall deformities, neuromuscular diseases or acute respiratory tract infections.
- An obstructive defect is one in which something obstructs the flow of air into or out of the lungs; it may occur with such disorders as asthma, chronic bronchitis, emphysema and cystic fibrosis.

Test	Implications
Tidal volume (V_T): amount of air inhaled or exhaled during normal breathing	Decreased V_T may indicate restrictive defect and indicates the need for further tests such as full chest X-rays.
Minute volume (MV): amount of air breathed per minute	Normal MV can occur in emphysema. Decreased MV may indicate other diseases such as pulmonary edema.
Inspiratory reserve volume (IRV): amount of air inhaled after normal inspiration	Abnormal IRV alone doesn't indicate respiratory dysfunction. IRV decreases during normal exercise.
Expiratory reserve volume (ERV): amount of air that can be exhaled after normal expiration	ERV varies, even in healthy people.
Vital capacity (VC): amount of air that can be exhaled after maximum inspiration	Normal or increased VC with decreased flow rates may indicate reduction in functional pulmonary tissue. Decreased VC with normal or increased flow rates may indicate respiratory effort, decreased thoracic expansion or limited movement of the diaphragm.
Inspiratory capacity (IC): amount of air that can be inhaled after normal expiration	Decreased IC indicates restrictive defect.
Forced vital capacity (FVC): amount of air that can be exhaled after maximum inspiration	Decreased FVC indicates flow resistance in the respiratory system from obstructive disorders, such as chronic bronchitis, emphysema and asthma.
Forced expiratory volume (FEV): volume of air exhaled in the first (FEV_1), second (FEV_2), or third (FEV_3) FVC manoeuvre	Decreased FEV_1 and increased FEV_2 and FEV_3 may indicate obstructive disease. Decreased or normal FEV_1 may indicate restrictive defect.

especially when evaluating a disorder for severity or progression, or when evaluating the effects of treatment.

Breathing on cue

PFTs require the child to cooperate and understand instructions. Most children aren't able to perform the testing until about 5 years of age because it requires manipulating equipment, holding their breath and exhaling on cue with directions.

Nursing considerations

Explain the test to the child and parents, stressing that there's no pain involved. Tell the child that their job will be to follow instructions related to holding equipment, holding their breath and inhaling on cue. Have them practice doing these things before the actual test. In addition:
• note that results may not be accurate because the young child may have difficulty following the necessary directions
• instruct the child and parents that only a light meal should be taken before the test
• withhold bronchodilators and intermittent positive-pressure breathing therapy before the test following medical advice.

Pulse oximetry

Pulse oximetry is a non-invasive monitoring technique used to estimate arterial oxygen saturation through a probe that measures saturation by the absorption of red and infrared light as it passes through tissue. It measures the amount of oxygen carried by haemoglobin by reading the amount of light that passes through a vascular bed and converting the amount of light absorbed by the oxygen-carrying haemoglobin, which gives a saturation value.

Sensing saturation

The sensor can be located on an extremity, a digit, a palm or an earlobe or wrapped around the foot (in an infant) and works best when there's adequate peripheral perfusion. A reading of 95% of greater is the target.

Nursing considerations

Explain this type of monitoring to the child and parents, and put the probe on a parent or nurse so the child can see that it's painless. Reassure them that even though it's used to measure oxygen in the blood, no needles are needed. In addition:
• Place the probe on a site with good perfusion, such as the finger, foot or toe.
• Periodically rotate sites for probe placement to prevent skin breakdown under the probe.
• To ensure that the value is accurate, make sure the pulse reading on the pulse oximeter matches the child's heart rate.

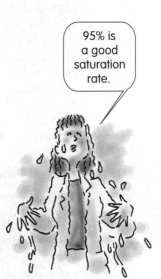

95% is a good saturation rate.

- Higher oxygen levels may be recorded even though there is poor blood flow or anaemia
- Carbon monoxide poisoning will affect oximeter readings.

Treatments and procedures

Respiratory treatments and procedures commonly used for children include aerosol therapy, assisted ventilation, chest physiotherapy (CPT), endotracheal (ET) intubation, oxygen administration and tracheostomy.

Aerosol therapy

The recommended way to use metered dose inhalers (MDIs) is with a spacer (and face mask if required) to ensure optimum drop size. Older children and adolescents not wish to use the spacer in which case breath actuated inhalers should be used.

Under-age aerosol

Nebuliser therapy is needed for children who are too young to use MDIs. A nebuliser aerosolises the medication, releasing it into a small mask that's placed over the child's face. The child can then breathe in the medication through his mouth by taking deep, slow breaths.

Nursing considerations

Before beginning treatment, show the child the MDI or nebuliser mask. Let the child place the MDI to their mouth or the mask to their face before the medication has been added.
- To determine the effectiveness of aerosol therapy, assess the child's breath sounds before and after treatment.
- Monitor the child's tolerance of the procedure. An infant or young child may fight the mask over their face during nebuliser therapy. (Calming techniques such as swaddling may be necessary.)
- After teaching the child and parents how to use the device correctly (which is necessary for optimal effectiveness), observe while they demonstrate their technique; provide support and correct technique as needed. (See *Using an MDI*.)

Assisted ventilation

Assisted ventilation can be administered to children via mechanical ventilation or nasal continuous positive airway pressure (CPAP).

Mechanical ventilation

Mechanical ventilation involves inflation of the lungs with compressed gas. It may be needed for children who are unable to maintain adequate

---

Using an MDI

To optimise treatment, make sure your patient (and his/her parents) know how to use a metered-dose inhaler (MDI) properly by providing them with the following instructions:

✊ Shake the canister while taking a deep breath in and out.

✌️ Hold the canister 1″ (2.5 cm) from the mouth.

🤟 Depress the button on the canister at the beginning of the next inhalation.

🖖 Breathe the mist in deeply and hold your breath for the count of 10, then exhale.

🖐️ Repeat as needed to complete the dosage. (Dosages are usually set in numbers of puffs or inhalations.)

gas exchange due to airway obstruction, neuromuscular disease or other pulmonary pathology.

Compress and pressurise

The compressed gas is pushed into the lungs with pressure, and the exhalation is then passive. Oxygen may also be administered. Mechanical ventilation requires the child to be intubated or to have a tracheostomy, whereas positive-pressure ventilations may also be given by a bag and mask apparatus.

Inflate and expand

Inflation pressures are limited to what's necessary to provide sufficient lung expansion for adequate ventilation and prevention of atelectasis, while keeping a careful watch for damage to airways and lung parenchyma.
• Pressure-cycled ventilators, most commonly used in infants, deliver an indefinite volume of gas at a fixed inflation pressure.
• Volume-cycled ventilators, most commonly used in children and adolescents, deliver a fixed volume of gas at whatever inflation pressure is necessary, up to a preset maximum.
 With any ventilator, the nurse must assess the child carefully and frequently for breathe sounds, chest wall excursion and ABG measurements and pulse oximetry.

Continuous positive airway pressure

CPAP is used to infuse oxygen or air under a preset pressure through nasal prongs or a small mask. The pressure increases the alveolar volume by preventing the alveoli from collapsing on expiration, which leads to an increased functional residual capacity and improves the diffusion time of oxygen.

Nasal fashion statement

Some CPAP systems come with small, triangular-shaped masks that fit only over the nose. These masks help prevent skin breakdown and irritation around and inside the nares that can occur with long-term use of nasal prongs and for preterm neonates whose nares are very small to begin with.

Nursing considerations

Before beginning assisted ventilation, explain the procedure to the parents and the child. If ventilation must be initiated in an emergent situation, tell the child (and parents) what's happening as it's being done.
• Place the child on a cardiorespiratory monitor and pulse oximeter during any form of assisted ventilation.
• Obtain blood gases to monitor gas exchange and oxygenation status as ordered. (Prepare the child if an arterial puncture must be performed.)

When there's no time to prepare a child before an emergency procedure, talk them through it – step-by-step – while it's being done.

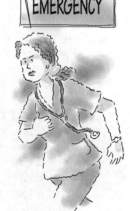

EMERGENCY

Suction secretions

- For infants who have an ET tube or tracheostomy, suction the airway as needed to prevent occlusion with secretions.
- Frequently assess breath sounds and watch for signs of ET tube or tracheostomy dislodgment. Make sure the ET or tracheostomy tube is appropriately secured to prevent dislodgment.

Assess for distress

- In children who are mechanically ventilated, observe for signs of pneumothorax, such as respiratory distress, absent or decreased breath sounds on one side (the affected side), hypotension, and oxygen desaturation on pulse oximetry.
- For children receiving CPAP via nasal prongs, cut and place a cushioning dressing over the edges of the nares and the tip of the nose to protect the skin.

Chest physiotherapy

CPT includes breathing exercises and postural drainage. These therapies help to strengthen respiratory musculature and develop more efficient patterns of breathing. Physiotherapy should be performed by, or under the direction of, a registered physiotherapist.

Drain and clear

Postural drainage is usually done in combination with other techniques to enhance the clearance of mucus from the airway. It can be done with manual percussion, vibration and squeezing of the chest followed by a cough or forceful expiration.

Percussion section

The most common technique involves manual percussion of the chest wall with the child placed in a postural drainage position with the head down, while the provider strikes the chest wall with a cupped hand or a special device for percussing small areas. CPT is contraindicated in children who have pulmonary haemorrhage, pulmonary embolism, increased intracranial pressure, osteogenesis imperfecta or minimal cardiac reserves. (See *Percussion devices*.)

Nursing considerations

Explain the purpose of physiotherapy to the child and parents. In addition, follow these steps:

- Administer bronchodilators, if prescribed, before CPT to enhance airway clearance.
- Perform percussion over the ribs only; don't percuss over the spine or the sternum.

Percussion devices

Percussion is done to clear secretions from the airway. It can be performed by striking areas over the child's lungs using either the hand (positioned as in the top illustration) or a percussion device (such as the one in the bottom illustration) that's used for infants.

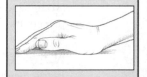

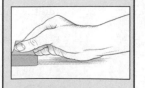

- Encourage the child to cough (which may be easier while sitting up) and give them a soft pillow or stuffed toy to hug while coughing to provide support.
- Encourage the child to perform deep breathing exercises; use techniques to make this fun, such as blowing soap bubbles, through a straw or blowing cotton balls or tissues across a table.

Endotracheal intubation

ET intubation is a short-term measure that may be needed in an emergency. It's used to stabilise the airway if a child is losing the ability to keep the airway open due to swelling or exhaustion that leads to a deteriorating level of consciousness. The ET tube can be inserted orally (orotracheal) or nasally (nasotracheal). The ET tube prevents vocal cord vibration; when the child is intubated they are unable to cry or talk. If long-term intubation is required, a tracheostomy may be necessary.

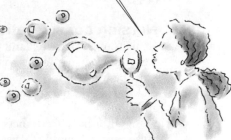

Soap bubbles and a bubble wand can do wonders for deep breathing – and it's fun too!

Nursing considerations

If there's time, explain the procedure before intubation. If the tube is inserted as an emergency measure, explain each step as it's taken. In addition, follow these steps:
- Suction the ET tube as needed to maintain patency.
- Securely tape the tube to the child's face as needed to prevent dislodgement.
- Monitor skin integrity around the tube, such as around the nares if nasotracheally intubated or on the lips and gums if orotracheally intubated.

Separate but equal

- Frequently monitor breath sounds to assess lungs and for positioning of the tube; breath sounds should be equal bilaterally.
- Observe for signs of tube dislodgement, such as audible crying or talking, oxygen desaturations on pulse oximetry and decreased breath sounds.

Silent cry

- Monitor the child's facial expressions. Although you may not hear them cry, their face will still make the grimaces of crying. Provide support, calming and comforting techniques, and pain medication as necessary.
- Because the tube passes through the child's vocal cords, facilitate communication with the child by providing alternatives, such as using sign language, allowing the child to write information or using a communication board.

Oxygen administration

Some children require more than the 21% oxygen that's present in room air to maintain an adequate oxygenation status. Oxygen is usually required for children who have a partial pressure of arterial oxygen (PaO_2) less than 60 mm Hg or an oxygen saturation range of 89% to 92% on pulse oximetry.

When oxygen therapy is used, the goal is usually to keep oxygen saturation above 92%. Because oxygen is a drug, it should be administered only in the prescribed dosage. It's administered in litres per minute (if via nasal cannula) or as a percentage (if via mechanical ventilation or a head box). Oxygen can be drying, so it must be humidified before it's delivered to the child.

Oxygen can be administered through an ET or tracheostomy tube during mechanical ventilation or via an anaesthetic bag and mask. For children breathing on their own, oxygen can be delivered via nasal cannula, a head box or mask.

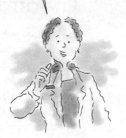

Always remember that oxygen needs to be administered as prescribed – just like any other drug.

Nursing considerations

Explain to the parents (and the child, if old enough) why oxygen is being administered and how it will help the child's condition. If an ET tube must be used, prepare the child for its insertion, explaining what they'll feel and reassuring them that they'll get used to the tube quickly. In addition:
• monitor the effectiveness of oxygen therapy by assessing the child's colour, pulse oximetry, and PaO_2 using ABG analysis
• make sure that the child is receiving the appropriate concentration of oxygen; also make sure that the oxygen is being humidified before delivery to the child.

Tracheostomy

Tracheostomy is a surgically created opening in the anterior neck at the cricoid cartilage leading directly to the trachea. This may be done in the emergency department, in the area where immediate intervention is necessary or in the more controlled setting of the operating theatre. A tracheostomy tube is inserted to keep the opening patent; the tube must be secured in place to prevent accidental extubation.

Tracheostomies are used for children requiring long-term ventilation, or they can be created urgently for epiglottitis, croup or foreign body aspiration. The tracheostomy is usually only needed short term for these urgent indications. (See *Tracheostomy*.)

Nursing considerations

If time permits, prepare the child and family before the procedure. Discuss how the tracheostomy will look and feel, and decide on a method of communication to be used after the procedure.

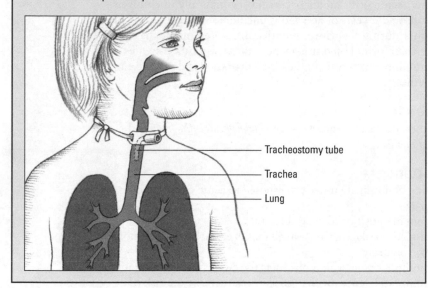

Tracheostomy

This illustration shows a tracheostomy tube in place in the trachea. Note how the tied cloth tapes keep the tube securely in place.

- Tracheostomy tube
- Trachea
- Lung

• After the procedure, monitor the child for complications such as haemorrhage, infection, oedema, extubation and tube obstruction.
• Frequently assess the child's breath sounds and monitor respiratory status with blood gases.
• Ensure prescribed oxygen is humidified.
• Suction the tracheostomy tube as needed to maintain patency. Use correct size suction catheters (Catheter diameter should be half the tracheostomy tube size).
• Provide stoma care as per unit policy. The skin around the stoma should be kept clean and dry. Monitor the skin for signs of breakdown.
• Keep the tracheostomy tube ties clean and dry, and change as needed.
• Keep the tracheostomy tube ties secured tightly, but with enough room to slip a fingertip between the ties and the neck to help prevent accidental extubation.

Respiratory disorders

Disorders of the respiratory system that can occur during childhood include acute otitis media, asthma, bronchiolitis, croup, cystic fibrosis, epiglottittis, pneumonia and tuberculosis (TB).

Acute otitis media

Acute otitis media is the most commonly diagnosed illness in childhood; it's an inflammation of the middle ear with a rapid onset of symptoms and clinical signs. Acute otitis media occurs most commonly in children between 6 months and 3 years of age and is uncommon after 8 years. The incidence is higher during the winter months. Breast-fed infants have a lower incidence than formula-fed infants because breast milk provides an increased immunity that protects the eustachian tube and middle ear mucosa from pathogens.

What causes it

The most common causative organisms are *Haemophilus influenzae* and *Streptococcus pneumoniae*.

How it happens

Infants and young children are more predisposed to acute otitis media because they have:
- short, horizontally positioned eustachian tubes
- poorly developed cartilage lining, which makes eustachian tubes more likely to open prematurely
- enlarged lymphoid tissue, which obstructs the eustachian tube opening
- immature humoral defence mechanisms, which increase the risk of infection. (See *Characteristics of a child's ear*.)

Characteristics of a child's ear

You'll recognise three major differences between an infant's or a young child's ear and an adult's ear. These anatomic differences make the infant and young child more susceptible to ear infection:

- A child's tympanic membrane slants horizontally, rather than vertically.
- A child's external canal slants upward.
- A child's eustachian tube slants horizontally; this causes fluid to stagnate and act as a medium for bacteria.

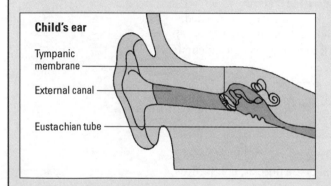

Child's ear

Tympanic membrane

External canal

Eustachian tube

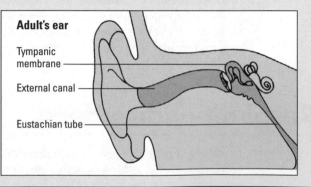

Adult's ear

Tympanic membrane

External canal

Eustachian tube

The great equaliser

The eustachian tube connects the middle ear to the nasopharynx and is normally closed and flat, thus preventing organisms in the pharyngeal cavity from entering the middle ear. The tube opens to allow drainage of secretions produced by the middle ear and equalises air pressure between the middle ear and the environment.

No escape

When swelling or other predisposing factors cause eustachian tube dysfunction, secretions are retained in the middle ear. Air is also unable to escape through the obstructed tubes and causes negative pressure within the middle ear. If the tube opens, the difference in pressure causes bacteria to be drawn into the middle ear chamber where they proliferate and invade the mucosa, causing infection.

Supine? Not this time

Bottle-feeding an infant in the supine position increases the risk of infection because this position promotes pooling of formula milk in the pharyngeal cavity, creating an excellent medium for the spread of infection.

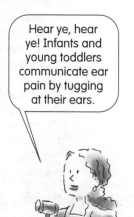

Hear ye, hear ye! Infants and young toddlers communicate ear pain by tugging at their ears.

What to look for

Common acute symptoms of acute otitis media include:
• ear pain that may present as pulling at the ears in younger children or difficulty eating or lying down due to ear pressure and pain
• fever
• irritability
• loss of appetite
• purulent drainage in the external ear canal
• nasal congestion and cough
• vomiting and diarrhoea.

The trouble with tympany

Otoscopy reveals:
• tympanic membrane injection (sometimes bright red)
• bulging tympanic membrane, which is dull, with no visible landmarks or light reflex
• diminished mobility of the tympanic membrane with air insufflation (pneumonic otoscopy).

What tests tell you

These tests are used for diagnosis and to guide treatment:
• A culture and sensitivity of any drainage may indicate what the organism is and which antibiotic is indicated for treatment.

- Tympanometry is used to measure the change in air pressure in the external auditory canal (from movement of the eardrum).
- Audiometric testing establishes a baseline or detects any hearing loss secondary to recurring infection. (Hearing evaluation is recommended for any child who has had bilateral acute otitis media that lasts 3 months or longer.)

Complications

Complications of acute otitis media include effusion (which may persist beyond 3 months), hearing impairment, spontaneous rupture of the tympanic membrane and mastoiditis.

How it's treated

Treatment now focuses on allowing, where possible, the child's immune system to deal with the infection and thus reduce the development of antibiotic-resistant organisms. This approach is intended for otherwise healthy children without underlying medical conditions that may complicate acute otitis media (such as cleft palate, Down's syndrome and other genetic or immune system disorders) and includes:

- using analgesics, such as ibuprofen and paracetamol to relieve pain, especially in the first 24 hours of infection (Parents should be aware that analgesics – not antibiotics – will relieve the ear pain of acute otitis media.)
- giving parents the option of allowing their child's immune system to fight the infection for 48 to 72 hours, then only starting antibiotics if the child's condition doesn't improve after that time. Up to 80% of children will get better within 2 to 3 days without treatment
- encouraging the prevention of acute otitis media by avoiding the use of a dummy and exposure to tobacco smoke.

Never fear, the antibiotics are here! We'll have the child feeling better in only 2 or 3 days.

But wait, there's more!

It is recommended that antibiotics should be used without a waiting period for infants younger than 6 months of age, children ages 6 months to 2 years with a confirmed diagnosis of acute otitis media and children ages 2 and older with severe symptoms.

Most children should receive amoxicillin as a first-line agent. With severe illness or if additional antibacterial coverage is necessary, amoxicillin-clavulanate may be initiated. In cases of allergic reaction to amoxicillin or penicillin, alternative therapies may include cephalosporins, erythromycin or co-trimoxazole (Bactrim). With antibiotic therapy, the child should experience symptom resolution within 48 to 72 hours.

If drugs don't do it

After antibiotic therapy is completed, the child should be re-evaluated to make sure that treatment was effective and there are no complications. Other treatments for repeated or complicated infections may include:

Ventilating tubes in the ear

This illustration shows where tubes are placed in the ear to equalise pressure on both sides of the tympanic membrane.

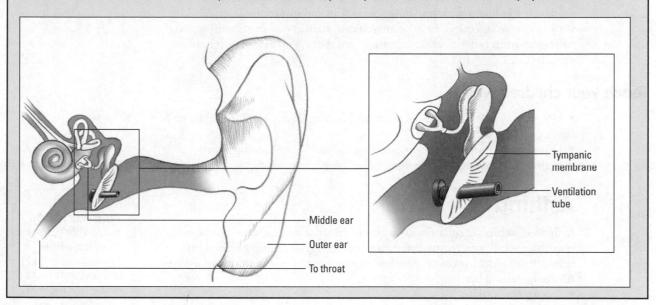

Middle ear

Outer ear

To throat

Tympanic membrane

Ventilation tube

• myringotomy, which is an incision in the posterior inferior aspect of the tympanic membrane and may be necessary to promote drainage of exudate and release pressure
• tympanoplasty grommets, or pressure-equalising tubes, which may be surgically inserted into the middle ear to create an artificial auditory canal that equalises pressure on both sides of the tympanic membrane. (See *Ventilating tubes in the ear.*)

What to do

To care for a child with acute otitis media, follow these steps:
• Relieve pain by administering analgesics, offering liquid or soft foods to limit the need for chewing and applying local warm or cool compresses over the affected ear.
• Reduce fever by administering antipyretics.
• Facilitate drainage by having the child lie with the affected ear in a dependent position.
• Help prevent skin breakdown by keeping the external ear clean and dry; apply zinc oxide or petroleum jelly to protect the skin if needed.
• Educate parents about the importance of completing the full course of any prescribed antibiotics.

Testing 1, 2

- Assess for hearing loss and refer for audiology testing if necessary.
- Administer prescribed medication as ordered, including prophylactic antibiotic treatment with low-dose amoxicillin and sulfisoxazole in a child with recurrent infection. Oral decongestants, such as pseudoephedrine, may be suggested to relieve nasal congestion, but there is no evidence that these are effective.

Teach your children well

- Provide appropriate pre-operative and post-operative teaching if the child requires surgical intervention.
- Educate parents about the indications for and use of earplugs post-operatively for bathing and swimming.

Asthma

Asthma is a chronic, inflammatory airway disorder that causes episodic airway obstruction and hyperresponsiveness of the airway to multiple stimuli. It results from bronchospasms, increased mucus secretion and mucosal oedema. It's characterised by:
- recurrent cough
- wheezing
- shortness of breath
- reduced expiratory flow
- exercise intolerance
- respiratory distress.

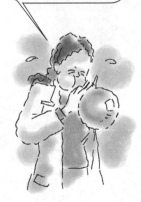

Asthma can take your breath away! That causes stress, which worsens asthma, which causes more stress, which ... well, you get the idea.

What causes it

Asthma exacerbations or attacks are caused by inflammation of the lungs, including the protective mechanisms of mucus formation, swelling and airway muscle contraction.

Over-reacting

The lungs react excessively in response to a stimulus (trigger), increasing anxiety and physical responses, in addition to releasing histamine and intracellular chemical mediators that result in bronchospasm. The result is a vicious cycle of anxiety and physiologic response to anxiety.

Gentleman, choose your triggers

Common asthma triggers include:
- exercise
- viral or bacterial agents
- allergens, such as mould, dust and pollen
- pollutants

- changes in weather
- food additives.

Many people with asthma, especially children, have intrinsic and extrinsic asthma.

Outside and sensitive

Extrinsic, or atopic, asthma begins in childhood. Children are typically sensitive to specific external (extrinsic) allergens and have a family history of asthma or other allergies. Extrinsic allergens that can trigger an asthma attack include such elements as pollen, animal scales, house dust or mould, feather pillows, food additives containing sulphites and other sensitising substances. Extrinsic asthma in childhood is commonly accompanied by other hereditary allergies, such as eczema and allergic rhinitis.

A look within

Children with intrinsic, or non-atopic, asthma react to internal, non-allergenic factors. Intrinsic factors that can trigger an asthma attack include irritants, emotional stress, fatigue, endocrine changes, temperature variations, humidity variations, exposure to noxious fumes, anxiety, coughing or laughing and genetic factors. Most episodes occur after a severe respiratory tract infection, especially in adults.

Exercise-induced asthma is a narrowing of the airways that makes it difficult to move air out of the lungs. Symptoms include coughing, wheezing, chest tightness and prolonged, unexpected shortness of breath after 5 to 20 minutes of exercise. These symptoms are commonly worse in cold, dry air.

Genetic messes

Asthma is associated with two genetic influences:
- ability to develop asthma because of an abnormal gene (atopy)
- tendency to develop hyperresponsive airways (without atopy).

A potent mix

Environmental factors interact with inherited factors to cause asthmatic reactions with associated bronchospasms.

How it happens

Asthma attacks follow a predictable course of bronchospasm, inflammation and airway narrowing. Here's how asthma develops:

The tracheal and bronchial linings over-react to various stimuli, causing episodic smooth-muscle spasms that severely constrict the airways.

Mucosal oedema and thickened secretions also block the airways.

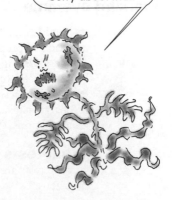

You can't always trust a pretty face. Exposure to my pollen makes mast cells in the lung release histamine. Sorry about that!

Immunoglobulin (Ig) E antibodies, attached to histamine containing mast cells and receptors on cell membranes, initiate intrinsic asthma attacks.

When exposed to an antigen such as pollen, the IgE antibody combines with the antigen.

On subsequent exposure to the antigen, mast cells degranulate and release mediators. These mediators cause the bronchoconstriction and oedema of an asthma attack.

Ready, set, spasm!

As a result, expiratory airflow decreases, trapping gas in the airways and causing alveolar hyperinflation.

Atelectasis may develop in some lung regions. The increased airway resistance initiates laboured breathing.

Repeat and damage

With repeated episodes of bronchospasm, swelling airways and mucus plugging, cells that line the airways suffer damage, leaving a chronically irritated and scarred lining that results in air trapping or hyperinflation.

What to look for

An acute asthma attack may begin dramatically, with simultaneous onset of multiple, severe symptoms or insidiously, with gradually increasing respiratory distress. Look for these signs and symptoms:
• sudden onset of breathing difficulty
• frequent coughing or frequent respiratory infections such as pneumonia or bronchitis (which may be an indication that the child's airway is overly sensitive to stimuli).

Working overtime

• rapid and laboured respirations and a tired appearance due to the ongoing exertion of breathing
• nasal flaring and intercostal retractions
• productive cough and expiratory wheezing
• use of accessory muscles, decreased air movement and respiratory fatigue
• barrel chest and use of accessory muscles after repeated acute exacerbations. (See *Four levels of asthma severity.*)

What tests tell you

Several tests are used to diagnose asthma, assess its severity and identify allergens:

Four levels of asthma severity

Four levels of asthma severity have been identified, based on the frequency of symptoms and exacerbations, effects on activity level and lung function study results. The four levels are mild intermittent, mild persistent, moderate persistent and severe persistent.

Level of severity	Clinical findings
Mild intermittent	• Symptoms occur less than two times per week. • The patient is asymptomatic with normal peak expiratory flow (PEF) between exacerbations. • Brief exacerbations (from a few hours to a few days) vary in intensity. • Nighttime symptoms occur less than two times per month. • Lung function studies show forced expiratory volume in 1 second (FEV_1) or PEF greater than 80% of normal values; PEF may vary by less than 20%.
Mild persistent	• Symptoms occur more than two times per week, but less than once per day; exacerbations may affect activity. • Nighttime symptoms occur more than two times per month. • Lung function studies show FEV_1 or PEF greater than 80% of normal values; PEF may vary by 20% to 30%.
Moderate persistent	• Symptoms occur daily. • Exacerbations occur more than two times per week and may last for days; exacerbations affect activity. • Bronchodilator therapy is used daily. • Nighttime symptoms occur more than once per week. • Lung function studies show FEV_1 or PEF 60% to 80% of normal values; PEF may vary by greater than 30%.
Severe persistent	• Symptoms occur on a continuous basis. • Exacerbations occur frequently and limit physical activity. • Nighttime symptoms occur frequently. • Lung function studies show FEV_1 or PEF less than 60% of normal values; PEF may vary by greater than 30%.

• PaO_2 and partial pressure of arterial carbon dioxide ($PaCO_2$) are usually decreased, except in severe asthma, when $PaCO_2$ may be normal or increased, indicating severe bronchial obstruction.

Function or obstruction?

• PFTs reveal signs of airway obstructive disease, low-normal or decreased vital capacity and increased total lung and residual capacities. (Pulmonary function may be normal between attacks.)
• Serum IgE levels may increase from an allergic reaction.
• Sputum analysis may indicate the presence of Curschmann's spirals (casts of airways), Charcot–Leyden crystals and eosinophils.
• Chest X-rays can be used to diagnose or monitor the progress of asthma and may show hyperinflation with areas of atelectasis.

- ABG analysis detects hypoxemia (decreased PaO_2; decreased, normal or increasing $PaCO_2$) and guides treatment.
- Skin testing may identify specific allergens.

Up to the challenge?

- Bronchial challenge testing evaluates the clinical significance of allergens identified by skin testing
- Electrocardiogram shows sinus tachycardia during an attack; during a severe attack, this test may show signs of cor pulmonale (right axis deviation, peaked P wave) that resolve after the attack.

Complications

Status asthmaticus, in which there's unrelenting, severe respiratory distress and bronchospasm, may occur despite pharmacologic and supportive interventions. Mechanical ventilation may be needed due to respiratory failure. Death may occur if a child in acute exacerbation isn't treated in a timely manner and proceeds to respiratory failure without intubation.

How it's treated

Prevention and treatment should follow the BTS/SIGN Asthma Guidelines (2009) and Stepwise Management. The best treatment of asthma is prevention of exacerbations. Management includes medications, and education and support of the child and parents. Choice of medications to promote optimal respiratory function is typically based on the asthma's level of severity.

Anti-inflammatory agents

Anti-inflammatory medications to reduce mucosal oedema in airways include cromolyn (Intal) and corticosteroids, such as beclomethasone, triamcinolone and prednisolone. These drugs are all preventive medications, usually taken on a daily basis to stop the release of chemicals such as histamine during the inflammatory process. They may be used to control seasonal, allergic and exercise-induced asthma or for unavoidable allergen exposure.

Anti-inflammatories must be taken consistently to be effective. These medications aren't effective after wheezing starts, but may help gain control and speed the resolution of an asthma attack.

> Anti-inflammatory medicines can help control seasonal allergies.

Corticoreactions

Adverse reactions of corticosteroids include glucose metabolism abnormalities, increased appetite, fluid retention, weight gain, moon face, mood alteration, growth suppression and hypertension, all of which may be severe if used daily for long-term therapy. Inhaled corticosteroids are being used more commonly in children because they're thought to have lesser adverse reactions.

Bronchodilators

Bronchodilators are used to relax smooth muscle in the airway for moderate to severe symptoms resulting in rapid bronchodilation within 5 to 10 minutes. These medications include beta2-adrenergic agonists, such as terbutaline and salmeterol as well as methylxanthines and theophylline.

Open wide

Bronchodilators relax the muscle bundles that constrict airways for airway dilation and relaxation and are used for acute or daily therapy, nocturnal symptoms and exercise-induced bronchospasm. When used for long-term control, they work best when a specific amount is maintained in the bloodstream, so serum level checks and dosage adjustments may be required. Adverse effects include tachycardia, nervousness, nausea and vomiting and headaches.

Leukotriene receptor antagonists (LRA)

Leukotriene receptor antagonists such as montelukast or zafirlukast may be used as a steroid-sparing adjunct for the prevention of bronchospasm in exercise-induced asthma. They improve pulmonary function and enhance the effect of corticosteroids, allowing for lower dosages of corticosteroids. Adverse reactions include diarrhoea, laryngitis, pharyngitis, nausea, otitis media, sinusitis or headache. Administering LRAs daily, at bedtime, may promote compliance.

Allergy injections and oxygen

The use of allergy injections for hyposensitisation – to reduce sensitivity to environmental allergens that may be unavoidable, such as mould or pollen – is controversial because their actual effect is questionable.

Oxygen is administered by nasal cannula or face mask for the child exhibiting difficulty breathing. The oxygen must be humidified to decrease drying and thickening of mucus secretions. Oxygen levels must be monitored often with a pulse oximeter.

What to do

Nursing interventions are focused on maintaining airway patency and fluid status, promoting rest and decreasing stress for the child and parents.
• On arrival evaluate the child's current respiratory status, remembering the ABCs (airway, breathing and circulation); move on to other activities only after establishing that the child doesn't need immediate intervention to promote oxygenation.
• If the child isn't moving air or is unable to talk, take emergency action following paediatric life support guidelines
• Continue to assess the quality of the child's breathing, obtain oxygen saturation via pulse oximeter and peak expiratory flow rate in an older child (the frequency of assessment is based on the severity of symptoms).

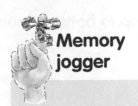

Memory jogger

To remember which drug should be inhaled *first*, think about your ABCs.
A *Bronchodilator* comes before a *Corticostesroid*.

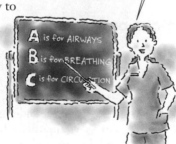

Always think about your ABCs when evaluating a child's respiratory status.

A is for AIRWAYS
B is for BREATHING
C is for CIRCULATION

Top to bottom, looking for problems

- Assess skin and intake and output, and perform a head-to-toe assessment to identify associated problems contributing to the asthma exacerbation.
- Assess the child's psychosocial status, looking for indications of anxiety or fear and promote comfort for the child and family. (Encouraging the parents' presence can be reassuring for the child and can decrease anxiety and fear.)
- Place the child in a sitting position to facilitate respiratory effort.
- Administer fluids, which are important for restoring and maintaining fluid balance as adequate hydration helps break up trapped mucus plugs in a narrowed airway. (IV fluids may be necessary if adequate fluid intake isn't possible due to compromised respiratory status and risk of aspiration with tachypnoea.)

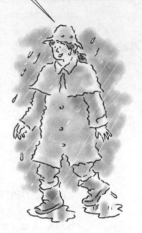

Good hydration is essential for a child with asthma.

Please do not disturb

- Promote rest and stress reduction by grouping nursing tasks and avoiding repeated disturbances.
- Support the family by encouraging them to rest and giving them the opportunity to assist with the child's treatments as they wish; give them frequent updates on the child's condition.
- Provide discharge planning and home care teaching that gives the parents a thorough understanding of the disease and how to prevent attacks and maintain the child's health to avoid illness that leads to hospitalisation. (Include education on medication therapy and stress the need for follow-up care.)

Smoke provokes

- Teach parents about the dangers of smoking around a child with asthma. Encourage them to quit or, at the very least, never smoke indoors, even if the child isn't in the home at the time.
- Refer the child to an asthma clinic/children's asthma nurse specialist.
- Teach the older child signs of early respiratory distress so they can seek treatment before the signs get more serious.
- Inform and involve the School Health Nurse so as to ensure optimal care when at school.

Smoking and asthma don't mix! Teach parents that being around cigarette smoke is particularly dangerous for a child with asthma.

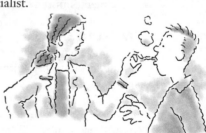

Bronchiolitis

Bronchiolitis is an illness that usually occurs after an upper respiratory infection causes inflammation and obstruction of the small airways (bronchioles) – either early in life as a single episode or with multiple occurrences in the first year of life. It most commonly affects toddlers and preschoolers, but can become severe in infants younger than 6 months old, causing life-threatening respiratory distress that requires hospitalisation.

What causes it

Respiratory syncytial virus (RSV) is the leading cause of bronchiolitis. Other causes exist, however, including viruses, bacteria and mycoplasmal organisms. Premature infants and those with bronchopulmonary dysplasia, immunodeficiency or congenital heart disease are at especially high risk.

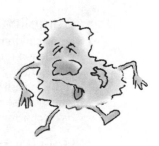

How it happens

Bronchiolitis occurs when viruses or other infectious agents invade the mucosal cells lining the bronchi and bronchioles, causing the cells to die. Cell death results in cell debris that clogs and obstructs the bronchioles and irritates the airway. The airway lining responds by swelling and producing excessive mucus resulting in partial airway obstruction and bronchospasm. The process continues as both lungs are invaded and the obstructed airways allow air in, but the swollen airways and build-up of mucous don't allow for expulsion of the air, creating wheezing and crackles in the airways.

Diminishing returns

Air trapped below the obstructed airways interferes with gas exchange, leading to decreased oxygen and increased carbon dioxide levels. Airflow continues to decrease and breath sounds diminish.

What to look for

The diagnosis of bronchiolitis is based on clinical findings, the child's age and the season. Clinical findings may include:
- recent history of upper respiratory symptoms, including nasal stuffiness or serous nasal discharge accompanied by mild fever and a cough in older toddlers and preschoolers
- wheezing, deep and frequent cough and laboured breathing
- rapid, shallow respirations accompanied by nasal flaring and retractions
- tachypnoea, paroxysmal cough and increasing irritability with increasing respiratory distress.

The child commonly appears ill, is less playful, and has little interest in feeding/eating or has a history of vomiting with thick, clear mucus being present.

What tests tell you

Bronchiolitis is diagnosed primarily by history and physical examination.
- Chest X-rays usually show non-specific findings of inflammation, but may show areas of consolidation that are difficult to differentiate from bacterial pneumonia.
- Viral cultures or antigen testing by nasal swab or a direct aspiration of nasal secretions or nasopharyngeal washings may indicate RSV.
- If the bronchiolitis is severe and advanced, there may be a rise in $PaCO_2$, leading to respiratory acidosis and hypoxaemia.

Complications

Some children with more severe cases require intubation and assisted ventilation if they become too fatigued to breathe effectively, and they progress to respiratory failure. Death may result due to severe RSV bronchiolitis in children with pre-existing cardiopulmonary disease. Bronchiolitis in infancy may increase the chances of childhood wheezing and asthma and is a major risk factor for chronic obstructive pulmonary disease later in life.

How it's treated

Usually, supportive management with high humidity, adequate fluid intake and rest is all that's needed when the bronchiolitis is mild to moderate in severity. The child with more severe bronchiolitis will need:
- monitoring with pulse oximetry
- postural drainage and possibly CPT to loosen trapped mucus.

Hydrate and humidify

- humidified oxygen therapy via nasal cannula or head box to alleviate dyspnoea and hypoxia
- IV hydration if the child is tachypnoeic and unable to maintain hydration status (due to decreased intake with respiratory distress or insensible fluid loss due to fever and increased respiratory rate).

Drugs to the rescue

Pharmacological therapy may include:
- aerosol medications such as bronchodilators, steroids and beta-adrenergic agonists to act directly on inflamed and obstructed airways; however, the evidence for these is limited and guidelines such as those from SIGN (http://www.sign.ac.uk/pdf/sign91.pdf) do not recommend them
- antipyretics to reduce fever
- antibiotics (only if a secondary bacterial infection such as otitis media is present)
- ribavirin (Virazole), an antiviral drug delivered via hood, tent or mask, to treat RSV. (Ribavirin's effectiveness is controversial, and is usually reserved for life-threatening cases.)

'Tis the season

Preventative vaccination may be indicated for RSV bronchiolitis in high-risk infants or children with congenital heart disease, bronchopulmonary dysplasia, chronic lung problems, cystic fibrosis or prematurity. Palivizumab is given for 5 consecutive months during RSV season (November to April).

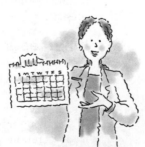

What to do

Nursing care focuses on careful attention to respiratory function:
- Assess airway and respiratory function carefully and frequently because it's important to intervene in a timely manner for worsening respiratory symptoms to prevent respiratory distress.

- Maintain respiratory function by administering prescribed humidified oxygen.

Head's up

- Elevate the head of the bed to ease the work of breathing and assist mucus to drain from upper airways.
- Use oxygen saturation level as an indicator of the severity of the disease and to spot early signs of deterioration.
- Maintain isolation in a separate room or cohort room for RSV infection and use meticulous hand washing to prevent spreading infection. (RSV is highly contagious and has the potential to spread during close contact.)

Assess and de-stress

- Perform psychosocial assessment by observing the child and parents for signs of fear and anxiety, which can worsen respiratory distress.
- Help to reduce anxiety by providing thorough explanations and updates and encouraging parents to participate in the child's care as able (to promote emotional security).
- Cluster nursing activities to promote rest and decrease stress as rest is required to improve the child's breathing and healing.
- Administer antipyretics to control temperature and promote comfort as needed.
- Assist in hydrating the child by encouraging oral fluid intake if possible or maintaining IV infusion.
- Assist in discharge planning and home care teaching when the child is able to go home; supportive therapies may be needed at home until resolution of all symptoms, which may take weeks.

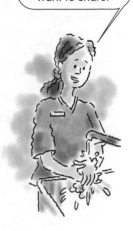

Never skimp on hand washing when caring for a child with RSV. The virus is one thing you definitely don't want to share.

Croup

Croup, also known as acute laryngotracheobronchitis, is a self-limiting upper airway obstructive disease that affects young children (usually younger than age 5). It involves severe inflammation and obstruction of the upper airway and is most common from the late fall to early spring, although it may occur throughout the year.

What causes it

Croup usually results from viral infection with common causative organisms, typically parainfluenza, RSV, *H. influenzae* or mycoplasma pneumoniae. It also may be of bacterial origin (diphtheria or pertussis). It affects more boys than girls, and is typically seen in children between 6 months and 3 years.

How it happens

Croup is usually preceded by an upper respiratory infection that proceeds to laryngitis and then descends into the trachea (and sometimes the bronchi), causing inflammation of the mucosal lining and subsequent narrowing of

How croup affects the upper airway

In croup, inflammatory swelling and spasms constrict the larynx, reducing airflow. This cross-sectional drawing (from chin to chest) shows the upper airway changes caused by croup. Inflammatory changes obstruct the larynx (which includes the epiglottis) almost completely and significantly narrow the trachea.

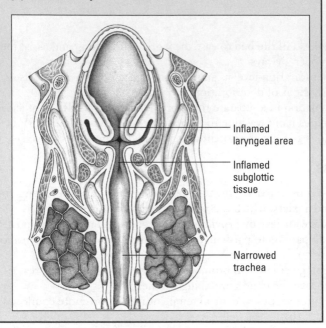

Inflamed laryngeal area

Inflamed subglottic tissue

Narrowed trachea

the airway. Profound airway oedema may lead to obstruction and seriously compromised ventilation. (See *How croup affects the upper airway*.)

If it barks like a seal ...

The flexible larynx of a young child is particularly susceptible to spasm, which may cause complete airway obstruction. When the child's airway is significantly narrowed, he struggles to inhale air past the obstruction and into the lungs, producing the characteristic inspiratory stridor and suprasternal retractions, and the classic barking or seal-like cough.

It's always darkest before the dawn

Croup is characterised by gradual onset of a low-grade fever. Worsening of symptoms at night and a cough is common. The airway obstruction increases, leading to retractions, restlessness, anxiety, tachycardia and tachypnoea. Severe obstruction leads to respiratory exhaustion, hypoxemia, carbon dioxide accumulation and respiratory acidosis.

What to look for
History and physical examination typically reveal:
- history of upper respiratory infection
- inspiratory stridor and substernal and suprasternal retractions

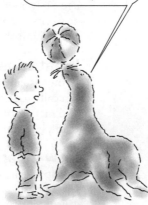

This child with croup has my bark down to pat! I guess imitation really is the sincerest form of flattery.

- barking cough and hoarseness
- pallor or cyanosis
- restlessness and irritability
- low-grade fever
- crackles, rhonchi, expiratory wheezing and localised areas of diminished or absent breath sounds
- retractions, wheezing and cyanosis (in severe cases).

What tests tell you

The diagnosis of croup is based primarily on history and clinical findings. Croup is differentiated from epiglottitis by a lateral neck radiograph that shows a normal epiglottis. X-rays show symmetrical narrowing of the subglottic space ('steeple sign').

Complications

If the child experiences obstruction that's severe enough to prevent adequate exhalation of carbon dioxide, respiratory acidosis results and the child eventually experiences respiratory failure.

How it's treated

The majority of children with croup don't require hospitalisation. The mainstays of home care are time, oral fluids and antipyretics. The major objectives of treatment are to maintain an airway and provide for adequate respiratory exchange. Croup is usually self-limiting and so treatment in hospital or with antibiotics is not needed. There is no real evidence for the effectiveness of increasing humidity so this is not advised.

Reading the signs

Parents must learn the signs of respiratory distress so they can seek medial attention if symptoms progress. Indications for hospitalisation include:
- dusky or cyanotic skin colour
- severe stridor
- significant retractions
- increasing agitation, restlessness, or exhaustion.

Epi for oedema

These medications are used to treat croup in severe cases:
- Nebulised adrenaline is used for its alpha-adrenergic properties, which decrease subglottic inflammation and oedema by causing mucosal vasoconstriction. This drug acts quickly – within 10 to 15 minutes – last about 2 hours, and can be administered as a nebulisation every 20 to 30 minutes for severe croup and every 4 to 6 hours for moderate croup.
- Corticosteroids reduce subglottic oedema and inflammation. Dexamethasone given once early in the course of croup results in a shorter hospital stay and reduces cough and dyspnoea and, commonly, the need for intubation.

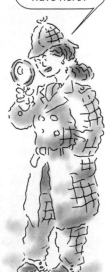

Careful monitoring is key. Hmmm... what do we have here?

• Paracetamol reduces fever, although there is limited evidence about its effectiveness when used for croup.

What to do

The most important nursing intervention for the child with croup is continuous observation and accurate assessment of respiratory status, including careful monitoring of colour, respiratory effort, evidence of fatigue and vital signs to assess for worsening of symptoms that would require further management.

Continually assess for possible respiratory failure, and have intubation equipment readily accessible at the bedside.
• Assess for airway obstruction by evaluating respiratory status.
• Administer prescribed medications, which may include oxygen and adrenaline via nebuliser, antibiotics if croup is bacterial or there is a secondary infection, and corticosteroids to reduce inflammation.
• Because oral hydration is essential to help loosen secretions, encourage the child to drink unless the respiratory rate is greater than 60 breaths/minute, putting them at risk for aspiration. If aspiration risk exists, fluids may need to be administered IV in the very ill child.
• Help the child find the most comfortable position for the best oxygenation. Most infants and small children prefer sitting upright and many want to be held by their parents.

A friend from home

• Help reduce the child's anxiety by maintaining a quiet environment, promoting rest and relaxation and minimising intrusive procedures. Encourage the parents to bring a favourite toy for their child.
• Support the parents, who may be frightened by the rapid progression of croup and the alarming sound of the cough and stridor, by answering questions and explaining treatments and procedures. Encourage them to be present and participate in their child's care as appropriate.
• Educate the parents about caring for the child at home. (See *Croup class*.)

Cystic fibrosis

Cystic fibrosis is a chronic, autosomal-recessive, inherited disorder of the exocrine glands that affects multiple organ systems. It's characterised by chronic airway infection that leads to bronchiectasis, bronchiolectasis, exocrine pancreatic insufficiency, intestinal dysfunction, abnormal sweat gland function and reproductive dysfunction. The disease is the most common fatal genetic disease in white children. Cystic fibrosis is accompanied by many complications. Life expectancy for the person with the disease is currently 32 years.

What causes it

The gene responsible for cystic fibrosis is located on chromosome 7q. It encodes a membrane-associated protein called the cystic fibrosis

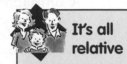

It's all relative

Croup class

Teach parents how to care for their child with croup at home by telling them:

• medication dosages, administration techniques and possible adverse reactions
• symptoms of croup to watch for and report
• how to manage home vaporiser or mist treatments
• how to alleviate symptoms (such as awakening with a barking cough) by putting the child in the bathroom and running hot water to produce steam (always with adult supervision).

transmembrane regulator (CFTR). The exact function of CFTR remains unknown, but it appears to help regulate chloride and sodium transport across epithelial membranes. Causes of cystic fibrosis include abnormal coding found on as many as 350 CFTR alleles and autosomal-recessive inheritance.

How it happens

Abnormally thick secretions affect the normal function of multiple organ systems, including the:
- bronchi, resulting in chronic bronchial pneumonia and obstructive emphysema
- small intestine, causing intestinal obstruction and failure of the neonate to pass meconium (meconium ileus)
- pancreatic ducts, leading to malabsorption syndromes
- bile ducts, leading to biliary cirrhosis and portal hypertension
- salivary and sweat glands, leading to increased sodium and chloride excretion
- autonomic nervous system, which may lead to hyperactivity.

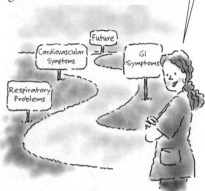

Parents of a child with cystic fibrosis may travel a difficult road; they need ongoing education, support and encouragement.

What to look for

Clinical manifestations may appear at birth or may take years to develop and can vary in severity. Respiratory assessment findings may include:
- dyspnoea
- dry, non-productive cough
- wheezing
- atelectasis and generalised obstructive emphysema due to mucoid obstruction as the disease progresses with the characteristic features of barrel-shaped chest, cyanosis and clubbing of fingers and toes
- chronic sinusitis
- bronchitis
- bronchopneumonia.

Eye on the GI

GI assessment findings include:
- meconium ileus in a neonate
- weight loss despite increased appetite
- malnourishment and vitamin deficiency
- obstruction of pancreatic ducts and absence of pancreatic enzymes, leading to malabsorption syndrome with chronic diarrhoea and large, frothy, foul-smelling stools
- abdominal cramping and distention; foul-smelling flatus
- cirrhosis leading to possible portal hypertension with resultant splenomegaly and oesophageal varices.

The legacy stops here

Reproductive system assessment findings include:
- decreased fertility due to increased viscosity of cervical mucus, blocking the entry of sperm in females

- sterility in males due to blockage of the vas deferens with abnormal secretions, preventing sperm formation.

To the heart of it all

Cardiovascular system assessment findings include:
- right-sided heart enlargement (cor pulmonale) and heart failure resulting from obstruction of pulmonary blood flow
- hyponatraemia, which may lead to circulatory collapse if sodium isn't replaced.

What tests tell you

Elevated sodium and chloride levels detected on a sweat test are used to establish a diagnosis. Stool analysis reveals steatorrhoea (fat in the stool). Chest X-rays show evidence of generalised obstructive emphysema.

Complications

One complication of cystic fibrosis is pneumothorax, which is most commonly caused by rupture of subpleural blebs through the visceral pleura. This condition occurs most commonly in children with more advanced disease. Other complications include bronchiectasis, intestinal obstruction, rectal prolapse, cor pulmonale, diabetes mellitus and nasal polyps.

How it's treated

Pulmonary treatment of cystic fibrosis is aimed at prevention and treatment of pulmonary infection by improving aeration, removing mucopurulent secretions and administering antimicrobial agents.

Twice per day keeps infection away

Prevention of infection is maintained with good pulmonary hygiene with a daily routine of CPT, which is usually performed twice daily and more often if needed during pulmonary infections.

Dilate and stimulate

Bronchodilators delivered in an aerosol help open the bronchi for easier expectoration and are administered before CPT if the child has reactive airway disease or wheezing. Recombinant human deoxyribonuclease can be used to decrease the viscosity of mucus. Physical exercise is also an important adjunct to daily physiotherapy as it stimulates mucus secretion and provides a sense of well-being. Oxygen is administered to children with acute episodes, as needed, but is used cautiously as many of these children have chronic carbon dioxide retention.

What to do

Nursing care will vary depending on where a child is in the disease process and whether they're being treated for an acute exacerbation of pulmonary infection or undergoing routine care.

Oil change not included

When PFTs are low or when children have difficulty breathing or experience a flare-up of infection, they may need to be hospitalised for a 'pulmonary tune-up'. This type of treatment may include:
• IV antibiotic therapy
• rigorous CPT
• inhalation therapy.

The deluxe treatment

Nursing care also involves:
• encouraging pulmonary hygiene (such as CPT, postural drainage, inhaled bronchodilators and breathing exercises) to aid in sputum expectoration
• monitoring respiratory status by evaluating breathing patterns and vital signs.

No dieting here

• promoting adequate nutrition by providing a diet high in calories and protein, with fats as tolerated and prescribed salt supplements during hot weather or febrile periods
• maintaining calorie counts, monitoring intake and output and recording daily weights
• administering medications as ordered, including aminoglycosides to prevent or treat infection, bronchodilators and pancreatic enzymes (Creon or Pancrease)
• administering vitamin supplements and iron and medium-chain triglycerides as dietary supplements.

Infection-free zone

• monitoring for signs of infection and limiting exposure to persons with respiratory infections
• promoting adequate rest by clustering nursing interventions and scheduling regular rest periods
• providing and encouraging activities according to the child's developmental level and physical capabilities, and arranging for a school tutor or help with schoolwork if a school-age child is hospitalised
• providing family support through education and referrals for counselling, support groups and other resources, such as a dietician, social worker, physiotherapist and community children's nurse.

Epiglottitis

Epiglottitis is an acute inflammation of the epiglottis that occurs most commonly in children between 2 and 5 years. Epiglottitis obstructs the airway and needs immediate attention.

What causes it

Epiglottitis commonly results from infection with *H. influenzae* type B but other possible causative organisms include pneumococci and group A streptococci.

How it happens

Epiglottitis is commonly preceded by a minor upper respiratory infection and sore throat of several days duration that rapidly progresses to severe respiratory distress. The child usually goes to bed with no symptoms and then awakens later complaining of a sore throat and difficulty swallowing. If untreated, it may rapidly progress to increasing upper airway obstruction that results in hypoxia, hypercapnia and acidosis, closely followed by decreased muscle tone, altered level of consciousness and, if obstruction becomes complete, sudden death.

What to look for

Health history and physical assessment typically reveal one or more of these signs and symptoms:
- sudden onset of symptoms, commonly preceded by upper respiratory infection
- sore throat, pain on swallowing and refusal to eat or drink due to dysphagia.

There's a frog in my throat

- muffled, thick voice; wheezy inspiratory stridor and snoring expiratory sound with a froglike croaking sound on inspiration (not hoarseness as with croup)
- characteristic positioning of sitting upright, leaning forward, with chin thrust out, mouth open and tongue protruding (tripod position)
- drooling because of difficulty or pain with swallowing.

Hot and toxic

- high fever, toxic appearance
- irritability, restlessness and an anxious, apprehensive, frightened expression
- suprasternal and substernal retractions
- tachycardia and thready pulse.

Hypoxia

Late signs of hypoxia include listlessness, cyanosis, bradycardia and decreased respiratory rate with decreased aeration. On inspection, the child's throat appears red and inflamed with a large, cherry-red, oedematous epiglottis.

A job for the experts

When symptoms of epiglottitis occur, throat inspection should be undertaken only by an ENT specialist or (paediatric) anaesthetist. In

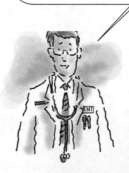

Give me a call if you suspect epiglottitis. Unless it's done by an expert, a throat inspection can make matters worse.

addition, equipment should be readily available for performing emergency ET intubation or tracheotomy because examination may precipitate complete airway obstruction.

What tests tell you
• A lateral neck film showing epiglottal enlargement confirms the diagnosis of epiglottitis.
• Elevated white blood cell (WBC) count and increased bands and neutrophils on differential count may also indicate the diagnosis.
• Identification of causative bacteria through blood cultures will assist with antibiotic selection.

Complications
Complications of epiglottitis include rapid progression of the illness to the point at which the airway is swollen shut, the child is unable to be intubated and may then suffer acute respiratory distress. This is a life-threatening situation and if the respiratory distress isn't reversed in a timely manner, the child can die or suffer from the long-term disabling results of brain anoxia.

How it's treated
The child is immediately transported to a hospital that's set up to manage this type of emergency. Life support measures must be initiated. The child is usually intubated or a tracheotomy is performed to maintain an airway and to allow for ventilation if necessary.

The best treatment of epiglottitis is prevention, and it's recommended that all children receive the *H. influenzae* type B conjugate vaccine beginning at age 2 months.

First by vein, then by mouth

Children with epiglottitis are treated with antibiotics, first IV and then orally, to complete a 7- to 10-day course. Sometimes, corticosteroids are used to reduce oedema during initial treatment. Most intubated children will be treated with corticosteroids for 24 hours before extubation.

The child continues to require intensive observation for the first 24 hours of antibiotic therapy, after which the epiglottal swelling usually decreases. By the third day, the epiglottis is near normal and most children can be extubated at that time.

What to do
Nursing care focuses primarily on maintaining airway patency and observing for any signs of respiratory distress or infection:
• Initiate paediatric life support.
• Closely monitor respiratory status to ensure airway patency; if the child presents with symptoms of epiglottitis, ensure that a throat examination is performed only by a trained professional with emergency equipment on hand.

• After the child is intubated, monitor closely and maintain a patent airway. Suction as needed, and provide oxygen therapy as ordered.
• Observe closely for signs of respiratory distress after extubation.
• Monitor for signs and symptoms of infection.
• Ensure adequate hydration by monitoring IV fluid administration and keeping strict intake and output records.
• Help relieve anxiety by maintaining a calm, relaxing atmosphere, limiting intrusive procedures, encouraging the parents to bring in security objects from home, providing age-appropriate play activities, assisting the child to the most comfortable position for breathing before intubation and administering sedative agents, as prescribed, after the child is intubated.
• Support the family by answering their questions and providing information about diagnosis and treatment. Allow the parents to be present to participate in their child's care, as appropriate.
• Administer prescribed medications, which may include ampicillin and chloramphenicol; sedation with diazepam, pentobarbital or chloral hydrate while the child is being intubated and corticosteroids to reduce oedema.

> Making sure a parent's questions are answered is the best prescription for stress reduction.

Pneumonia

Pneumonia is an acute inflammation or infection of the respiratory bronchioles, alveolar ducts and sacs and alveoli (the parenchyma) of the lungs that impairs gas exchange. It occurs in about 4% of children younger than 4 years; the incidence decreases with advancing age.

What causes it

Infection can result from viruses, bacteria, mycoplasma or aspiration of foreign substances. Viral pneumonia is the most common type, with RSV the most common causative organism. Other viral causes include influenza and parainfluenza viruses, rhinovirus and adenovirus.

Major causative organisms in bacterial pneumonia include pneumococci, streptococci and staphylococci. Children with bacterial pneumonia appear more ill than those with viral pneumonia and have more localised physical findings.

How it happens

Bacterial and viral pneumonia begin as upper respiratory infections:
• Bacterial pneumonia typically begins as a mild upper respiratory infection in which bacteria circulate through the bloodstream to the lungs, leading to cell damage throughout one or more lobes of a single lung.
• Viral, or mycoplasma, pneumonia begins as an upper respiratory tract infection. The virus infiltrates the alveoli near the bronchi of one or both lungs, where they replicate and burst out to kill cells and send out cell debris.

Invasion of the cell snatchers

Invasion of the virus, bacteria or mycoplasma results in exudate from cell death. This exudate fills the alveolar spaces, with pooling and clumping in dependent areas of the lung to create areas of consolidation. Bacterial pneumonia most commonly causes lobular involvement and sometimes consolidation. Viral pneumonia most commonly results in inflammation of interstitial tissue. (See *Types of pneumonia*.)

What to look for

Regardless of the causative agent, symptoms of pneumonia may include:
* raised temperature
* rhonchi
* crackles
* wheezes
* dyspnoea
* tachypnoea
* restlessness
* decreased breath sounds if consolidation exists.

Fretful and feverish

Infants may also demonstrate vomiting, seizures, poor feeding, fretfulness, fever, stiff neck, bulging anterior fontanelle, circumoral cyanosis, respiratory distress, diminished breath sounds and crackles and pleural friction rub.

Headache and hacking

Older children usually experience headache, abdominal or chest pain, high fever with chills, intermittent drowsiness and restlessness, tachycardia, tachypnoea, hacking non-productive cough, expiratory grunting, circumoral cyanosis, diminished breath sounds and disappearance of crackles (indicating consolidation) and moist crackles and cough that produce copious, blood-tinged mucus (as the disease resolves). Some children exhibit only minimal signs which can delay diagnosis.

What tests tell you

Diagnosis of pneumonia is made by chest X-ray, which shows abnormal density of tissue such as lobar consolidation. Other tests include:
* sputum specimen, Gram stain and culture and sensitivity tests help differentiate the type of infection and the drugs that are effective against it
* blood cultures reflect bacteraemia and are used to determine the causative organism
* WBC count reveals leucocytosis in bacterial pneumonia; the WBC count is normal or low in viral or mycoplasmal pneumonia
* ABG levels vary, depending on the severity of pneumonia and the underlying lung state
* pulse oximetry may show a reduced oxygen saturation level.

Complications

Hospitalisation is reserved for seriously ill children. Complications of pneumonia include pleural effusion, empyema and tension pneumothorax. Some effusions require surgical drainage.

Types of pneumonia

Pneumonia is classified according to location and extent of involvement:

* *Lobar pneumonia* involves a large segment of one or more lung lobes; if it involves both lungs it's known as *bilateral* or *double pneumonia*.
* *Bronchopneumonia* begins in the terminal bronchioles and involves nearby lobules, which become clogged to form consolidated patches.
* *Interstitial pneumonia* is confined to the alveolar walls and peribronchial and interlobular tissues.
* *Aspiration pneumonia* is caused by aspiration of fluid or food substance in a child who has difficulty swallowing; who's unable to swallow due to paralysis, weakness, congenital anomalies or who has an absent cough reflex. It can also occur if the child is fed while crying or breathing rapidly.

How it's treated

Treatment of all types of pneumonia consists mainly of symptomatic therapy, such as pain and fever control, supportive care of the airway and hydration status and rest promotion.
• Bacterial pneumonias are treated with organism-sensitive antibiotics; mycoplasma pneumonias may also be treated with antibiotics to prevent secondary bacterial infection.
• Some children may also be treated with anti-inflammatory medications.
• Immunisation against pneumococcal bacteria is recommended for children older than 2 years who are immunosuppressed or have chronic diseases, such as asthma and sickle cell disease.

> Thanks for elevating the head of the bed. It makes my work a lot easier when I'm dealing with pneumonia.

What to do

The goal of nursing care is to restore optimal respiratory function:
• Ease respiratory effort by administering oxygen therapy as prescribed.
• Perform ongoing respiratory assessment, watching for respiratory distress by monitoring vital signs and respiratory status.
• Use a humidifier to increase oxygen humidity.
• Perform CPT as directed, postural drainage and suctioning as needed to remove mucus from airways.
• Reposition the child frequently and elevate the head of the bed to prevent pooling of secretions and ease respirations.
• Provide relief from pain when coughing and deep breathing with such medications as paracetamol and ibuprofen.
• Administer prescribed medications including antibiotics and antipyretics.

What goes in must come out

• Monitor intake and output, and weigh the child daily.
• Encourage adequate oral intake or administer IV fluids to prevent dehydration.
• Promote rest by clustering nursing care to minimise disturbances, and maintain bed rest as necessary to conserve energy.
• Provide a diet of high-calorie foods in small amounts in a relaxed atmosphere.

Keeping parents in the loop

• Provide support to the child and his family by answering questions, providing updates and encouraging the parents to participate in the child's care.
• Begin discharge planning early, providing teaching on medications, especially antibiotics that must be taken at prescribed intervals for the full course.

Tuberculosis

The rates of TB in the UK overall have been decreasing for many years. In 2006 there were 8000 cases reported. Over 70% occurred in people born outside the UK, and nearly half occurred in London.

Individuals at highest risk include the homeless, those with weakened immune systems (such as those with HIV infection or leukaemia or those on corticosteroid therapy), young infants and children with immature immune systems. Cases of TB are mostly found in urban and low-income areas, although the increase in asylum-seeking families may impact on the incidence.

Lying in wait

TB is considered latent when the child is asymptomatic and can't spread the disease to others, but has a positive purified protein derivative (PPD) test result. In these individuals, the body has been able to prevent the infection from growing; however, the infection retains the ability to become active disease in the future, especially if the individual becomes immunocompromised. Active TB occurs when the body can't prevent the bacteria from multiplying and the individual becomes symptomatic.

What causes it

TB is caused by *Mycobacterium tuberculosis*. The main source of infection in children is an infected adult or young person in the household.

How it happens

The lung is the usual portal of infection for human beings. Transmission occurs as the child inhales the microorganisms into the respiratory tract after an infected individual coughs or sneezes. Epithelial cells proliferate around multiplying bacilli of *M. tuberculosis* in an attempt to wall off the invading organisms. This forms the typical tubercle. There's progressive tissue destruction as the primary lesion extends and spreads within the lung, which can produce pneumonia and erode blood vessels.

One kid sneezed and another inhaled. It's into the respiratory tract we go to spread, destroy and erode.

What to look for

Contact with an infected individual is the most important finding of the history. A child may be asymptomatic, but if signs and symptoms do occur, they may include:
- chronic cough
- anorexia
- weight loss or failure to gain weight
- fever.

What tests tell you

The tuberculin test is used to determine if the child has been exposed to the tubercle bacillus. The Mantoux test, which uses PPD injected intradermally, is the recommended procedure. A positive reaction (defined as 10 mm or more induration in 48 to 72 hours) indicates that the child has been exposed and his/her body has developed sensitivity to the protein of the tubercle bacillus; it doesn't, however, confirm the presence of active disease.

Once positive, always positive

After a child has a positive reaction, they'll continue to have positive reactions. A previously negative reaction that converts to a positive indicates that the child has been exposed since the last skin test.

Chest X-rays may be helpful in diagnosis as they may demonstrate hilar lymphadenopathy in active disease or calcification if the disease is in the healing phase.

Complications

Very young children (younger than 2 years), young people and children who are HIV-positive are more affected by the disease and have a higher incidence of disseminated disease. Death seldom occurs in treated children but may be an outcome in those who contract TB meningitis.

How it's treated

Treatment of TB lesions in children consists of drug therapy, general supportive care and prevention of unnecessary exposure to other infections that may further compromise the body's defences. Hospitalisation isn't usually necessary except for needed diagnostic tests or, when indicated, surgery.

Teaming up to treat TB

The use of two or more drugs simultaneously has been found to be optimal, with isoniazid and pyrazinamide given in a 6- to 9-month regimen. Rifampin is used in children who are found to have isoniazid resistance. The guidelines for drug therapy are based on chest X-ray findings after a positive skin test has been verified.

Removing the source

Rarely surgery may be required to remove the source of infection in tissues that aren't affected by drug therapy or tissue that has been destroyed by the disease. Bronchoscopy for removal of a tuberculous granulomatous polyp or resection of a portion of a diseased lung may also be performed.

What to do

Hospitalisation is not usually necessary and so nursing care for children with TB is provided in the outpatient's department or at the GP and can include:

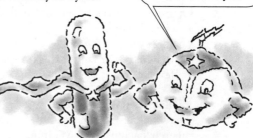

Two or more are better than one when it comes to treating TB – and we're the team for the job!

• Assist with radiographic examinations, perform skin tests and obtain specimens for laboratory examination.
• Encourage the child to attend school and continue life activities as usual. However, older children should be restricted from vigorous activities, such as competitive games and contact sports, during the active stage of TB.
• Encourage compliance with the drug regimen to optimise treatment success. (Parents must be instructed to give the medication at the correct times and for the length of time it's ordered.)

Quick quiz

1. In which anatomical structure does gas exchange take place?
  A. Nasopharynx
  B. Trachea
  C. Bronchioles
  D. Alveoli
Answer: D. The exchange of oxygen for carbon dioxide occurs in the alveoli.

2. A child with difficulty breathing and a 'barking cough' is displaying signs associated with which condition?
  A. Cystic fibrosis
  B. Asthma
  C. Epiglottitis
  D. Croup
Answer: D. A 'barking cough' and difficulty breathing indicate croup. These signs arise as the child attempts to inhale air around a laryngospasm that obstructs the airway.

3. The nurse is assessing the lung sounds of a child with asthma. Which sound is the nurse most likely to hear?
  A. Murmur
  B. Wheezing
  C. Crackles
  D. Pleural friction rub
Answer: B. When listening to the lung sounds of a child with asthma, the most commonly heard adventitious sound is wheezing, which sounds like a musical note.

4. Which condition can rapidly obstruct the airway, requiring immediate attention?
  A. Tonsillitis
  B. Bronchiolitis
  C. Epiglottitis
  D. Tuberculosis
Answer: C. Epiglottitis is an acute inflammation of the epiglottis that can rapidly progress to upper airway obstruction. It requires immediate attention

because, if the obstruction becomes complete, death can result unless emergency treatment such as tracheotomy is initiated.

5. Which sign or symptom suggests cystic fibrosis?
   A. Steatorrhea (fat in the stool)
   B. Decreased appetite
   C. Decreased respiratory rate
   D. Early passage of meconium in the neonatal period

Answer: A. Cystic fibrosis causes thick secretions that block the pancreatic ducts and prevent essential pancreatic enzymes from reaching the duodenum. This condition causes stools that are greasy, foul-smelling and frothy from undigested fats.

Scoring

☆☆☆ If you answered all five items correctly, excellent work! You can breathe easy about your knowledge of respiratory problems.

☆☆ If you answered four items correctly, good job! Your knowledge of respiratory problems in children is unobstructed.

☆ If you answered fewer than four items correctly, don't hyperventilate! Take a deep breath, review the chapter and move on.

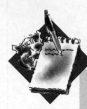

10 Urinary problems

Just the facts

In this chapter, you'll learn:
♦ anatomy and physiology of the urinary tract
♦ assessment of the child with a urinary problem
♦ diagnostic tests and treatments used for urinary problems
♦ specific acquired and congenital urinary disorders.

Anatomy and physiology

The key structures of the genitourinary system are the kidneys and urinary tract.

Kidneys

The kidneys are bean-shaped organs located near the middle of the back. Their primary functions are to filter waste products from the blood and form urine and send it to the bladder through the ureters. Other functions of the kidneys include regulation of volume, electrolyte concentration, acid–base balance of body fluids and blood pressure and support of red blood cell (RBC) production (erythropoiesis).

The kidney is divided into two distinct areas:

🖐 renal cortex – the outside, superficial area of the kidney

🖐 renal medulla – the internal portion of the kidney in which the nephrons are located.

Nephrons

Nephrons are the kidney's functional units. These microscopic structures form urine. (See *A closer look at a nephron*, page 332.)

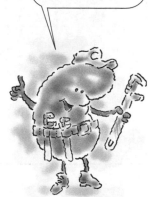

I filter waste from the blood and form urine. It's a dirty job, but someone's gotta do it.

A closer look at a nephron

The nephron is the kidney's basic functional unit and the site of urine formation:

☝ The renal artery, a large branch of the abdominal aorta, carries blood to each kidney.

✌ Blood flows through the interlobular artery (running between the lobes of the kidneys) to the afferent arteriole, which conveys blood to the glomerulus.

🤟 Blood passes through the glomerulus into the efferent arteriole, and into the peritubular capillaries, venules, and the interlobular vein.

🖐 The peritubular capillary network of vessels then supplies blood to the tubules of the nephron.

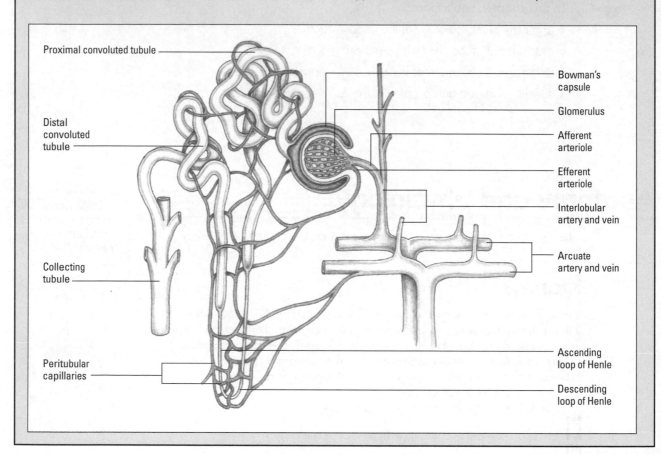

A child acquires the adult number of nephrons shortly after birth, although these structures continue to mature throughout early childhood. The renal corpuscle within the nephron filters blood plasma. The renal tubules within the nephron allow the filtered fluid to pass through on its way to the bladder.

Multitasking kidneys

To produce urine, the various parts of the kidney perform three basic functions:

glomerular filtration (the process of filtering blood as it flows through the kidneys)

tubular resorption

tubular secretion.

While waste products and excess fluids are filtered out of the blood for elimination, necessary fluids, electrolytes, proteins and blood cells are retained (reabsorbed) into the bloodstream.

Urinary tract

The urinary tract consists of the bladder, urethra and ureters.

The bladder is a balloon-shaped pouch of a thin, flexible muscle, in which urine is temporarily stored before being eliminated from the body through the urethra. Urine is produced by the kidneys and passed into the bladder through two ureters, one from each kidney.

A friendly nudge

Peristaltic contractions within the ureters push urine from the kidneys towards the urinary bladder. A valve mechanism prevents urine from backing up into the kidneys as the bladder fills. When the bladder is full:
• the micturition reflex is triggered and nervous innervation causes relaxation of the internal sphincter muscle
• relaxation of the internal sphincter muscle sends a message to the person's conscious mind to indicate the need to void
• the person then releases the external sphincter, and urine passes through the urethra and out of the body.

Any volunteers?

Voluntary control of these urethral sphincters usually occurs in a child between 18 and 24 months. However, the psychological readiness to initiate toilet training may develop much later.

Urine

Urine is a liquid waste product that's filtered out of the blood by the kidneys, stored in the bladder and expelled from the body through the urethra during urination. About 96% of urine is water, and the other 4% is waste product.

A child's bladder can hold 30–45 ml of urine for every year of age. Average urine output will vary according to age (See *Urine output in children*.) and is measured as mls/kg/hour.

Urine output in children

This chart shows the average volume of urine output per 24 hours for children according to age.

Age-group	Urine output
Neonate	50 to 300 ml/day
Infant	300 to 550 ml/day
Preschool	500 to 800 ml/day
School-age	600 to 1,400 ml/day
Adolescent	1,000 to 1,500 ml/day

Diagnostic tests

Diagnostic tests commonly used to assess urinary system problems in children include:
• urinalysis and urine culture
• blood urea nitrogen (BUN) and creatinine levels
• X-ray of the kidneys, ureters and bladder (KUB)
• Ultrasonography
• DMSA (dimercaptosuccinic acid) scan
• micturating cystourethrogram (MCU)
• renal biopsy.

Urinalysis and urine culture

Urinalysis determines urine characteristics, such as specific gravity, pH and physical properties (colour, clarity, odour), and detects the presence of RBCs, white blood cells (WBCs), casts and bacteria.

Culture on a plate

In a urine culture, the urine specimen is placed on a medium and bacteria that may be present are allowed to grow and are then counted. As soon as bacteria are identified, sensitivity testing can determine which antibiotics would be most effective for treating the infection.

Catch 'em while you can

Specimens for urinalysis and urine culture are typically obtained as clean-catch specimens, but may also be obtained from an infant's nappy (urinalysis only), a urine collection bag for infants and young children, bladder catheterisation or a suprapubic bladder tap.

Nursing considerations

Nursing considerations differ according to the child's age and gender. For boys, the head of the penis must be cleaned. For girls, the urinary meatus must be cleaned, carefully washing between the labia.

Lather up, rinse away

For both boys and girls, lukewarm water, which is then rinsed away, is usually used for cleaning. In addition, follow these steps:
• Instruct the child or parents on how to clean the penis or meatus.
• Instruct the child or parents on how to collect the urine specimen by starting to urinate into the toilet bowl to clear the urethra of contaminates, and then catching 90–180 ml (or as much as possible) of urine in a sterile container.
• For neonates and infants, apply a urine bag to obtain a clean specimen; the bag fits over the perineum in females, and the penis (and perhaps the

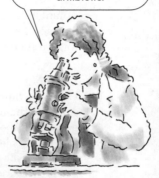

After bacteria are identified with a urine culture, sensitivity testing can be done to choose the best antibiotic.

scrotum) in males to catch urine as the infant voids (instruct the parents to inform you as soon as the child voids, so the container can be removed and faecal contamination can be avoided).
• When obtaining a urine specimen from a catheterised child, don't take the specimen from the collection bag; aspirate a specimen through the collection port in the catheter with a sterile needle and syringe.

Keep it clean

A clean-catch specimen may be needed to diagnose a urinary tract infection (UTI). In addition to the procedures used for routine urinalyses, it's useful to:
• instruct the child or parents to clean the urethral meatus with lukewarm water; the urethral meatus should be cleaned at least three times, using a new wipe or cotton ball each time
• stress to the child and parents the importance of not touching the inside of the sterile container to maintain its sterility.

Blood urea nitrogen and creatinine

Serum BUN and creatinine levels are obtained from blood samples drawn from venepuncture.
• BUN levels can provide a great deal of information about kidney function; they measure the blood nitrogen that's part of the urea resulting from catabolism of amino acids (proteins). When the glomerular filtration rate (GFR) reduces suddenly and severely, the BUN level rises suddenly.
• Plasma creatinine levels become elevated when there's catabolism of creatinine phosphate in skeletal muscles. An elevation in these levels indicates poor renal function.

Nursing considerations

Nursing considerations are aimed at making venepuncture less stressful for the child.
• Use of a surface anaesthetic cream or some other form of topical anaesthetic to make it easier and less traumatic; remember to apply it at least 1 hour before taking blood.
• Allow the parent to be present, and allow the child to hold a comfort object, such as a stuffed animal or blanket, during the venepuncture.
• Follow dietary orders as necessary; sometimes, when BUN levels are elevated, protein intake may need to be limited.

Kidney ureter bladder (KUB) radiography

KUB assesses the size, shape, position and possible areas of calcification of the kidneys, ureters and bladder. A KUB may be required as a first step if a problem with these structures is suspected.

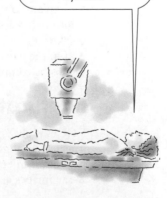

For a child, the hardest part of a KUB is holding still. It's a painless first step towards sorting out a problem in the urinary system.

Nursing considerations

The nurse should help the child remain quiet and lie still during the X-ray. Tell the child that this is their 'job' and that there's no 'hurting part' involved.

Depending on facility policy, parents may be able to remain in the radiology room with the child. The radiographer will instruct them that they must be shielded from radiation by wearing a lead apron.

Ultrasonography

This is a non-invasive scan that can provide information about the structure of the renal tract and possible dilatation of the collecting system.

Nursing considerations

The child and family should have the procedure described to them, assuring them that it will not hurt. The parents should be encouraged to stay with the child during the procedure.

DMSA scan

DMSA scan is a form of X-ray of the lower urinary tract, during which a dye is injected IV A series of X-rays is taken as the dye passes through the bloodstream, is filtered through the kidneys, passed on through the ureters into the bladder and then through the urethra to be eliminated from the body.

Nursing considerations

Begin by explaining the reason for the test to the child and parents, and telling them what to expect.
• Prepare the child for insertion of the IV line and reassure that it's the only injection to be given.
• Assess for a history of allergies to dyes, iodine, shellfish or eggs because of the use of an iodine-based contrast medium.
• Administer a bowel preparation if prescribed; the colon must be emptied because a full bowel won't allow proper visualisation of the urinary tract.
• Following application of surface anaesthetic insert an IV line to allow for the injection of the dye.
• Explain to the child that they may feel warm or a bit woozy when the dye is injected; reassure them that this is normal and that the feeling will pass quickly.
• On the day of the test, allow only clear liquids to be consumed until after the test is completed.

Micturating cystourethrogram

VCUG is an X-ray of the bladder and the lower urinary tract. A catheter is inserted through the urethra into the bladder, and a water-soluble contrast medium is injected through the catheter. The catheter is then withdrawn, and X-ray images are taken as the bladder is emptied.

This test is performed to determine if there are abnormalities of the lower urinary tract, particularly vesicoureteral reflux, a condition that increases the risk of or prolongs a UTI. Sedation is rarely required, nor is it desirable, because the child must urinate during the test.

Nursing considerations

VCUG can be a difficult and uncomfortable test for children and stressful for parents. Insertion of a catheter can also be uncomfortable and embarrassing. The child will be asked to urinate during the test, and to do so without going into the bathroom, which can be confusing to a child who has recently been toilet trained. What's more, the thought of voiding in the X-ray room in full view of the staff can be embarrassing. Reassure the child that the hospital staff understand he/she knows how to use the toilet, and that 'weeing' in a different way is just for the test (explain why this is necessary).

In addition, follow these steps:
• Explain the reason for the test and prepare the child for insertion of the catheter.
• Before the test, make sure the child is dressed in comfortable clothing and is wearing no metal objects.
• Assess for a history of allergies to dyes, iodine, shellfish or eggs because of the use of an iodine-based contrast medium.
• Tell the parents of infants and young children that the child may be wrapped tightly in a blanket to help them lie still during the procedure.
• Assure the parents that the amount of radiation received by the child is minimal.
• Inform the parents that an MCUG can't be performed while the child has an active UTI.

Behind closed doors

• Insert a urinary catheter just before the test; provide as much privacy as possible by closing the door or drawing curtains, and allow a parent to remain in the room if the child desires.
• After the procedure, remove the urinary catheter and encourage the child to drink fluids to reduce burning on urination and to flush out residual dye; pouring a glass of very cold water over the genital area during the first few voids after catheter removal helps to minimise the burning sensation.

Renal biopsy

Although renal biopsy isn't performed routinely in children, it may be used to evaluate decreased kidney function, persistent blood in the urine or protein in the urine. It may also be performed to evaluate the functioning of a newly transplanted kidney.

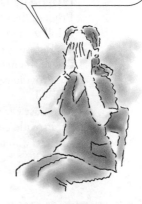

Before a VCUG, reassure the child that the radiographer won't be watching while you're peeing; they'll be looking at the X-ray instead.

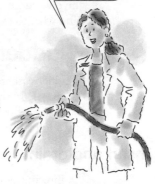

A little cold water can put out the "fire" during a postcatheter void.

In renal biopsy, a needle is inserted through the child's flank under ultrasound guidance. A small specimen of kidney tissue is withdrawn and sent for microscopic study. The child's blood clotting levels should be assessed before the procedure as bleeding can occur afterwards.

The biopsy is performed under a general anaesthetic or by the child using Entenox.

Nursing considerations

Prepare the child and parents for the procedure, which can be frightening. Use a doll to show the child how it will be done. In addition, follow these steps:

• Reassure the parents that ultrasound will allow the doctor to see exactly where the needle will be inserted and thus prevent damage to other organs.

• Provide care and support based on the anaesthetic or analgesia/sedation utilised.

• Assist with positioning and holding the child throughout the procedure.

• Provide education to the parents and child where appropriate about signs to watch for when at home such as infection, bleeding from the site. Immediate help should be sought.

Treatments and procedures

Common treatments and procedures used in the care of a child with a urinary disorder include bladder catheterisation, haemodialysis, kidney transplantation, and peritoneal dialysis.

Always prepare children for treatments and procedures with an age-appropriate explanation of what to expect. When treatments and procedures involve surgery, preparation should include an explanation of the anaesthesia and what to expect post-operatively.

Bladder catheterisation

Bladder catheterisation may be performed for diagnostic or treatment purposes. In this procedure, the urethral meatus is thoroughly cleaned, local anaesthetic gel is inserted and an appropriate-sized catheter is inserted through the urethra into the bladder.

Insert and drain

In intermittent catheterisation, a straight catheter is inserted and a urine specimen may be taken; the catheter is removed after the bladder is drained.

Insert and inflate

If the catheter is to remain in place, an indwelling catheter, also called a Foley catheter, may be used and attached to a drainage bag for urine collection. An indwelling catheter has an inflatable balloon near its tip to hold the catheter in place in the bladder.

Nursing considerations

Remember that catheterisation can be uncomfortable and embarrassing for a child. The older child may feel more comfortable when a same-sex nurse inserts the catheter. The younger child may be confused and fearful if they have been told it's wrong for anyone to touch their 'private parts'. Have the parents explain to the child that this situation is different.

To minimise trauma, follow these steps:
• Educate the child and parents about the purpose of the catheterisation; if it's being done to obtain a sterile specimen, explain why this is preferable to a clean-catch specimen.
• Prepare the child to facilitate the procedure and ease the child's fears; use a doll to show them what will happen.
• Be sure to choose the appropriate-sized catheter. (For a premature neonate, a size 5 French feeding tube may be used; for a larger infant or a small toddler, use a size 8 French feeding tube; for children ages 4 and older, use a size 8 French to 14 French catheter.)
• Provide as much privacy as possible; close the door, draw the room divider curtain and allow the child to keep on as much clothing as possible.
• Allow the parent to be present if the child desires.
• Give the child coping mechanisms to deal with discomfort (such as 'Squeeze your mother's hand if it hurts', or, 'Count to 10 and the hurting part will be over').

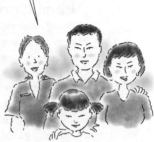

A young child may need their parents' okay for a doctor or nurse to touch parts of the body that are otherwise off-limits to adults.

Generous and gentle

When inserting the catheter:
• Clean the urethral meatus three times, using a different swab each time.
• Generously lubricate the tip of the catheter and gently insert it through the urethra into the bladder until urine returns and is collected in the sterile specimen container.
• If the catheter doesn't easily enter the meatus, use a smaller catheter; never force it into the urethral meatus.
• If performing an intermittent catheterisation, gently remove the catheter after the bladder is drained, clean off the lubricant with water.
• If inserting an indwelling urinary catheter, insert the inflatable balloon with sterile water and gently pull on the catheter to make sure it inflated; next, connect the catheter to the closed drainage system.
• Record the amount of fluid inserted into the balloon in the health records

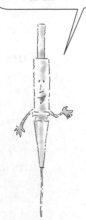

When it comes to children and catheters, one size doesn't fit all.

Haemodialysis

Haemodialysis involves the use of a machine to clean waste products from the bloodstream if the kidneys are severely damaged or have failed. The blood travels through tubes to an artificial kidney in the machine, and waste products and excess fluid are removed from the body. The purified blood then flows back to the body through another set of tubes.

To stick or not to stick

The child on haemodialysis may have a double-lumen central catheter in place in his chest to serve as a site for blood removal. Children needing long-term dialysis may have a subcutaneous graft, anastomosing a vein and an artery. This graft reduces the risk of infection but means the child will need two venepunctures each time dialysis is performed. EMLA cream should be used to reduce discomfort.

Nursing considerations

Provide diversional activities to prevent boredom, such as computer games, music, drawing or colouring materials and DVDs; encourage a family member to stay with the child. In addition, follow these steps:
• Weigh the child before beginning haemodialysis.
• If the child has a subcutaneous graft, check the blood access site every 2 hours for patency and signs of clotting; don't use the arm with this site for taking blood pressure or drawing blood.
• During dialysis, monitor vital signs, clotting times, blood flow, the function of the vascular access site, and arterial and venous pressures.

Look out for losses

• Watch for complications, such as septicaemia, embolism, hepatitis and rapid fluid and electrolyte loss.
• After dialysis, monitor vital signs and the vascular access site; weigh the patient and watch for signs of fluid and electrolyte imbalances.
• Use standard precautions when handling blood and body fluids.

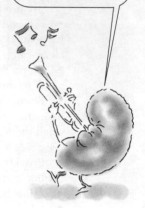

A set of headphones and a mp3 player can be a great antidote to boredom during haemodialysis.

Kidney transplantation

Kidney transplantation involves replacing a diseased kidney with a healthy kidney from another person. The donor kidney may come from a living donor or a cadaver donor. Although haemodialysis and peritoneal dialysis are life-preserving procedures and may even be carried out in the home, kidney transplantation is the preferred method of renal replacement therapy for children because it offers the opportunity for a normal life.

Nursing considerations

By the time a child undergoes kidney transplantation, they most likely have a long history of procedures and hospitalisations. The child should be given as many choices as possible; a choice as simple as which arm to use for venepuncture can help to give the child a sense of control.
    In addition, follow these steps:
• Provide emotional support and guidance to the child and parents; prepare them for the procedure, including what will occur pre-operatively, during the procedure, and post-operatively.
• Arrange for the child and parents to tour the children's intensive care unit and meet the nursing staff before the transplantation.

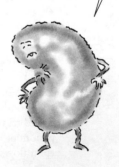

When I can't do my job, the professionals send in a replacement – a healthy kidney from a living person or a cadaver.

- Administer immunosuppressive medications as prescribed; a child who will have or has had a kidney transplant will be taking immunosuppressive medications to decrease the risk of organ rejection.
- Monitor for signs and symptoms of infection; while immunosuppressed, the child is at increased risk for infection.

You sneeze, you leave

- Make sure that no one with obvious infection takes care of the child.
- Prepare the child (and parents) for the possibility of continuing to need haemodialysis temporarily after the transplant because the transplanted kidney might not work effectively right away.

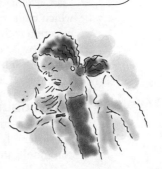

It isn't worth the risk. Even the common cold can pose a major threat to an immunosuppressed child.

Peritoneal dialysis

In peritoneal dialysis, the blood is cleaned of waste products and excess fluids using the lining of the abdomen as a filter. Peritoneal dialysis is especially useful for children who are poor risks for vascular access and for those who live far from a medical centre. This procedure includes these steps:
- With the child under a general anaesthetic a peritoneal dialysis catheter is inserted through a small abdominal incision or a puncture hole into the peritoneal cavity. The catheter is then connected to fluid bags and tubing.
- A cleaning solution is drained from a bag into the abdomen.
- Fluids and waste products flow through the lining and are 'caught' by the dialysis fluid.
- This fluid is then drained from the abdomen, taking the extra fluids and waste products with it.

Nursing considerations

Prepare the child and parents for the insertion of the catheter into the abdominal cavity. Make sure a valid informed consent form has been signed and included in the health records. In addition, follow these steps:
- Monitor the child's reaction to the sedation, anaesthesia and pain management regimen.
- Make sure strict sterile technique is used at all times during catheter placement and peritoneal dialysis.
- Monitor the child's response to the therapy.
- Make the child as comfortable as possible and provide sufficient rest periods.
- Assess for bleeding from the catheter insertion site.
- Maintain patency of the peritoneal dialysis catheter; keep it in place, without kinks or pulling, and with the fluid bags at the correct level.
- Monitor for signs of infection at the insertion site.

Urinary disorders

Urinary disorders that may affect children include acute post-streptococcal glomerulonephritis, chronic glomerulonephritis, congenital urologic anomalies, haemolytic uraemic syndrome, nephrotic syndrome, renal failure (acute and chronic) and Wilms' tumour.

Acute post-streptococcal glomerulonephritis

Glomerulonephritis is an inflammation of the tubules of the kidneys (glomeruli), which filter waste products from the blood. When this inflammation follows an infection with streptococcal bacteria (most commonly via strep throat), it's called acute post-streptococcal glomerulonephritis. It's most commonly seen in boys between 3 and 7 years but can occur at any age. Up to 95% of children recover fully; the rest may progress to chronic renal failure.

What causes it

Acute post-streptococcal glomerulonephritis typically follows a group A beta-haemolytic streptococcal infection of the respiratory tract. Less commonly, it may follow a skin infection such as impetigo.

How it happens

The disease usually begins about 1 to 6 weeks after a streptococcal infection, although 2 weeks is the most common time of onset.

Clumping with the enemy

In this immunologic disorder, antigens from streptococci clump together with the antibodies that killed them, and become trapped in the tubules of the kidneys. The tubules become inflamed, and oedema of the capillary walls decreases the amount of glomerular perfusion. The kidneys then become incapable of filtering and eliminating body wastes.

What to look for

Oedema may initially appear in the face, especially around the eyes. Later, oedema may occur in the legs. Changes in urination may include low urine output (oliguria), blood in the urine (haematuria), protein in the urine (proteinuria) and cola-coloured (smoky) urine. Other signs and symptoms may include:
- high blood pressure
- mild anaemia, pallor
- joint pain and stiffness
- malaise, lethargy
- anorexia
- fever
- headache.

What tests tell you

Urinalysis reveals the presence of protein, RBCs and WBCs in the urine. Blood studies show elevated levels of urea and creatinine.
- Antistreptolysin-O test confirms that the child has had a streptococcal infection.

- Throat culture, if performed during an acute infection, confirms the presence of group A beta-haemolytic streptococci.
- Renal ultrasound shows slightly enlarged kidneys bilaterally.
- Renal biopsy may be performed to assess the renal tissue or confirm the diagnosis.

Complications

No complications are typically associated with acute post-streptococcal glomerulonephritis. Generally, a full recovery can be expected within a matter of weeks to months. If complications occur, they may include:
- hypertensive encephalopathy
- chronic or progressive problems of kidney function
- renal failure (in rare instances)
- pulmonary oedema and heart failure (occasionally).

How it's treated

Treatment may involve antibiotics for 7 to 10 days to treat infections contributing to the ongoing antigen-antibody response. Other medications may include:
- antihypertensives to control high blood pressure
- diuretics to reduce fluid retention and oedema
- corticosteroids to decrease antibody synthesis and suppress the inflammatory response.

A child with acute poststreptococcal glomerulonephritis might have to wait a while for chips and pepperoni pizza.

Lay low

The child may be placed on bed rest to reduce metabolic demands. In the acute phase, a low-sodium, low-protein diet may be required to prevent fluid retention, and fluid restrictions to decrease oedema. In rare instances, dialysis may be necessary.

What to do

Nursing care of the child with acute post-streptococcal glomerulonephritis focuses on monitoring and education.
- Check vital signs; monitor intake and output and measure the child's weight daily.
- Assess urea and electrolytes regularly
- Assess renal function daily through serum creatinine, BUN and urine creatinine clearance levels; watch for and immediately report signs of acute renal failure (oliguria, azotaemia and acidosis) and monitor for ascites and oedema.

Battle the boredom

- Provide quiet, age-appropriate activities that the child can enjoy while on bed rest; allow them to gradually resume normal activities as symptoms subside.
- Monitor for signs of complications, such as sudden major changes in vital signs, a change in the amount or appearance of urine output, significant weight gain, changes in vision, changes in motor abilities, seizure activity, severe pain or behavioural changes.

Medication education

- Teach the child and parents about medications the child will be taking; tell them that the child should continue taking the prescribed medications even if feeling better, and to report adverse effects.
- Teach the child and parents about necessary dietary restrictions.

Strep alert

- Advise the child and parents to immediately report signs of a streptococcal throat infection, such as sore throat and fever.
- Teach the parents to monitor the child's weight and blood pressure on a regular basis; instruct them to report changes in the child's condition, such as increased oedema, changes in appetite, signs of infection, abdominal pain, headaches, lethargy or changes in urine output.

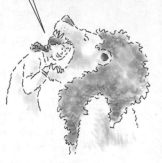

After a child has had acute poststreptococcal glomerulonephritis, a sore throat can take on gigantic significance!

Chronic glomerulonephritis

Chronic glomerulonephritis results from slow, progressive destruction of the glomeruli of the kidney with progressive loss of kidney function. It may eventually result in renal failure.

What causes it

Most cases of chronic glomerulonephritis are thought to be caused by an abnormality of the immune system. Other causes may include:
- systemic lupus erythematosus (SLE)
- bacteremia associated with a ventriculoperitoneal shunt
- exposure to organic solvents, mercury or certain non-steroidal anti-inflammatory drugs
- human immunodeficiency virus infection.

How it happens

Because chronic glomerulonephritis may go undetected for years until renal function declines markedly, it's more commonly diagnosed during adolescence than in early childhood.

Damage, changes, impairment

Damage to the glomeruli of the kidneys is caused by abnormal immune responses – possibly a direct attack on the kidney itself or accumulated immune complexes in the glomerular filter. Chronic changes to the structure of the glomeruli result. These changes impair renal function – specifically, inefficient filtering of the blood. Blood and protein then spill into the urine.

What to look for

In chronic glomerulonephritis, symptoms of declining renal function may be present along with haematuria, proteinuria and hypertension that doesn't respond to routine treatment. Nephrotic syndrome may develop.

What tests tell you
• Urinalysis shows a high specific gravity and the presence of blood, casts and protein.
• Blood chemistry shows hyperkalaemia and anaemia.
• Ultrasound, computerised tomography (CT) scan or excretory urography may show small kidneys.
• Renal biopsy may show one of the forms of chronic glomerulonephritis or non-specific scarring of the glomeruli.

Complications
Complications of chronic glomerulonephritis may include nephrotic syndrome, chronic renal failure, end-stage renal disease, chronic hypertension, malignant hypertension, heart failure, pulmonary oedema, chronic or recurrent UTI and increased susceptibility to other infections.

How it's treated
Treatment of chronic glomerulonephritis is largely symptomatic and may include:
• antihypertensive medications to control blood pressure
• corticosteroids or immunosuppressive medications to suppress inflammatory and immune responses
• restricted dietary intake of salt, fluids and proteins to help in the control of hypertension
• dialysis or kidney transplantation if renal failure develops.

What to do
Care of the child with chronic glomerulonephritis includes careful monitoring and long-term follow-up. Provide emotional support and reassurance to the child and parents and be sure to include clear explanations of procedures. In addition, follow these steps:
• Weigh the child daily at the same time of day. Carefully measure and record intake and output.
• Monitor vital signs and watch for and report signs of inadequate renal perfusion (hypotension) and acidosis.

Strike a balance

Maintain proper electrolyte balance by:
• strictly monitoring potassium levels
• watching for symptoms of hyperkalaemia (malaise, anorexia, paraesthesia or muscle weakness)
• monitoring for and immediately reporting electrocardiogram (ECG) changes (tall, peaked T waves; widening QRS segment and disappearing P waves)
• avoiding medications containing potassium. (See *Managing the child with hyperkalaemia*, page 346.)

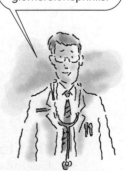

A good relationship with the health care team is essential to help the child and family deal with chronic glomerulonephritis.

Advice from the experts

Managing the child with hyperkalaemia

Emergency treatment is needed for the child with acute hyperkalaemia (a serum potassium level higher than 7 mmol/L or electrocardiogram changes). Hypertonic glucose, insulin, and calcium gluconate may be administered because they provide a rapid, although temporary, reduction in potassium. However, these infusions won't remove potassium from the body. They may be used until a slower-acting agent, such as sodium polystyrene sulfonate (Kayexalate), can be administered. Kayexalate can be administered orally or rectally to bind potassium and remove it from the body.

During emergency treatment to lower potassium levels, assess the patient frequently.

- If the child receives hypertonic glucose and insulin infusions, monitor potassium and glucose levels.
- If the child receives calcium gluconate, monitor calcium and potassium levels.
- If Kayexalate is given rectally, make sure the child doesn't retain it and become constipated (to prevent bowel perforation).

Follow through on the follow-up

In addition, the importance of long-term medical follow-up should be stressed to the parents. They should also be informed that follow-up renal biopsies will be needed every 2 to 5 years. If renal failure occurs, the child and parents should be prepared for the possibility of an eventual kidney transplant.

Congenital anomalies of the ureter, bladder and urethra

Congenital anomalies of the ureter, bladder and urethra are among the most common birth defects, occurring in about 5% of births. Some of these abnormalities are obvious at birth; others are recognised only after they produce symptoms.

What causes it
Causes of these congenital anomalies are unknown.

How it happens
The most common malformations include duplicated ureter, retrocaval ureter, ectopic orifice of the ureter, stricture or stenosis of the ureter, ureterocele, exstrophy of the bladder, congenital bladder diverticulum, hypospadias and epispadias. Their pathophysiology, signs and symptoms, diagnosis and treatments vary. (See *Congenital urologic anomalies*.)

What to look for
Signs and symptoms will vary. (See *Congenital urologic anomalies*.)

Congenital urologic anomalies

Three congenital urologic anomalies are described here, along with their pathophysiology, clinical features and diagnosis and treatment.

Duplicated ureter	Retrocaval ureter (preureteral vena cava)	Ectopic orifice of ureter

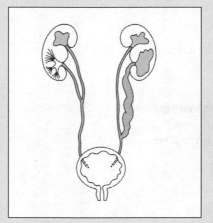 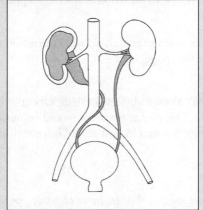 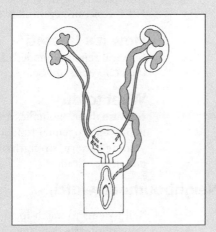

Duplicated ureter

Pathophysiology
- Most common ureteral anomaly
- Complete—double collecting system with two separate pelves, each with its own ureter and orifice
- Incomplete—two separate ureters that join before entering the bladder.

Clinical features
- Persistent or recurrent infection
- Frequency, urgency or burning on urination
- Diminished urine output
- Flank pain, fever and chills.

Diagnosis and treatment
- DMSA scan
- Voiding cystoscopy
- Cystoureterography
- Retrograde pyelography
- Surgery for obstruction, reflux or severe renal damage.

Retrocaval ureter (preureteral vena cava)

Pathophysiology
- Right ureter that passes behind the inferior vena cava before entering the bladder (with compression of the ureter between the vena cava and the spine that causes dilation and elongation of the pelvis; hydroureter, hydronephrosis and fibrosis and stenosis of the ureter in the compressed area)
- Relatively uncommon; higher incidence in males.

Clinical features
- Right flank pain
- Recurrent urinary tract infection
- Renal calculi
- Haematuria.

Diagnosis and treatment
- DMSA scan demonstrating superior ureteral enlargement with spiral appearance
- Surgical resection and anastomosis of the ureter with the renal pelvis, or reimplantation into the bladder.

Ectopic orifice of ureter

Pathophysiology
- Ureters single or duplicated in females (ureteral orifice usually inserting in urethra or vaginal vestibule, beyond external urethral sphincter)
- In males, in prostatic urethra, seminal vesicles or vas deferens.

Clinical features
- Symptoms rare if ureteral orifice opening between trigone and bladder neck
- Obstruction, reflux and incontinence (dribbling) in 50% of females
- In males, flank pain, frequency, urgency.

Diagnosis and treatment
- DMSA scan
- Urethroscopy, vaginoscopy
- Voiding cystourethrography
- Resection and ureteral reimplantation into the bladder for incontinence.

What tests tell you

With the exception of bladder exstrophy, hypospadias and epispadias (which can be diagnosed on clinical examination), diagnostic tests are used to visualise the defect.

Complications

Complications will vary according to the specific anomaly but may include UTI, vesicoureteral reflux, voiding dysfunction and hydronephrosis.

How it's treated

Surgical repair is needed. The specific procedure will depend on the anomaly. (See *Congenital urologic anomalies*, page 347.)

What to do

Because these anomalies aren't always obvious at birth, carefully evaluate the neonate's urogenital function. Document the amount and colour of urine, voiding pattern, strength of stream and indications of infection, such as fever and urine odour.

Neighbourhood watch

Tell parents to watch for these signs at home. In all children, watch for signs of obstruction, such as dribbling, oliguria or anuria, abdominal mass, hypertension, fever, bacteriuria or pyuria.

When caring for the hospitalised child, follow these steps:
• Monitor renal function daily; record intake and output accurately; weigh nappies if necessary.
• Follow strict sterile technique in handling cystostomy tubes or indwelling urinary catheters.
• Make sure that ureteral, suprapubic or urethral catheters remain in place and don't become contaminated; document type, colour and amount of drainage.
• Apply cling film to protect the exposed mucosa of the neonate with bladder exstrophy; don't use heavy clamps on the umbilical cord and avoid dressing or putting nappies on the infant.
• Provide reassurance and emotional support to the parents and, when possible, allow them to participate in their child's care to promote normal bonding.
• As appropriate, suggest or arrange for genetic counselling.

Haemolytic uraemic syndrome

Haemolytic uraemic syndrome is a complex of symptoms that includes acute renal failure, haemolytic anaemia and thrombocytopenia. It's an acute renal disease that occurs mostly in infants and children from 6 months to 3 years. It's one of the main causes of acute renal failure in the young child.

What causes it

The tendency to develop haemolytic uraemic syndrome may be genetically determined by an autosomal mode of inheritance.

The usual suspects

Haemolytic uraemic syndrome usually follows an attack of infectious bacterial diarrhoea caused by *Escherichia coli*, Shigella, Salmonella, Yersinia or Campylobacter. Viral infections, such as varicella, echovirus and coxsackie A and B, may also cause it. Haemolytic uraemic syndrome may follow an upper respiratory infection, and may be associated with such long-term illnesses as acquired immunodeficiency syndrome and cancer.

> We cannot tell a lie. One of us is usually the culprit in a case of haemolytic uraemic syndrome.

How it happens

The bacterial infection causes endothelial cell injury in the lining of the small glomerular arterioles. The endothelial cell damage triggers microvascular lesions with platelet-fibrin microthrombi that occlude the arterioles and capillaries. This platelet aggregation results in thrombocytopenia, and the kidneys become swollen and pale.

Although damage occurs mainly in the endothelial lining of the glomerular arterioles, other organs may be involved. Heart failure and arrhythmias may occur from cardiac involvement. Pancreatitis or type 1 diabetes mellitus may occur from pancreatic involvement. Retinal or vitreous haemorrhage may occur from ocular involvement.

What to look for

The history typically shows a recent episode of diarrhoea. Less commonly, there may be a history of upper respiratory tract infection or viral infection. Signs and symptoms may include:

- irritability, weakness, lethargy
- pallor
- ecchymosis and petechiae, purpura
- decreased or absent urine output (oliguria or anuria)
- hypertension
- GI bleeding with blood in stool
- seizures
- heart failure.

What tests tell you

A urinalysis shows the presence of protein and RBCs, haemosiderin, WBCs and casts.

In the blood

> Blood work is the mainstay of diagnostic testing in a child with suspected haemolytic uraemic syndrome.

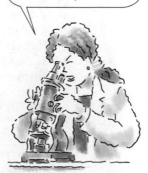

Blood studies show:
- microangiopathic haemolytic anaemia (severe) and mild-to-moderate thrombocytopenia
- prothrombin time, activated partial thromboplastin time and fibrinogen levels within normal ranges
- elevated lactate dehydrogenase and indirect bilirubin levels
- markedly elevated BUN and creatinine levels
- increased reticulocyte count

- negative Coombs' test
- moderately elevated WBC count
- plasma containing free haemoglobin, the concentration of which coincides with the degree of the anaemia.

I got cultcha

Other studies may include a stool culture, which may be positive for a specific type of *E. coli*. Bone marrow biopsy shows hyperplasia. Renal biopsy would clinically establish the diagnosis but is rarely required.

Complications

Complications of haemolytic uraemic syndrome may include:
- hypertension
- acute renal failure
- chronic renal failure
- need for haemodialysis
- neurological deficits with seizures and coma
- stroke
- bleeding complications such as disseminated intravascular coagulation (DIC).

How it's treated

Antibiotics aren't effective in treating haemolytic uraemic syndrome, except when caused by *Shigella dysenteriae*. Treatment of haemolytic uraemic syndrome is mainly supportive and may include:
- maintenance of adequate fluid and electrolyte balance and correction of acidosis to prevent seizures and azotaemia
- management of hypertension with antihypertensive medications and, if needed, fluid and salt restriction
- early dialysis if acute renal failure occurs
- daily plasma exchange until remission is achieved (rarely and in very severe cases).

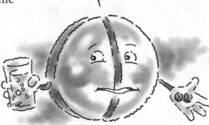

Sorry. Antibiotics aren't effective for haemolytic uremic syndrome unless *Shigella dysenteriae* is to blame.

What to do

Monitoring and maintaining fluid and electrolyte balance is important. Intake and output should be accurately recorded, and the child's weight should be recorded once or twice daily during the acute phase.
- Monitor blood pressure and pulse pressure at least every 4 hours.
- Assess hydration status at least every 4 to 6 hours.
- Monitor the child's nutritional status.
- Observe and report signs and symptoms of complications, such as seizures, shock, infection and DIC.
- Prepare the child and family for the possibility of haemodialysis or peritoneal dialysis.
- Teach the parents and child to avoid eating raw or partially cooked meat or drinking untreated water to decrease the risk of infection with *E. coli*.

Nephrotic syndrome

Nephrotic syndrome is a condition in which the kidneys lose a significant amount of protein in the urine, resulting in low blood levels of protein. The syndrome is characterised by proteinuria, hypoalbuminaemia, hyperlipidaemia and oedema. The prognosis is highly variable depending on the underlying cause.

Preschool predominance

Primary nephrotic syndrome occurs predominantly in preschool children; the incidence peaks between ages 2 and 3, and the syndrome is rare after age 8. It's more common in boys than in girls. Some forms of nephrotic syndrome may eventually progress to end-stage renal disease.

What causes it

Causes of nephrotic syndrome include:
* lipid nephrosis
* glomerulonephritis
* metabolic diseases such as diabetes mellitus
* collagen-vascular disorders such as SLE
* circulatory diseases, such as heart failure, sickle cell anaemia and renal vein thrombosis
* nephrotoxins, such as mercury, gold and bismuth
* allergic reactions.

How it happens

In nephrotic syndrome, the injured glomerular filtration membrane allows the loss of plasma proteins, especially albumin and immunoglobulin, resulting in decreased levels of serum albumin (hypoalbuminemia). Hypoalbuminemia results in decreased colloidal osmotic pressure and fluid accumulation in the interstitial spaces. Oedema subsequently results from sodium and water retention. (See *What happens in nephrotic syndrome*, page 352.)

What to look for

Signs and symptoms of nephrotic syndrome include:
* oliguria with dark, concentrated urine
* oedema starting around the eyes (periorbital) and then becoming more generalised
* weight gain
* abdominal distension, which may be so severe that it causes respiratory difficulty, abdominal pain, anorexia and diarrhoea
* irritability
* lethargy, easy fatigability and activity intolerance
* pallor
* hypertension (in later stages).

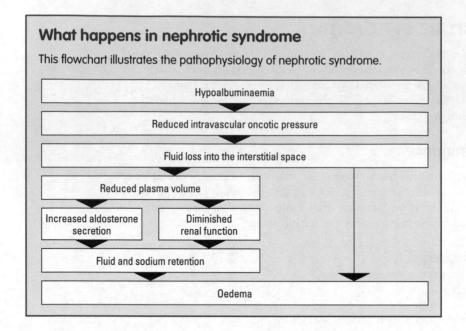

What happens in nephrotic syndrome

This flowchart illustrates the pathophysiology of nephrotic syndrome.

Hypoalbuminaemia

Reduced intravascular oncotic pressure

Fluid loss into the interstitial space

Reduced plasma volume

Increased aldosterone secretion

Diminished renal function

Fluid and sodium retention

Oedema

What tests tell you

Urinalysis shows severe proteinuria, haematuria and casts; it also shows an elevated specific gravity because of the proteinuria. When performed, renal biopsy identifies the type of nephrotic syndrome the child has, and can be used to monitor response to medical management.

Highs and lows

Blood studies show:
- high levels of lipids, especially cholesterol (hypercholesterolemia)
- low levels of protein, especially albumin
- normal to high haematocrit and haemoglobin level
- high platelet levels.

Complications

Complications of nephrotic syndrome may include:
- hypovolaemic shock
- venous thrombosis
- respiratory difficulties
- impaired skin integrity from severe oedema
- infection
- loss of proteins required to fight infections, resulting in increased risk of infections
- loss of proteins that prevent blood from clotting, resulting in clot formation within the blood vessels
- adverse effects of steroid therapy.

How it's treated

Prednisone commonly produces a rapid improvement in symptoms (remission). IV administration of albumin may be used, followed by IV furosemide to induce diuresis. If marked hypertension exists, antihypertensive medications may be used. Other medications may include:
- pain medication to lessen discomfort
- prophylactic antibiotics to control and prevent infection
- immunosuppressive medications for children who don't respond to steroids.

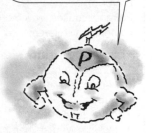

Prednisilone is my name – nephrotic syndrome remission is my game!

Hold the salt

Dietary changes may include some restriction of salt (sodium) intake. Bed rest may be required during the acute phase, especially if the child is hypertensive.

What to do

The child with nephrotic syndrome is likely to require multiple hospitalisations. Because these hospitalisations interrupt the child's normal routine, it's important to provide activities that support their continued development, and simply allow them to have some normal fun.

A delicate balance

Other interventions focus on monitoring and assessment:
- Maintain fluid balance and monitor for signs of fluid volume excess, such as oedema, ascites, weight gain, decreased and concentrated urine and pulmonary congestion.
- Assess for signs of electrolyte imbalance including cardiovascular, neurological, GI and skin changes and report these.
- Assess general nutritional status and work, with dietetic advice, to improve it by providing a diet the child will eat (with sufficient protein and other nutrients, and without excess sodium).
- Assess for adverse effects of medications, and report them to medical staff as soon as possible.

Protection from infection

- Assess for signs of infection and work to prevent it; if infection occurs, report it as soon as possible.
- Monitor for pain and provide appropriate pain relief measures.
- Provide emotional support and education to the child and parents.

Renal failure, acute

Renal failure is a general term used to describe what happens when the kidneys aren't functioning at an optimum level. In acute renal failure, the kidneys suddenly stop filtering waste products from the blood.

Causes of acute renal failure

The causes of acute renal failure may be classified as prerenal, intrarenal, or postrenal.

Prerenal

Prerenal causes, which are most common in children, may include:

- arrhythmias that cause reduced cardiac output
- heart failure
- burns
- dehydration
- diuretic overuse, hemorrhage, hypo-volemic shock
- disseminated intravascular coagulation
- sepsis.

Intrarenal

Intrarenal causes of acute renal failure include:

- poorly treated prerenal failure
- nephrotoxins
- transfusion reaction
- acute glomerulonephritis, acute interstitial nephritis, or acute pyelonephritis
- sickle cell anemia
- systemic lupus erythematosus.

Postrenal

Postrenal causes of renal failure are uncommon in children older than age 1 year. They may include:

- bladder obstruction
- ureteral obstruction
- urethral obstruction.

What causes it

Most commonly, acute renal failure in children is a temporary condition resulting from dehydration or other condition that causes poor renal perfusion (which can be resolved by increasing the child's fluid volume). The causes of acute renal failure may be classified as prerenal, intrarenal or postrenal. (See *Causes of acute renal failure*.)

How it happens

The pathophysiology of acute renal failure varies depending on whether the cause is prerenal, intrarenal or postrenal.

Prerenal failure

Prerenal failure ensues when a condition that diminishes blood flow to the kidneys leads to hypoperfusion.

It's rude to interrupt

When renal blood flow is interrupted, so is oxygen delivery. The ensuing hypoxemia and ischemia can rapidly and irreversibly damage the kidney. The renal tubules are most susceptible to hypoxemia's effects.

Azotaemia (excess nitrogenous waste products in the blood) develops in 40% to 80% of patients with acute renal failure and is also a consequence of renal hypoperfusion. The impaired blood flow results in a decreased GFR and increased tubular resorption of sodium and water. Usually, restoring renal blood flow and glomerular filtration reverses azotaemia.

Intrarenal failure

Intrarenal failure, also called intrinsic or parenchymal renal failure, results from damage to the filtering structures of the kidneys. Causes of intrarenal failure are classified as nephrotoxic, inflammatory or ischaemic.

Damage in the basement

When the damage is caused by nephrotoxicity or inflammation, the delicate layer under the epithelium (the basement membrane) becomes irreparably damaged, typically leading to chronic renal failure.

Severe or prolonged lack of blood flow caused by ischemia may lead to renal damage (ischaemic parenchymal injury) and excess nitrogen in the blood (intrinsic renal azotaemia).

Totally radical

Acute tubular necrosis is the precursor of intrarenal failure; it can result from ischaemic damage to renal parenchyma during unrecognised or poorly treated prerenal failure. The ischaemic tissue generates toxic, oxygen-free radicals, which cause swelling, injury and necrosis.

Postrenal failure

Bilateral obstruction of urine outflow leads to postrenal failure. The obstruction may be in the bladder, ureters or urethra.

What to look for

Acute renal failure is a critical illness in children. Its early signs are oliguria, azotaemia and, rarely, anuria.

System alert

Electrolyte imbalance, metabolic acidosis and other severe effects follow as the child becomes increasingly uraemic and renal dysfunction disrupts other body systems:
• GI – anorexia, nausea, vomiting, diarrhoea or constipation, stomatitis, bleeding, haematemesis, dry mucous membranes, uraemic breath
• central nervous system – headache, drowsiness, irritability, confusion, peripheral neuropathy, seizures, coma
• cutaneous – dryness, pruritus, pallor, purpura and, rarely, uraemic frost
• cardiovascular – hypotension (early in the course of the disease), hypertension (later in the course of the disease), arrhythmias, fluid overload, heart failure, systemic oedema, anaemia, altered clotting mechanisms
• respiratory – pulmonary oedema, Kussmaul's respirations.

What tests tell you

• Blood studies show elevated BUN, serum creatinine and potassium levels; decreased sodium, calcium, bicarbonate and haemoglobin levels, decreased haematocrit and low blood pH.

• Urine studies show casts, cellular debris and decreased specific gravity; in glomerular diseases, proteinuria and increased urine osmolality.
• ECG shows changes associated with electrolyte imbalance and heart failure.
• Ultrasound of the kidney shows the size of the kidneys and may reveal the presence of a tumour, cyst or urinary tract obstruction.
• Excretory urography demonstrates the appearance of the kidney structure and, possibly, the presence of obstruction.

Complications

Renal failure affects many body processes. Complications may include fluid volume overload, arrhythmias or seizures from electrolyte imbalance, heart failure, hypertension or hypotension, tachypnea, pulmonary enema, infection, skin breakdown, malnutrition or development of chronic renal failure.

How it's treated

The key to managing acute renal failure is prevention. For children with dehydration or any type of fluid loss, fluid volume should be restored as soon as possible to prevent disruption of perfusion to the kidneys. Caution should be exercised whenever nephrotoxic drugs are used in children. Treatment of acute renal failure may include:
• diet high in carbohydrates and fats and low in protein, sodium and potassium to meet metabolic needs
• fluid restriction
• careful monitoring of electrolytes and fluid status; IV therapy to maintain and correct fluid and electrolyte balance
• diuretic therapy with furosemide or mannitol to treat oliguria
• calcium resonium by mouth or enema to reverse hyperkalaemia with mild symptoms (malaise, loss of appetite, muscle weakness); hypertonic glucose, insulin and sodium bicarbonate IV for more severe hyperkalemic symptoms (numbness and tingling and ECG changes)
• antihypertensives to control elevated blood pressure
• blood products as needed to control anaemia or reverse effects of bleeding
• haemodialysis or peritoneal dialysis (occasionally required).

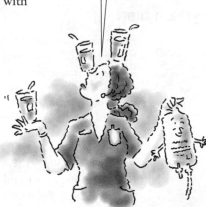

Fluid and electrolyte balance is essential for the child with renal failure.

What to do

Care of the child with acute renal failure includes careful monitoring and dietary education. The child and parents will need emotional support and reassurance, with clear explanations of all procedures.

No fluid shall go unmeasured

Measure and record intake and output, including body fluids, such as wound drainage, nasogastric output, and diarrhoea; weigh the child daily.

Monitor vital signs; watch for and report signs of inadequate renal perfusion (hypotension) and acidosis.

Maintain proper electrolyte balance by:
- strictly monitoring potassium levels
- watching for symptoms of hyperkalaemia (malaise, anorexia, paresthesia or muscle weakness)
- monitoring for and immediately reporting ECG changes (tall, peaked T waves; widening QRS segment and disappearing P waves)
- avoid administering medications containing potassium.

Monitor and maintain

Other interventions focus on monitoring and maintaining nutritional status and preventing infection:
- Maintain nutritional status; provide a high-calorie, low-protein, low-sodium and low-potassium diet with vitamin supplements. (Give the anorexic child small, frequent meals.)
- Use sterile technique because the child with acute renal failure is highly susceptible to infection; don't allow personnel with upper respiratory tract infections to care for the child.
- Use guaiac (Haemoccult) tests to monitor stools for occult blood, a sign of GI bleeding.

Renal failure, chronic

Chronic renal failure is usually the end result of gradual tissue destruction and loss of renal function. It can also result from a rapidly progressing disease of sudden onset that destroys the nephrons and causes irreversible kidney damage.

Few symptoms develop until less than 25% of glomerular filtration remains. The normal parenchyma then deteriorates rapidly and symptoms worsen as renal function decreases. End-stage renal disease is the final stage of chronic renal failure. This disorder is fatal without treatment, but maintenance on dialysis or kidney transplantation can sustain life.

What causes it
Chronic renal failure may be caused by:
- chronic glomerular disease (glomerulonephritis)
- chronic infection (such as chronic pyelonephritis)
- congenital anomalies (renal hypoplasia and dysplasia, obstructive uropathy)
- vascular disease (hypertension, nephrosclerosis)
- collagen disease (SLE)
- nephrotoxic agents (long-term aminoglycoside therapy).

How it happens
Chronic renal failure commonly progresses through four stages:

When renal reserve is reduced, GFR is 35% to 50% of normal function.

✌️ With renal insufficiency, GFR is 20% to 35% of normal function.

✌️ In renal failure, GFR is 20% to 25% of normal function.

✌️ In end-stage renal disease, GFR is less than 20% of normal function.

The point of no return

Nephron damage is progressive; damaged nephrons can't function and don't recover. The kidneys maintain relatively normal function until about 75% of the nephrons are non-functional. Surviving nephrons hypertrophy and increase their rate of filtration, reabsorption and secretion. Compensatory excretion continues as GFR diminishes.

Toxin takeover

Eventually, the healthy nephrons and glomeruli are so overburdened that they become sclerotic, stiff and necrotic. Toxins accumulate and potentially fatal changes ensue in all major organ systems. (See *Effects of chronic renal failure*.)

What to look for

In the early stages, the child may be asymptomatic (until normal kidney function has declined to 20% or less). The first signs are usually lethargy and fatigue. Progressing signs and symptoms may include:
- hypertension
- growth retardation evidenced by the child falling behind on growth charts
- oedema
- signs of fluid overload, evidenced by abnormal heart and breath sounds and shortness of breath
- 'uraemic' odour on the breath
- anorexia, nausea and vomiting
- general malaise
- headache
- generalised pruritus
- increased or decreased urine output, nocturia, enuresis
- easy bruising or bleeding
- decreased level of alertness, poor school performance
- muscle cramps and twitching
- seizures
- decreased sensation, especially in the hands or feet.

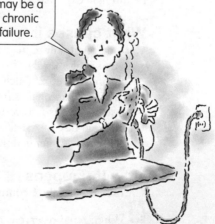

Decreased sensation in the hands may be a sign of chronic renal failure.

What tests tell you

Blood tests reveal:
- anaemia that doesn't respond to oral iron therapy
- reduced levels of platelets
- elevated serum creatinine and BUN levels

Effects of chronic renal failure

In addition to the retention of waste products, chronic renal failure may produce other physiologic changes; the presence and severity of these manifestations depend on the duration of renal failure and its response to treatment.

Hyperkalaemia and acidosis

In early renal insufficiency, acid excretion and phosphate reabsorption increase to maintain normal pH. When the glomerular filtration rate decreases by 30% to 40%, progressive metabolic acidosis ensues (characteristic of chronic renal failure) and tubular secretion of potassium increases. Total-body potassium levels may increase to life-threatening levels, requiring dialysis.

Bone demineralisation

Demineralisation of the bone (renal osteodystrophy or renal rickets) manifested by bone pain and pathologic fractures is due to several factors:

- Decreased renal activation of vitamin D decreases absorption of dietary calcium.
- Retention of phosphate increases loss of calcium in urine (which decreases serum calcium levels).
- Decreased urinary excretion causes an increase in parathyroid hormone circulation.

Anaemia

Anemia and platelet disorders with prolonged bleeding time ensue as diminished erythropoietin secretion leads to reduced red blood cell (RBC) production in the bone marrow. Uremic toxins associated with chronic renal failure shorten RBC survival time. The patient may experience lethargy and dizziness.

Growth and hormonal alterations

Growth retardation induced by renal failure is one of the most profound effects on children. Its cause isn't clearly understood.

All hormone levels are impaired in excretion and activation, which may delay sexual maturation or prevent it from occurring. This impairment may also cause anovulation or amenorrhea in females and impaired spermatogenesis in males.

Skin changes

The skin of a child with chronic renal failure acquires a grayish yellow tint as urine pigments (urochromes) accumulate. Inflammatory mediators released by retained toxins in the skin cause pruritus. Uric acid and other substances in the sweat crystallise and accumulate on the skin as uremic frost. High plasma calcium levels are also associated with pruritus.

Infection

Chronic renal failure increases the risk of death from infection. Children with chronic renal failure are at high risk for infection related to suppression of cell-mediated immunity and a reduction in the number and function of lymphocytes and phagocytes.

- elevated potassium, sodium, calcium and phosphorus levels
- metabolic acidosis.

What's in urine

Urine tests reveal:
- RBCs or casts in the urine
- alterations in urine electrolyte levels and specific gravity.

The also-rans

Other studies may include:
- ECG, which shows changes associated with electrolyte imbalances
- KUB, excretory urography, nephrotomography, renal scan or renal arteriography (all of which show reduced kidney size)

- renal biopsy to identify underlying disease
- EEG to identify metabolic encephalopathy.

Complications

Possible complications of chronic renal failure include:
- fluid and electrolyte imbalances
- arrhythmias
- heart failure, pulmonary oedema
- respiratory failure
- seizures
- altered level of consciousness
- malnutrition, faltering growth
- altered growth and sexual maturation
- bone pain and fractures
- skin breakdown
- progressive renal insufficiency.

How it's treated

Treatment of chronic renal failure involves:
- sodium and potassium limitations
- protein restricted only to the recommended daily allowance for children (because further protein restrictions may impede growth and neurodevelopment)
- fluid restrictions and diuretics to maintain fluid balance
- antihypertensives to control blood pressure and oedema
- calcium carbonate (Caltrate) or calcium acetate (PhosLo) to treat renal osteodystrophy by binding to phosphate and supplementing calcium
- antiemetics to relieve nausea and vomiting
- iron and folate supplements and an iron- and folic acid-rich diet for anaemia and, possibly, transfusion of RBCs if needed
- synthetic erythropoietin to stimulate the bone marrow to produce RBCs
- antipruritics such as diphenhydramine to relieve itching
- supplementary vitamins, particularly B and D, and essential amino acids
- dialysis for hyperkalaemia and fluid imbalances
- oral or rectal administration of cation exchange resins, such as Kayexalate, and IV administration of calcium gluconate, sodium bicarbonate, 50% dextrose or regular insulin to reverse hyperkalaemia
- peritoneal dialysis or haemodialysis to help control end-stage renal disease
- kidney transplantation (usually the treatment of choice if a donor is available).

What to do

Provide emotional support to the child and family and help them deal with the diagnosis and prognosis. They should be encouraged to express their feelings and to ask questions.

Because chronic renal failure has such widespread clinical effects, it requires meticulous and carefully coordinated supportive care.

In with the moisture, out with the itch

Good skin care is important. Bathe the child daily using superfatted soaps and use skin lotion without alcohol to ease pruritus. Glycerin-containing soaps shouldn't be used because they cause skin drying.

Good oral hygiene is also important. Brush the child's teeth often with a soft brush or sponge tip to reduce breath odour. Mouthwash can help to minimise the metallic taste in the mouth and alleviate thirst.

The child should be given small, palatable meals that are also nutritious; try to provide favourite foods within dietary restrictions.

A watchful eye

Other interventions focus on careful monitoring.
- Watch for hyperkalaemia; observe for diarrhoea and cramping of the legs and abdomen.
- As potassium levels rise, watch for muscle irritability and a weak pulse.
- Monitor for ECG changes.
- Assess hydration status carefully; measure daily intake and output carefully, including drainage, emesis, diarrhoea and blood loss. (Record daily weight, presence or absence of thirst, dryness of tongue, hypertension and peripheral oedema.)
- Monitor for bone or joint complications.
- Maintain strict sterile technique and watch for signs of infection (high fever, leukocytosis).
- Observe for signs of bleeding. Monitor haemoglobin levels and haematocrit and check stools, urine and vomit for blood.

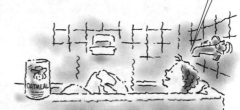

It's not just for breakfast anymore! A little oatmeal in the bath water keeps skin moist and eases the itch.

Wilms' tumour

Wilms' tumour, also called nephroblastoma, is the most common form of kidney cancer in children. The average age at diagnosis is 2 to 4 years. The tumour is more common in the left kidney and is usually unilateral. It can remain encapsulated for a long time, and prognosis is excellent if metastasis hasn't occurred.

What causes it

Studies have shown an increased risk in children with specific chromosomal abnormalities. Wilms' tumour has also been associated with several congenital anomalies including hypospadias and cryptorchidism.

How it happens

Wilms' tumour is an embryonal cancer of the kidney originating during foetal life. In the early stages, the tumour is well encapsulated, but it may later spread into the lymph nodes, renal vein or vena cava; metastasis to the lungs or other sites may occur.

Life is but a stage

The tumour is staged to determine the best treatment:
- Stage I – The tumour is limited to one kidney.
- Stage II – The tumour extends beyond the kidney but can be completely excised.
- Stage III – The tumour has spread but is confined to the abdomen and lymph nodes.
- Stage IV – The tumour has metastasised to the lung, liver, bone and brain.
- Stage V – The tumour involves both kidneys.

What to look for

The child usually has a non-tender abdominal mass, commonly first identified by the parents during bathing or dressing, or by a health professions during a routine assessment. The mass can be palpated in the region of the lower abdomen, and is usually confined to one side. Other signs and symptoms may include an enlarged abdomen, hypertension, vomiting, haematuria, anaemia and constipation.

What tests tell you

- Ultrasound will determine if the mass originated within the kidney, and if the mass is a solid tumour.
- CT scan or magnetic resonance imaging will determine the extent of the tumour and whether it has spread to other organs.
- Excretory urography assesses function of the unaffected kidney.
- Chest X-ray and CT scan of the chest will determine if the tumour has metastasised to the lungs.

Complications

Recurrence of Wilms' tumour may occur in several sites, such as the lungs, liver and the surgical area. Other complications may include:
- musculoskeletal defects from radiation therapy
- possible development of other (metastatic) cancers in the bones, breast and thyroid
- decreased fertility, especially after radiation therapy
- renal failure.

How it's treated

Most commonly, treatment involves surgical removal of the entire affected kidney (radical nephrectomy). Exploratory surgery of the lymph nodes and the liver may be performed at the same time to determine if the tumour has spread outside the kidney.

Keep the kidney

If the tumour is bilateral, neither kidney is removed during the initial surgery. Rather, a biopsy of the tumour is taken to help determine the tumour type.

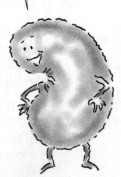

Phhhew! That was close. After surgery for bilateral Wilms' tumour, my partner and I were spared!

Chemotherapy will reduce the size of bilateral tumours. Later, with bilateral tumours, the child has further surgery, removing just the tumours and a portion of the kidneys, saving most of both kidneys to maintain kidney function.

Chemotherapy with agents such as actinomycin, vincristine doxorubicin or etoposide are used after nephrectomy, usually for 6 months. Radiation therapy may be used to improve survival rates.

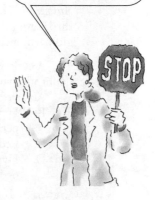

Stop-don't palpate! Abdominal palpation can rupture the surrounding capsule of Wilms' tumour, causing distant metastasis.

What to do

A great deal of emotional support is needed for the child and parents dealing with this diagnosis. The child should be thoroughly prepared for treatments and procedures, including surgery, chemotherapy and radiation, and their adverse effects. The nurse should serve as an advocate for the child and parents, making certain that questions are answered and concerns are addressed in a timely fashion.

In addition, follow these steps:
• Keep in mind that a Wilms' tumour is very soft, and the capsule can easily rupture before or during surgery; if this happens there can be rapid metastasis to other organs.
• Make sure that after the diagnosis is suspected or confirmed, there's absolutely no further palpation of the abdomen because this can cause rupture of the capsule.
• Tell the parents and the child that frequent imaging of the remaining kidney to detect recurrence of the tumour will be required.

Quick quiz

1. The main functioning unit of the kidney is the:
    A. renal cortex.
    B. renal medulla.
    C. nephron.
    D. ureter.

Answer: C. The nephron, located within the renal medulla, is the main functional unit of the kidney; it filters out waste products and excess water, forming urine.

2. An X-ray done with IV contrast media to show the structure of the urinary system is called:
    A. KUB.
    B. DMSA scan.
    C. VCUG.
    D. renal biopsy.

Answer: B. DMSA scan, IV contrast medium is injected, then X-rays are taken to visualise the structures of the entire urinary elimination system.

3. A child has decreased output of pink-tinged urine, facial oedema and a history of a sore throat 'a little while ago'. The nurse anticipates the medical staff will be evaluating the child for:
   A. cryptorchidism.
   B. adverse effects of haemodialysis.
   C. haemolytic uraemic syndrome.
   D. acute post-streptococcal glomerulonephritis.

Answer: D. Pink-tinged urine, facial oedema and a history of a sore throat are the typical signs and symptoms of acute post-streptococcal glomerulonephritis.

4. A child is admitted to the children's unit with a new diagnosis of nephrotic syndrome. Which set of symptoms would the nurse expect to see?
   A. Periorbital oedema, polyuria, proteinuria and hyperproteinaemia
   B. Hypercholesterolemia, hypoproteinaemia, proteinuria and periorbital oedema
   C. Pedal oedema, hypolipidaemia, haematuria and oliguria
   D. Hyperlipidaemia, glycosuria, hyperproteinaemia and generalised oedema

Answer: B. The four classic signs and symptoms of early stages of nephrotic syndrome are hypercholesterolaemia, hypoproteinaemia, proteinuria and periorbital oedema.

5. A child on the children's unit has a Wilms' tumour. One of the most important nursing functions for this child is to:
   A. prepare the parents for the loss of the child.
   B. maintain the child's fluid volume.
   C. ensure the child's nutritional status.
   D. make sure that no abdominal palpation is performed.

Answer: D. Remember that a Wilms' tumour is very soft and the capsule surrounding it can rupture easily, causing distant and potentially devastating metastasis to other organs.

Scoring

☆☆☆ If you answered all five items correctly, bravo! Your knowledge of urinary problems flows unobstructed.

☆☆ If you answered three or four items correctly, good for you! Take a potty break and read on.

☆ If you answered fewer than three items correctly, go with the flow! You'll breeze through the remaining five quizzes.

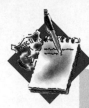

(11) Musculoskeletal problems

Just the facts

In this chapter, you'll learn:

♦ basic anatomy and physiology of the musculoskeletal system

♦ common diagnostic tests for musculoskeletal problems

♦ orthopaedic treatments and procedures

♦ selected musculoskeletal disorders in children.

Anatomy and physiology

The musculoskeletal system is one of the most complex systems within the body. The muscles and bones allow the body to move and function. If a problem occurs in the musculoskeletal system, mobility and general activities of daily living may be impaired.

Bones

The body's form and function are supported by the skeletal system. The human skeleton is made up of 206 bones that are shaped according to their function. The skeletal system:

• enables movement of the body by supporting soft tissues
• provides support and allows a person to stand erect
• protects underlying organs
• serves as a reservoir for storing such minerals as calcium and phosphorus
• serves as a site for red blood cell formation.

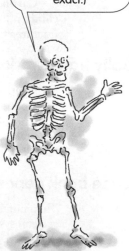

I support the body's form and function – no bones about it! (Actually, 206 bones, to be exact.)

The long and short of it

Long bones are found in the upper and lower extremities. They're responsible for carrying the body's weight and helping make ambulation possible. Short bones are found in the hands and feet and are shaped to provide strength in a compact area. Some bones, such as the ribs and sternum, are flat and thin; they provide structure. Other bones are large and irregularly shaped (e.g. the pelvic bone).

Universal coverage

The composition of bone differs depending on the type of bone, but all are covered by a double layer of connective tissue, called the periosteum, which helps provide nourishment to the bone. In children, the periosteum is thick and vascular, so a child's bone tends to heal faster than that of an adult with the same injury.

Bone growth and formation

The epiphysis is the growth end of the long bones. The epiphyseal plate, or growth plate, is located in the epiphysis.

A plate of cartilage

The epiphyseal plate is composed of cartilage cells that grow and develop, thereby causing the bone to lengthen. The growth plate is gradually replaced by bone until only the epiphyseal line remains. When the plate is completely replaced by bone, the bones can no longer lengthen; they can only increase in breadth. Injury to the growth plate may seriously impede bone growth. Children are particularly susceptible to growth plate injuries.

Cartilage serves as a smooth surface for articulating bones. Because young children have a more cartilaginous skeleton, they may be less prone to severe fractures than adults.

Salty framework

Ossification is the process of developing new bones from tissue. Osteoblasts form bone cells that lay down a framework for the new bone. Calcium and phosphorus combine to form salts, which are then deposited into the framework. The thyroid and parathyroid glands regulate this deposition. (See *Bone growth and remodelling*.)

Bone bank deposit

To maintain equilibrium, bone is deposited where it's needed within the skeletal system. If increased stress is placed on a certain bone, more bone is deposited. If there's no stress on the bone, part of the bone mass is reabsorbed.

Resorption is the process by which old bone is dissolved. The bone cells known as osteocytes and osteoclasts are responsible for the resorption of bone in this framework. This process can release calcium into the circulation.

Bone growth and remodeling

The ossification of cartilage into bone, or *osteogenesis*, begins at about week 9 of foetal development. The diaphyses of long bones are formed by birth, and the epiphyses begin to ossify around that time. The stages of growth and remodeling of the epiphyses of a long bone are shown in these illustrations.

Creation of an ossification centre

At about the ninth month of foetal development, an ossification centre develops in the epiphysis. Some cartilage cells enlarge and stimulate ossification of surrounding cells. The enlarged cells die, leaving small cavities. New cartilage continues to develop.

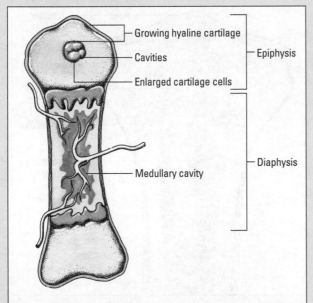

Growing hyaline cartilage
Cavities
Enlarged cartilage cells
Epiphysis

Medullary cavity
Diaphysis

Osteoblasts form bone

Osteoblasts begin to form bone on the remaining cartilage, creating the trabeculae network of cancellous bone. Cartilage continues to form on the outer surfaces of the epiphysis and along the upper surface of the epiphyseal plate.

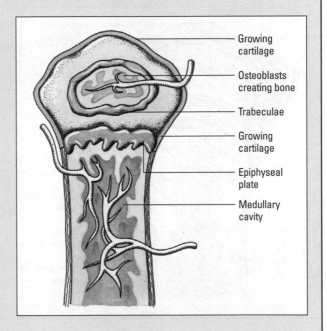

Growing cartilage
Osteoblasts creating bone
Trabeculae
Growing cartilage
Epiphyseal plate
Medullary cavity

(continued)

Muscles

Muscles are the major organs that enable movement. They're fibrous bundles covered with thin connective tissue. They also serve as repositories for some metabolites. Muscles are attached at each end directly to the bone or to a tendon, ligament or fascia:

• Tendons hold muscles to bones and are formed by strong, non-elastic collagen cords.

Bone growth and remodeling (continued)

Bone growth

Cartilage is replaced by compact bone near the outer surfaces of the epiphysis. Only cartilage cells on the upper surface of the diaphyseal plate continue to multiply rapidly, pushing the epiphysis away from the diaphysis. This new cartilage ossifies, creating trabeculae on the medullary side of the epiphyseal plate.

Remodeling

Osteoclasts produce enzymes and acids that reduce trabeculae created by the epiphyseal plate, thus enlarging the medullary cavity. In the epiphysis, osteoclasts reduce bone, making its calcium available for new osteoblasts that give the epiphysis its adult shape and proportion. In young adults, the epiphyseal plate completely ossifies (closes) and becomes the epiphyseal line; longitudinal growth of bone then ceases.

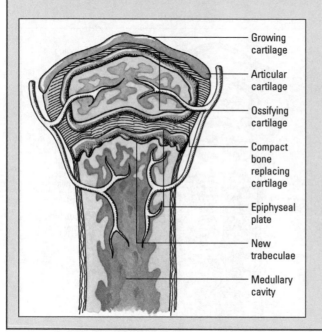

- Growing cartilage
- Articular cartilage
- Ossifying cartilage
- Compact bone replacing cartilage
- Epiphyseal plate
- New trabeculae
- Medullary cavity

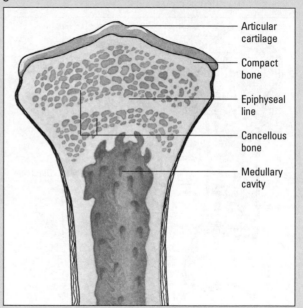

- Articular cartilage
- Compact bone
- Epiphyseal line
- Cancellous bone
- Medullary cavity

- Ligaments hold bones to other bones; they encircle the joints and add strength and stability.
- The fascia is a fibrous membrane of supporting, connective tissue.

Muscles in opposition

The movement enabled by muscles occurs through the contracting and lengthening of opposing muscle groups. As a muscle shortens on contraction, it pulls the bones to which it's attached, bringing the bones closer together. Most muscles are attached to two bones that articulate (join or work together as a single unit) at an intervening joint.

Taking turns

For the most part, movement happens when one bone moves while the other is held stable. The body of the muscle that produces movement of the extremity usually lies proximal to the bone that's moved.

Six hundred volunteers

There are more than 600 voluntary muscles (muscles we control) in the body. These muscles are called striated or skeletal muscles. Other types of muscles include visceral muscles (also called smooth or involuntary muscles) and the cardiac muscle.

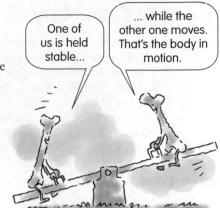

One of us is held stable...

... while the other one moves. That's the body in motion.

Joints

Joints are formed when two surfaces of bones come together and articulate.

Joints on the move

There are three types of joints, classified by the degree of movement:
• Synarthrodial (immovable) joints separate bone by a thin layer of cartilage – for example, the skull and various bones of the cranium.
• Amphidiarthrodial (semi-movable) joints separate bone with cartilage or a fibrocartilaginous disk – for example, the joints between the vertebral bodies.
• Diarthrodial (freely movable) joints are commonly called synovial joints. Most joints in the body are synovial joints. They're lined with a membrane that secretes and lubricates the joint with synovial fluid – for example, the knees, shoulders and hips. They're encased by the joint capsule, which is strengthened by ligaments that surround the capsule.

Flex or extend

Muscles are categorised according to the type of joint movement produced when the muscle is contracted. They're designated as flexor or extensor muscles depending on whether the joint is flexed or extended. Range of motion (ROM) is determined by the degree of movement in a joint. (See *Types of joint movement*, page 370.)

Diagnostic tests

Tests used to assess the musculoskeletal system and guide treatment include arthroscopy, bone scans, electromyography (EMG), muscle and bone marrow biopsy and X-rays.

Arthroscopy

Arthroscopy is a surgical procedure used to visualise, diagnose and treat problems inside a joint. It involves placing a fibre-optic instrument into the joint and then visualising the area. Corrective surgery can be done at the same time, which helps eliminate the need for more extensive surgery.

The knee is the most common joint evaluated and treated with arthroscopy. It's most commonly done under a general anaesthetic with younger children, but can also be performed with a local or spinal anaesthetic depending on the joint and the suspected problem.

Lean on me

There may be some swelling and pain after arthroscopy. With knee arthroscopy, the child may need to use crutches for 2 to 4 weeks after a surgical repair. It's important for the crutches to be the right size for the child and for the child to be instructed in their use, and safety issues. This instruction is best given by someone from the physiotherapy department. The child can usually return to school within a few days.

Nursing considerations

Prepare the child for the procedure by explaining the general anaesthesia or the anaesthetic, what the child will experience in the operating theatre (if to be awake), and how they'll feel after the procedure. In addition, follow these steps:
• Note any allergies because of the use of anaesthesia.
• Tell the child they may feel a thumping sensation as the cannula is inserted into the joint capsule (if during the procedure).
• Cover the site with a small dressing after the procedure.

Bone scans

Bone scans are used to diagnose osteomyelitis and metastatic bone disease. They can also be used to aid diagnosis of joint infections and certain fractures. Special radiographic techniques can help diagnose a musculoskeletal problem. These techniques include computed tomography (CT) scans and magnetic resonance imaging (MRI).

Nursing considerations

The tube-like structures that house the imaging equipment can be frightening to a child. Whenever possible, show the child a picture of the scanning equipment, or the equipment itself, before the procedure. Reassure the child that the parent will be allowed to remain in the room.
• Explain the procedure to the parents and child. Tell the child that they'll be placed in a tube so that pictures may be taken.
• Instruct the child to remain still during the procedure; sedation may be necessary. Distraction techniques may help to calm the child.
• Remove metallic objects.

Types of joint movement

There are seven types of joint movement:

• *Flexion* is a bending forward of the joint; this decreases the angle between the bones that are connected.
• *Extension* is an increase in the joint angle that occurs with straightening of the limb.
• *Abduction* is the movement of the limb away from the midline, or *central axis*, of the body.
• *Adduction* is the movement of the limb towards or beyond the midline, or *central axis*, of the body.
• *Internal rotation* is the turning of the body part inward, towards the midline, or *central axis*, of the body.
• *External rotation* is the turning of the body part away from the midline, or *central axis*, of the body.
• *Circumduction* is the movement of the body part in a circular motion.

Electromyography

EMG measures muscle response to nervous stimulation (the electrical activity within the muscle fibres). Needle electrodes are inserted into the muscle to be tested, and electrical activity is recorded when the muscle is at rest and during contraction.

A sign of weakness

EMG is used when there are symptoms of muscle weakness and decreased muscle strength. It can differentiate primary muscle conditions from weakness caused by neurological disorders or a lack of use of the particular muscle. Conditions that may be diagnosed by EMG include muscular dystrophy, nerve dysfunction, and Guillain–Barré syndrome.

Nursing considerations

EMG can be frightening and uncomfortable for a child. When explaining the procedure to the child and parents, prepare the child for insertion of the needle and the feeling in the muscle when the electrical impulses are sent through (like a hard hit to the 'funny bone'). Let them know that residual bruising may occur.

In addition, follow these steps:
• Explain that the child may be asked to voluntarily contract the muscle; help them practice the different positions or movements.
• Use deep breathing exercises and play preparation to help lessen the fear and anxiety the child may experience.
• Reassure the child that their parents can stay with during the procedure.

Muscle and bone marrow biopsy

Biopsy of the muscles and bones involves the removal of a small specimen of muscle or bone marrow for analysis. In most cases, these are undertaken when the child has a general anaesthetic. Although older children (young people) may have this under local anaesthetic/sedation and analgesia. The puncture site may remain tender for a few weeks. For bone marrow biopsy, the proximal tibia is the most commonly used site in young children. In older children, the vertebral bodies T10 through L4 are preferred.

Nursing considerations

Biopsy and the anaesthetic can be an extremely frightening procedure for a child and their parents. Thoroughly prepare the child and his parents. Allowing the child to 'perform' the procedure on a doll (using correct positioning, a syringe and a bandage) will enhance their understanding of the procedure and may help to ease fears.

In addition, follow these steps:
• Clarify the meaning of biopsy in context; many parents (and older children) automatically think of cancer when they hear the word biopsy.

A child who cries more when a parent is present probably does so because they feel safe. Feeling safe is the best antidote to emotional trauma.

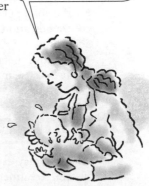

- Provide analgesics as ordered.
- Assist the child into the desired position depending on the site to be used. If necessary, assist in holding the child still during the procedure. (Allow a parent to be present in a comforting capacity only, leaving the positioning and restraint of the child to the health care professionals.)
- When the specimen is obtained, apply direct pressure to the site for 5 to 10 minutes.
- Cover the site and make sure the child remains still for approximately 30 minutes after the procedure.

X-rays

Radiography is the most widely used diagnostic test in the assessment of children with bone abnormalities or other conditions affecting the bones. X-rays can show pathology, such as a fracture, and can show bone density and irregularities. X-rays are used not only for initial evaluation but also for monitoring and evaluating the effectiveness of treatment.

Invisible bone

Normally, the calcium deposits in bones will make skeletal structures appear radiopaque, or white, on X-rays. However, in the infant and young child (whose skeleton is composed mostly of growth cartilage), structures are radiolucent and may not appear on X-ray. Thus, X-rays are less reliable in this population. High-resolution ultrasound may provide a more accurate picture.

Nursing considerations

Always explain to the child the reason for obtaining an X-ray. Explain that an X-ray simply takes pictures (of whatever part of the body is being X-rayed). Reassure the child that the X-ray itself doesn't hurt, but keep in mind that a child with an injury may experience discomfort during positioning for the X-ray.

It's common to allow the parents to remain with the child during the procedure as long as appropriate precautions are taken. In addition, follow these steps:

- Tell the child that it's their job to remain still during the procedure.
- Obtain previous X-rays if possible, which may be useful for comparison.
- If a young person is sexually active, assess for possible pregnancy, a contraindication for radiography. Be careful how you ask the young person about this!
- Remove metallic objects, such as jewellery or snaps on gowns, before the X-ray because metallic objects may be mistaken for pathology.

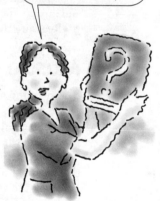

Where did they go? The skeletal structures of an infant or young child are radiolucent, meaning they may not be visible on X-ray.

Treatments and procedures

Children may experience dysfunction in any part of the musculoskeletal system. Treatment depends on a thorough assessment and appropriate interventions based on findings. These interventions are typically designed to promote healing and lessen the impact of the condition on mobility. Principles of body mechanics are used to maintain the integrity of the musculoskeletal system.

Prevent and restore

Nursing care of orthopaedic conditions involves the correction of alterations in the musculoskeletal system. These preventive and restorative measures include:
• casting and traction, which are used to help correct, maintain and support the body part in a functional position
• limb amputations, which may be necessary in some circumstances.

Casting

Casts may be required when a child has a fractured bone, weakness, paralysis or spasticity. They're also used following corrective orthopaedic surgery.

The cast may be made of plaster or, more commonly, of synthetic material such as fibreglass or plastic. Polyester and cotton impregnated with water-activated polyurethane resin may also be used. (See *Types of casts for children*, page 374.)

Depending on the type of material that's used, drying time for the cast may be as little as 7 minutes or as much as 48 hours. Weight-bearing on the affected part of the body is typically avoided until the cast has dried.

A wash and a blow dry

Some synthetic casts may be immersed in water. If appropriate, instruct the child and family to dry the cast after bathing or immersion by using a blow-dryer on a cool setting.

Nursing considerations

Explain each step of the procedure to the child before the procedure, and again as the cast is being applied. If plaster will be used, explain that the child will experience a sensation of warmth when it's first applied. As it dries, the cast – and the child – will feel cold. If applied after a fracture, the child will probably feel immediate some relief!

In addition, follow these steps:
• If a closed reduction is necessary, explain to the child that there will be some pain. Allow the parents to remain close to the child and hold their hand to help lessen anxiety.
• Assess the casted area every 30 minutes for the first few hours, then every hour for 24 hours, then every 4 hours for an additional 48 hours. Drainage from a wound under the cast should be noted.
• If there are signs and symptoms of compromise in the affected area, notify the medical staff immediately. Also notify if cracks are noted in the cast.

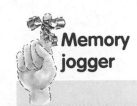

Memory jogger

Remember the five 'Ps' when checking for signs of compromised blood supply in a child with a cast.

Pain
Pallor
Paraesthesia
Paralysis
Pulselessness.

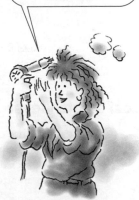

In addition to drying your hair, blow dryers can be set on cool and aimed at the edges of the child's cast. It's a great itch reliever!]

Types of casts for children

These illustrations show the types of casts commonly used for children.

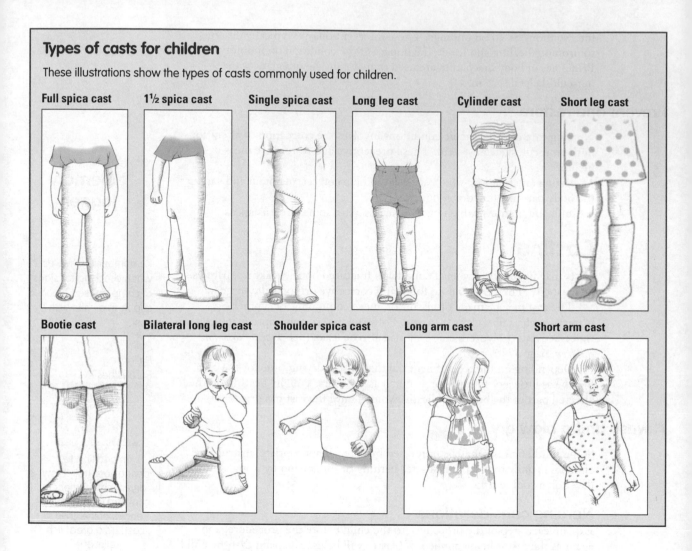

Full spica cast

1½ spica cast

Single spica cast

Long leg cast

Cylinder cast

Short leg cast

Bootie cast

Bilateral long leg cast

Shoulder spica cast

Long arm cast

Short arm cast

• Assess for signs of skin breakdown, a common occurrence. The area around the cast edges will typically become pink and warm and swelling may also occur. (Provide skin care to prevent further breakdown.)

Cast scratch fever

• Because cool air can relieve the itchiness that accompanies casting, instruct the parents (not the child) to blow cool air down into the cast using a blow-dryer on a cool setting. Also advise against putting an object down the cast in an attempt to scratch.

Fluorescent green, shocking pink or gothic purple???

Casts come in different colours so the child is usually asked which one they want.

May I have your autograph?

- Ask the child if they would like anyone to sign the cast although they will probably ask first.
- Explain to the child and parents that the cast must be worn as recommended. It shouldn't be removed and overly rigorous activities should be discouraged (to prevent dislodgment or misalignment of a fracture).

The cut stops here – promise!

- When the fracture is healed, prepare the child for cast removal with the cast cutter. Let them hear the noise and feel the vibrations, and show them (on your body) how the cutter stops when it touches skin and won't, therefore, cut anything except the cast.
- Inform the child that their skin will look, and smell, different after cast removal, especially if it has been in the cast for weeks. Reassure them that this is temporary, apply baby oil, then gently wash the area to remove the dead skin. (See *Cast care*.)
- Instruct the child and parents in an exercise regimen to help regain muscle strength and function following the injury.

Traction

Traction can be continuous or intermittent. It's used to:
- stabilise or immobilise a certain body part
- reduce muscle spasms
- realign fractures or joint dislocations.

Just hanging out

Traction uses weights and pulleys to exert a pulling force and maintain the body part in correct alignment. Weights must hang freely and the ropes shouldn't have knots that could interfere with free movement.

Serial X-rays are taken while the child is in traction in order to monitor progress and determine the need for changes in the direction and amount of traction pull.

Central location

The child should be kept in the centre of the bed to maintain countertraction and prevent complications, although children naturally want to move around! Traction can cause muscle spasms that may require analgesics or muscle relaxants. The child is in bed for extended periods; therefore, circulatory and skin assessment is vital.

It's all relative

Cast care

Be sure to include these points in your teaching plan for the child with a cast and their parents:

- mechanism of bone healing and necessity for casting
- cast care, including air exposure, elevation and movement
- measures to protect the cast
- measures for skin care
- methods to relieve itching
- measures to keep the cast dry
- ways to test for sensation, movement and circulation
- measures for coping with swelling
- ways to relieve skin irritation
- monitoring for wound drainage
- exercises for the casted extremity.

Types of skin traction

This chart describes the various types of skin traction.

Traction	Purpose	Patient positioning
Buck's extension	Used for a fractured hip to prevent muscle spasms and dislocation	• Child lies flat in bed. • Head of the bed is elevated only for activities of daily living.
Cervical traction	Used for neck strain and arthritic or degenerative conditions of the cervical vertebrae	• Child lies flat in bed or with the head of the bed elevated 15 to 20 degrees.
Dunlop's traction	Used for a fractured humerus	• Child lies flat in bed. • Arm is suspended horizontally.
Pelvic girdle	Used for muscle spasms, lower back pain or a herniated disc	• Child lies with head and knees raised to keep the hips flexed at a 45-degree angle.
Russell traction	Used for older children with a femur fracture or certain knee injuries	• Child lies with the head of the bed elevated 30 to 45 degrees.
Bryant's traction	Used for children younger than 2 years and who weigh less than 14 kg, with a fractured femur	• Hips are flexed at a 90-degree angle. • Buttocks are raised 1″ (2.5 cm) above the mattress.

Traction in twos

There are two basic types of traction:

 skin

 skeletal.

Skin traction

Skin traction is a non-invasive traction that's especially useful for a child who may not require continuous traction. It's applied by placing foam rubber straps against the affected part and then securing the straps with elastic bandages.

Sometimes, the straps have an adhesive backing. If this type of strap is used, the nurse should protect the skin by first applying compound benzoin tincture or other skin protectant. Traction should be applied and removed by two people. (See *Types of skin traction*.)

Skeletal traction

Skeletal traction exerts a greater force than skin traction by using wires or pins inserted into the bone. They're usually placed under anaesthesia. Skeletal traction is continuous. (See *Types of skeletal traction*.)

Types of skeletal traction

This chart describes the different types of skeletal traction.

Traction	Purpose	Special considerations
Thomas leg splint with Pearson attachment	Used for bone alignment and as a more effective line of pull	• Child is placed in the supine position with the knee flexed.
External fixation devices (Ilizarov)	Used to manage open fractures that have soft tissue damage, or to provide stability for severe comminuted fractures	• Child is on bed rest (however, early mobility and active exercise of other joints are necessary).
Halo	Used to provide immobilisation of the cervical spine and to support the neck following injury	• Early ambulation is recommended. • The anterior metal bars maintain traction. • The posterior bars can be used to position the patient.
Skeletal tongs (Crutchfield, Vinke, Gardner-Wells)	Used to maintain alignment of the cervical spine, for immobilisation, and for reduction in cervical roll fractures	• Child is on bed rest. • Special frames may be used for turning.

Nursing considerations

The sight and idea of a body part in skeletal traction can be frightening to a child and parents. Explain what the child will see and feel before the traction is applied. Use dolls and toy traction devices to show the child what's about to happen and help familiarise them with the equipment and reduce fear.

In addition, follow these steps:
• Involve the family as much as possible to reduce anxiety, alleviate boredom, encourage cooperation with the recommended treatment and minimise disruption of the family structure.
• Maintain the traction system and frequently check the ropes, pulleys and weights for proper function.
• Maintain correct alignment of the affected body part.
• Monitor neurovascular function in the splinted limb.

Don't fall behind

• Provide age-appropriate activities to help maintain the child's developmental level, prevent developmental delay and alleviate boredom. This includes school work!
• Frequently assess for signs of skin breakdown
• Encourage regular foot movements especially on the affected side to prevent footdrop.

Pin and skin

• For the child in skeletal traction, assess the pin insertion sites for signs of infection or tenting (new skin that has attached to the insertion site, creating

a tent-like configuration); tenting may cause the skin to tear, which can promote infection.
• Clean the area around the pin insertion sites frequently, and cover the tips of the pins to prevent injury to the skin or other parts of the child's body. Notify medical staff immediately if the pins become loose, and keep the child immobilised until skeletal traction is assessed.

Amputation

Unfortunately, amputations occur in children as well as adults. An amputation may be needed because of a disease process, such as osteosarcoma, or it may have occurred prenatally due to teratogens, metabolic diseases in the mother or small pieces of the amnion that cut off circulation to a certain body part (known as an amniotic band). Only rarely is a congenital amputation genetically determined.

A loss that lasts

Limb amputation that isn't congenital is very traumatic to a child, young person and their family. It may be particularly damaging to the child's self-image. Everyone deals with feelings of loss in their own way and their own time; there's no right or wrong way to grieve. Families need extra time and support to deal with the grief and loss they feel when they're given the news that amputation is required. This will be exacerbated if associated with the discovery of a carcinoma.

Something in common

It may be helpful to introduce the child and family to another family who has gone through an amputation and has learned to cope successfully with day-to-day activities and enjoy life.
Many amputations are treated with a prosthesis. Sometimes, stump shrink bandages are used to apply pressure, reduce swelling and help mould the stump for fitting a prosthesis, which usually can be done within 4 to 6 weeks after the amputation.

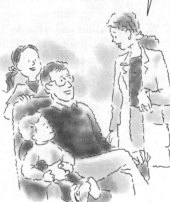

The best prescription for feelings of fear, loss, and grief is a nurse who simply listens and validates those feelings.

Quick studies

Children quickly learn how to function with a prosthesis and can lead very active, normal lives. They should be reassured that amputation doesn't have to mean permanent disability. Many children participate in sports and other strenuous activities while using a prosthesis. The nurse can play an essential role in helping the child and his/her family cope with this traumatic situation.

Nursing considerations

After the surgery, the nurse should provide basic post-operative care while keeping in mind some special considerations:

- Provide care to prevent contractures and perform ROM exercises to keep the stump from becoming permanently flexed or abducted. (These exercises also increase muscle strength and improve mobility of the stump.)

Let's get physical

- Depending on the site and extent of the amputation, the child should begin to move and start physiotherapy as quickly as possible.
- Teach the child and parents about proper care of the stump and application and maintenance of the prosthesis.
- If the amputation is on a lower extremity, teach the child how to walk with crutches, then how to ambulate using a prosthetic device. Refer the child for physiotherapy as they will need extensive training.
- Assess for phantom limb pain, which is real pain and should be treated with analgesics as appropriate. (Tell the child and parents that this pain should gradually fade.)

Musculoskeletal disorders

Musculoskeletal disorders that may occur in children include congenital talipes equinovarus, developmental dysplasia of the hip (DDH), Ewing's sarcoma, fractures, juvenile rheumatoid arthritis (JRA), Legg–Calvé–Perthes disease and scoliosis.

Congenital talipes equinovarus

Congenital talipes equinovarus (talipes) is a deformity that occurs in utero in approximately 1 of every 1,000 births. Boys are twice as likely to be affected as girls. If a family has one child with talipes, the chances of having another affected child increase markedly.

Although talipes equinovarus is the most commonly occurring type of talipes, other variations may be present and are identified according to the orientation of the deformity. (See *Recognising talipes*, page 380.)

What causes it

Talipes may be caused by a mechanical force (the position in utero), through prenatal exposure to drugs or infections or by an inherited factor. It can be a singular birth defect or associated with certain syndromes. An infant with a talipes should be carefully examined for additional anomalies.

How it happens

Regardless of the cause of the talipes, the result is a non-functional position of the foot and ankle due to abnormal muscles and joints and contracture of soft tissue. The position of the foot determines the classification of the talipes.

Recognising talipes

Talipes may have various names, depending on the orientation of the deformity, as shown in these illustrations

Talipes equinus

Talipes calcaneus

Talipes cavus

Talipes varus

Talipes equinovarus

Talipes calcaneovarus

Talipes valgus

Talipes calcaneovalgus

Talipes equinovalgus

The classic definition of talipes equinovarus requires these three components:

plantar flexion of the foot at the ankle joint

inversion deformity of the heel

turning in of the forefoot.

What to look for

The deformity is usually obvious at birth. The foot is usually inverted (turned in), also known as a varus position. An everted (turned outward) foot is known as a valgus position. A single foot or both feet may be affected. The deformity may be mild with some flexibility noted, or severe with the foot completely rigid. In the most severe form, the foot has a club-like appearance.

What tests tell you

Early diagnosis of talipes is usually relatively simple because the deformity is obvious. However, X-rays may show superimposition of the talus and calcaneus and a ladder-like appearance of the metatarsals.

Complications

If identification and treatment of talipes isn't instituted early on, chronic impairment may result. The prognosis is good, however, for infants who receive treatment.

How it's treated

Treatment of talipes consists of manipulation of the foot to stretch the contracted tissues. Splinting is then applied to maintain that correction. If treatment is begun shortly after birth, the correction is fairly rapid. If treatment is delayed for any reason, the foot quickly becomes more rigid, which can occur in a matter of days. Straps and splints are applied and are quite effective until formal casting can be done.

Casting call

Casts are applied sequentially by first correcting the forefoot adduction, then the heel inversion and then the flexion of the ankle. Casts are usually changed at 1- to 2-week intervals to allow the infant's foot to grow and to manipulate the foot gradually. To maintain the long-term correction, exercises and a night brace are commonly prescribed.

Please release me

In approximately one-half of children with talipes, corrective surgery is required to release the tightened structures around the foot. The outcome of this surgery is usually good; the foot appears normal and is adequate for normal footwear and sports. For infants, surgery is usually limited to soft tissue to prevent interference with bone growth.

From designer wedges ...

For the older child or the child with severe talipes, the bones of the foot may need to be realigned by using bone wedges. Casts are worn for months following surgery. A specialised splint called the Denis Browne splint is commonly used.

... to designer shoes

This splint consists of specially made shoes attached to an adjustable bar that provides the eversion, rotation and dorsiflexion needed to achieve a slight overcorrection. It's worn for several weeks, and then worn only at night to help maintain this position.

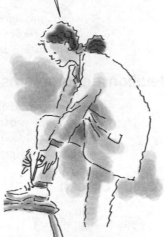

Successful surgery for congenital talipes is usually followed by successful shoe shopping!

What to do

The primary concern related to talipes is the need for early recognition, preferably during the neonatal period. Look for exaggerated attitudes in the infant's feet. Apparent talipes (resulting from positioning in utero) can be differentiated from true talipes because an apparent talipes will easily move back to normal position.

When caring for a child with talipes, follow these steps:
- Don't use excessive force when assessing a talipes.
- Stress to the parents the importance of prompt treatment; talipes demands immediate therapy and orthopaedic supervision until growth is completed.

Put up your feet and relax

• After casting, elevate the child's feet with pillows; check the toes every 1 to 2 hours for temperature, colour, sensation, motion and capillary refill time and watch for oedema.
• Before discharge, teach parents to recognise signs of circulatory impairment, such as numbness or tingling of the toes, coldness in the toes or lack of capillary refill.
• Emphasise the need for long-term orthopaedic care to maintain the correction.

The agony of de feet

• Help the parents (and child) deal with grief or other emotional issues that arise from this problem.
• Teach parents the prescribed exercises that the child should do at home.
• Urge parents to make sure the child wears their corrective shoes and splints during naps and at night. Make sure they understand that treatment of talipes continues throughout the entire growth period.

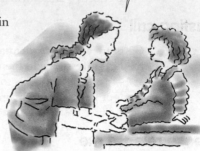

It takes a gentle touch to examine a child with talipes.

Developmental dysplasia of the hip

The hip joint develops early in utero. By the end of the first trimester, the shape of the joint is recognisable and the cartilage, ligaments, capsule and vascular pattern are formed.

Relationship problems

DDH is a spectrum of conditions in which there's an abnormal relationship between the proximal femur and the acetabulum. It occurs in approximately 1.5 of every 1,000 live births. Females are six times more likely to be affected as males. A positive family history of DDH increases the risk fivefold.

Frankly breech

Another important risk factor for DDH is a breech presentation at birth. Children who present in a frank breech position have a risk of DDH almost 20 times higher than children who have a cephalic presentation.

Other associated abnormalities include oligohydramnios (decreased amniotic fluid in utero) torticollis and metatarsus adductus (a form of talipes).

What causes it

Dislocation of the hip is usually a developmental problem in an otherwise normal child. It isn't always clear when it occurs. A child who develops a deformity in utero is usually more severely affected than the child who has a hip that dislocates after birth.

What's in a name?

Although congenital dislocation of the hip is a common term for DDH, it implies that the dislocation occurs at birth. However, the problem may occur over several months after birth. Therefore, DDH is a more accurate description of the hip pathology that exists in this disorder.

How it happens

There are three typical forms of DDH:
*   Dysplasia is a result of the femoral head failing to exert appropriate pressure against the acetabulum. As a result, the femoral head becomes small and flattened and the acetabulum becomes shallow and eventually flat. A dysplastic hip may progress to a subluxated or dislocated hip. The abductor muscles of the hip will also shorten and contract.
*   The hip is considered subluxated when the femoral head (the ball) is in contact with the acetabulum (the socket) but not deeply cantered within it.
*   Dislocation occurs when the femoral head (the ball) is no longer in contact with the acetabulum (the socket). (See *Forms of DDH*.)

What to look for

A dislocation diagnosed in the first few weeks of life can be treated conservatively. If the diagnosis is delayed until walking age, reconstructive surgery is usually required for correction, which greatly increases the likelihood of complications.

Forms of DDH

These illustrations show a normal hip and the three presentations of developmental dysplasia of the hip (DDH).

Normal hip	Dysplasia	Subluxation	Dislocation
	The acetabulum is more flattened than cup-shaped.	The femoral head is in contact with the acetabulum but isn't deeply centered within it.	The femoral head is no longer in contact with the acetabulum.

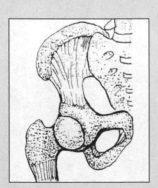 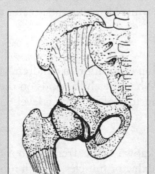 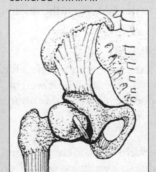 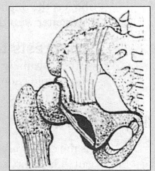

It's important for the nurse to be aware of risk factors for DDH and to assess the infant and child carefully for signs of a hip problem. Physical signs of DDH include asymmetrical skin folds, Galeazzi (or Allis) sign, limited hip abduction and hip instability.

Asymmetrical skin folds

When the infant is lying on his back with his hips and knees flexed at a 90-degree angle, the same number of skin folds should appear in the medial (inner) aspect of both thighs. If a hip is dislocated, the soft tissues of the thigh may fold down on each other like an accordion, producing a larger number of skin folds on the affected side.

Galeazzi or Allis sign

If there's a dislocation, the femoral head may be placed superior to the acetabulum when the hips and knees are flexed at 90 degrees. This malpositioning will cause the knee on the affected side to be significantly lower than the other knee, a sign known as the Galeazzi or Allis sign.

Limited hip abduction

The normal range of hip abduction in an infant is from 0 degrees (with thighs perpendicular to the table) to almost 90 degrees (with thighs resting on the table). In DDH, a shortening of the adductor muscle on the medial aspect of the thigh while the femoral head is displaced superiorly causes the thigh to be limited in its range. This sign may not be apparent in the neonate because, at this age, there hasn't been enough time for muscle spasms and contractures to develop.

Hip instability

Testing hip stability is important in the diagnosis of DDH. In neonates, this test is usually the only clue to a problem.

A clunky diagnosis

Barlow test and Ortolani's test are used to evaluate hip stability.
• A positive Barlow test is noted when a 'clunk' is heard as the examiner adducts the thigh towards the midline while trying to displace or dislocate the femoral head posteriorly.
• A positive Ortolani's test occurs when a 'clunk' is felt as the examiner abducts the thigh to the table from the midline while lifting up the greater trochanter with the finger.

What tests tell you

A Trendelenburg test can be used to assess for hip dislocation in children who are old enough to stand and bear weight. When the child stands on the affected leg, the opposite hip slants downward instead of remaining level.

A limp or a waddle

As the child walks, there's a characteristic limp known as the Trendelenburg gait. This limp is due to a weakness of the hip abductor muscles. If both hips are dislocated, the child will have lordosis and a waddling gait.

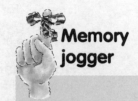

Memory jogger

Here's an easy way to keep adduction and abduction straight.

- *Adduction* is moving a limb towards the body's midline; think of it as *adding* two things together.
- *Abduction* is moving a limb away from the body's midline; think of it as taking something away like *abducting*, or kidnapping.

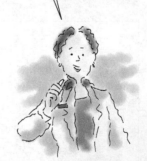

In neonates, a 'clunk' during thigh adduction and abduction may be diagnostic of DDH.

X-rays will show the location of the femoral head and a shallow acetabulum. X-rays are also used to monitor treatment or deterioration.

Complications

For children who don't receive treatment before 7 years, treatment is very unsatisfactory. Delayed treatment may have lifelong implications for walking, development of back problems, and self-esteem. DDH may cause:

- degenerative hip changes
- abnormal acetabular development
- lordosis (abnormally increased concave curvature of the lumbar and cervical spine)
- joint malformation
- sciatic nerve injury (paralysis)
- avascular necrosis of the femoral head
- soft tissue damage
- permanent disability.

How it's treated

Treatment of DDH depends on the severity of the dysplasia, how quickly the diagnosis is made and the child's age and includes a Pavlik harness, spica cast and surgical correction.

Pavlik harness

If treatment is instituted early, the success of treatment with a Pavlik harness is between 80% and 90%. As the child ages and treatment is delayed, the prognosis worsens. (See *Two views of the Pavlik harness*.)

Whoa, Nellie!

In a child younger than 6 months, careful positioning to maintain the hip in abduction with the head of the femur in the acetabulum is achieved with a Pavlik harness. This harness is worn at all times until the hips are stable on examination. When the hips are stable, usually in 1 to 3 weeks, the harness may be removed for bathing.

Harness hip hooray!

If DDH is diagnosed during the neonatal period, the harness may be needed for only 2 to 3 months. The older infant may need to wear it for 4 or 5 months.

Don't double up

Parents should be taught how to apply the harness correctly and to avoid double and triple layers of nappies (which can cause extreme abduction, leading to avascular necrosis). The harness doesn't interfere with the child's ability to receive immunisations as the thighs remain exposed.

Two views of the Pavlik harness

These illustrations show an infant in a Pavlik harness. The Pavlik harness maintains the hip in abduction, with the femoral head in the acetabulum.

Front view

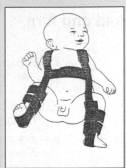

Back view

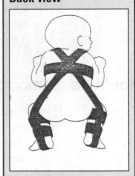

Spica cast

For the child older than 6 months, a Pavlik harness can't reliably treat the dysplasia. These children require a spica cast to hold the hips in a flexed and abducted position. Traction is commonly used before the application of the cast to gently stretch out the soft tissues around the hip that have contracted. Traction is usually used for 2 to 3 weeks before placement of the cast. Sometimes the traction can be done at home.

A temporary setback

When the cast has been applied, it usually remains on for several months, and is removed and reapplied to accommodate growth. It may delay walking for a few months, but the child usually learns quickly how to walk when the cast is removed.

Hold and turn

Care for a child in a spica cast is essentially the same as that for a child in a Pavlik harness. Parents should be encouraged to hold the child as much as possible. The infant should be turned frequently to prevent skin breakdown.

Surgical correction

For the child older than 18 months, surgical correction is usually required. Surgery enables the removal of tissues that block reduction and positioning of the femoral head into the acetabulum under direct visualisation. Occasionally, a bone graft is required.

What to do

Listen sympathetically to the parents' expressions of anxiety and fear. Explain possible causes of DDH, and reassure them that early, prompt treatment will probably result in complete correction.

You'd be cranky too

During the child's first few days in a cast or harness, they may be prone to irritability due to the unaccustomed restriction of movement. Encourage parents to stay with them as much as possible and try to calm and reassure their child. Assure parents that their child should adjust to this restriction and return to normal sleeping, eating and playing behaviour in a few days.

   If treatment requires a spica cast, follow these steps:
• Position the child on a Bradford frame (a rectangular frame of pipe with attached sheeting used for immobile children) elevated on blocks with a bedpan under the frame, or on pillows to support the child's legs. Be sure to keep the cast dry and change the child's nappies often.
• Turn the child every 2 hours during the day and every 4 hours at night. Check colour, sensation and motion of the infant's legs and feet. (Be sure to examine their toes, and notify the medical staff of dusky, cool or numb toes.)

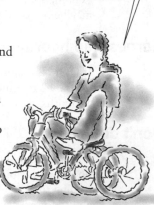

Children with DDH still need to be children – and a tricycle is the perfect fit for hips that are abducted in a frog-like position.

Investigate the itch

• If the child complains of itching, they may benefit from diphenhydramine or you may aim a blow-dryer set on cool at the cast edges to relieve itching. (Don't scratch or probe under the cast; investigate persistent itching.)
• Provide adequate stimuli to promote growth and development. If the child's hips are abducted in a frog-like position, tell parents that their child may be able to fit on a tricycle that the parent can push (if the child can't pedal) or an electric child's car.

A change of scenery

• Encourage parents to let the child sit at a table (by sitting on pillows on a chair), sit on the floor for short periods of play and play with other children their age.
• Tell parents to watch for signs that the child is outgrowing the cast (cyanosis, cool extremities or pain).

Ewing's sarcoma

Ewing's sarcoma is the second most common bone tumour in children and adolescents. It's fairly rare, with only approximately 30 new cases reported in the UK each year. It affects primarily young, white males younger than age 20. The tumour usually develops in the midshaft of the long bones of the arms and legs, although it's occasionally found in the pelvis, ribs, spine and, rarely, in the soft tissues or other bones.

What causes it

A consistent, chromosomal abnormality has been identified in the cells responsible for Ewing's sarcoma. The cause of this chromosomal problem hasn't yet been identified. It doesn't appear to be inherited, and it isn't thought to be due to exposure to chemicals or radiation, or to an environmental factor.

How it happens

Although Ewing's sarcoma is considered a form of bone cancer, it arises from a type of primitive nerve cell, which explains why the tumour can be found in the soft tissues.

Off to a bad start

Ewing's sarcoma is a cancer that spreads quickly. The tumour is aggressively malignant and approximately 25% of children diagnosed with the disease have experienced metastasis. The most common sites of metastasis include the lungs, other bones and the bone marrow.

What to look for

Signs and symptoms of Ewing's sarcoma include pain and swelling over the affected site (even causing wakening at night), possible tenderness over the affected area and weight loss. Fever occurs in 25% of children. If the tumour is over the leg bone, a limp may be present. If it's on one of the ribs, shortness of breath may be evident. In physically active children, the disease may be initially diagnosed as a sports injury.

Pelvic prognosis

Prognosis is good in children with a small, localised primary tumour. For children with significant pelvic involvement or metastatic disease, survival rates are poor. New treatment options for these high-risk children include autologous bone marrow transplants.

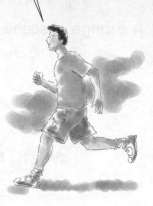

In athletes like me, the signs and symptoms of Ewing's sarcoma might initially be diagnosed as a sports injury.

What tests tell you
- Serology reveals the cells of Ewing's sarcoma (the cells stain a characteristic blue colour), which are described as small and round; they're tightly packed and arranged into compartments by bands of fibrous tissue.
- X-rays reveal the tumour and, commonly, an area of bone destruction around the tumour.
- CT scanning and MRI should be performed to determine as precisely as possible the extent of local disease.
- A chest X-ray, bone scan, and bone marrow biopsy may be performed to determine the extent of metastasis, if any.

Complications
As with any cancer, some complications arise due to treatment. Metastasis may result from the cancer itself. Children receiving prolonged, intensive treatments are forced to endure frequent venepuncture. Access devices are helpful to lessen the need for repeated venepuncture.

When chemo gets complicated

Complications of chemotherapy include nausea and vomiting, anorexia, weight loss and bone marrow suppression. Hair loss is a noticeable adverse effect of chemotherapy. The child and family should be reassured that the hair will grow back after therapy, although the texture and colour may be different. With prompt treatment, the prognosis is generally very good.

How it's treated
Treatment includes chemotherapy, radiation and surgery. Chemotherapy continues for 1 year. When surgery is performed, the tumour is usually removed without needing to amputate the limb, although this will depend on the stage of the growth. The site of tumour excision is then filled in with a graft or prosthesis to allow for normal limb function.

What to do
Caring for a child with cancer can be a difficult, yet rewarding part of nursing. By offering support, assisting with necessary treatments and helping

the family adjust to the diagnosis, the nurse can have a significant impact on the lives of a child and his/her family during this time.

• Because of the severity of the disease, be available to help the family and child cope with the diagnosis.

Nurse in shining armour

• Assure the child and parents that you're there to be their advocate; make sure their questions are answered promptly and facilitate communication between the family members and the health care team.
• Prepare the child and parents for treatments and procedures.
• Allow the child to make as many choices as possible during their day-to-day care; this helps give the child a sense of control in a situation that's likely to make them feel helpless.
• Clarify the prognosis and help the child and family deal with their fears; to many people a diagnosis of cancer is viewed as a death sentence.

Growing up too fast

• Help the child be a child while dealing with a very 'adult' diagnosis; provide play activities and encourage interaction with peers.
• If needed, refer the child and family (including siblings) to support groups and other professionals with expertise in helping families cope with a cancer diagnosis.

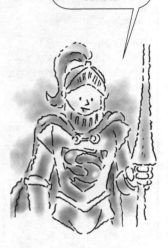

A nurse can be a superhero to a child with cancer.

Fractures

Bones are designed to withstand stress; however, when increased stress and traumatic force are exerted on the bone, a fracture will occur. Fractures can occur in almost any bone, but the long bones are the most commonly fractured. Other common sites of fracture include the wrists, fingers, toes and skull.

What causes it

Fractures commonly occur during athletic activities and accidents. They may also result from child abuse (suspected in the case of multiple, repeated episodes or specific fractures), bone tumours or metabolic disease.

How it happens

Fractures occur when traumatic forces are exerted on the bone. Because children are more flexible than adults, they may not be as prone to fractures.

Sticks and stones may bend my bones

Rather than fracturing completely, children's bones tend to simply bend, buckle or sustain an incomplete fracture.

Common fractures in children

Bends, buckle fractures, greenstick fractures and complete fractures commonly occur during childhood. Each of these fractures is described and illustrated below.

Bends

Bends are common in childhood because of the flexibility of children's bone. Children's bones can be bent up to 45 degrees, or possibly more, before breaking.

Buckle (torus) fractures

Buckle fractures occur due to compression of the porous bone, causing a raised area or bulge at the fracture site.

Greenstick fractures

Greenstick fractures occur when the bone is bent beyond its limits, causing an incomplete fracture.

Complete fractures

Complete fractures occur when the bone is broken into separate pieces.

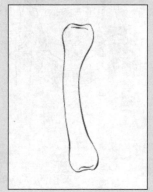 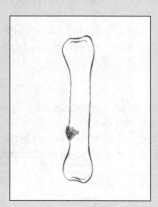 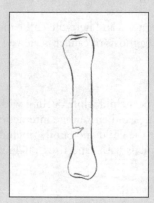 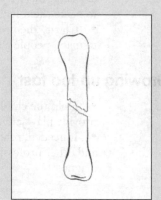

A stressful situation

Stress fractures are associated with unusually strong physical stress and are commonly seen in children who suddenly begin a vigorous training program. (See *Common fractures in children*.)

The remodelling team

After a fracture occurs, the body quickly begins a repairing process. A blood clot is formed at the site of the fracture. Osteoblasts and fibroblasts then converge on the site and begin to lay down an organic matrix. This forms a callus into which calcium salts are deposited, evolving into bone tissue that connects the pieces of the original bone. After that happens, the callus is remodelled into a strong, permanent bone.

What to look for

Bone fractures are classified according to:
• type of injury to the bone or surrounding tissue

- whether they're open (in which the skin has been broken due to penetration of bone fragment or external trauma) or closed (in which the fracture is contained under the skin's surface)
- whether there's involvement of the epiphyseal (growth) plate.

Sudden and sharp

Fractures usually cause sudden, sharp pain at the fracture site. Pain increases with movement and limits motion in the affected part. Swelling, bruising or discoloration around the site may occur. There may be obvious deformity or abnormal positioning of the affected part.

What tests tell you

X-rays provide the definitive diagnosis for a fracture. Occasionally, an incomplete fracture isn't seen initially on the X-ray, and appears only after the film has dried after several hours. Serial X-rays are taken to monitor healing and check the alignment of the bone.

Complications

Complications of fractures include infection, particularly in open fracture. A fracture that affects the growth plate can interrupt and alter growth. The impact of this alteration depends on the area of the epiphyseal plate that's affected.

The Salter–Harris classification system is used to determine the severity of the injury on the epiphyseal plate. Type I injuries typically don't affect growth. Injuries identified as type III and above require intervention to prevent future dysfunction in the bone and affected body part. (See *Salter–Harris classification system*, page 392.)

From bone to lung

Fat embolism is a major, life-threatening complication of a fracture. Fat globules are released into the circulation and can become lodged in the capillaries of the lung, thereby decreasing the exchange of oxygen and carbon dioxide. Signs of an embolism are increasing blood pressure, dyspnoea and other signs of respiratory compromise.

How it's treated

Reducing or realigning the bone into proper placement and allowing it to heal is the treatment required for a fracture. The reduction may be closed (through external manipulation of the body part) or open (done through surgery).

Closed reductions are usually treated with casting. Surgical repair of a fracture involves the use of either internal or external fixation devices.

Permanent hardware

Internal devices (rods, pins or wires) are permanent; they remain in the child unless a problem develops. External devices are pins or wires that are inserted

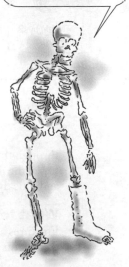

A cast is usually applied after a closed reduction. It's a little easier on the eyes when there's clothing involved – not to mention skin.

Salter–Harris classification system

The Salter–Harris classification system divides growth plate fractures into five categories. These categories are based on the type of damage to the growth plate.

Type I	Type II	Type III	Type IV	Type V
The epiphysis is completely separated from the metaphysis or end of bone. Although a type I fracture generally requires casting, it rarely requires manipulation. Growth disturbance isn't common unless the blood supply has been injured.	Type II is the most common type of fracture. The epiphysis and the growth plate are separated from the cracked metaphysis. This type of fracture must be manipulated and casted for normal growth to continue. Minimal shortening of the bone may occur but usually doesn't result in functional limitations.	Type III is a rare fracture that usually involves the lower tibia, or a long bone of the lower leg. It occurs when the fracture runs completely through the epiphysis and separates part of the epiphysis and the growth plate from the metaphysis. Surgery may be necessary. Growth usually isn't affected as long as the blood supply to the bone is intact.	A type IV fracture runs through the epiphysis, across the growth plate and into the metaphysis. It occurs most commonly in the humerus near the elbow. Perfect alignment must be achieved for normal growth to occur.	A crush or compression injury, a type V fracture most likely occurs in the knee or ankle. Stunting of growth is possible and prognosis is poor. Surgery is required as well as future reconstructive or corrective surgery.

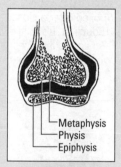

- Metaphysis
- Physis
- Epiphysis

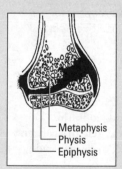

- Metaphysis
- Physis
- Epiphysis

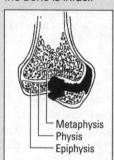

- Metaphysis
- Physis
- Epiphysis

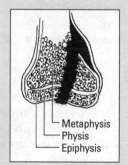

- Metaphysis
- Physis
- Epiphysis

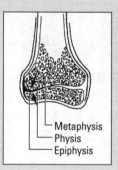

- Metaphysis
- Physis
- Epiphysis

through the bone and then attached to an external frame. When the bone heals, the devices are removed. Follow-up evaluation is essential to prevent and quickly treat complications that may arise.

What to do

Fractures are usually treated in an emergency setting. Formal preparation for treatments and procedures may not be possible.

Prepare on the go

Tell the child (and parents) everything that's being done as it's happening and provide as much support as possible to help ease the child's fears and enhance cooperation.
• Provide emergency care to the child with a fracture; steps should be taken to quickly assess the injury, prevent further damage and promote comfort.
• Ensure analgesia or sedation is given as prescribed.
• Frequently check for neurological and circulatory compromise to the affected area.

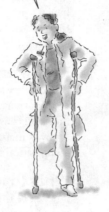

Telling the child his classmates will think his crutches are 'cool' – priceless!

Cast caution

• After the cast or splint has been applied, continue to assess the area around the cast.
• When a fracture requires long-term immobilisation with traction, reposition the patient often to increase comfort and prevent pressure ulcers, assist with active ROM exercises to prevent muscle atrophy and encourage deep breathing and coughing to prevent pneumonia.

Are you shocked?

• Watch for signs of shock in the child with a severe open fracture of a large bone such as the femur.
• Assist the child to regain normal function as quickly as possible; encourage them to start moving around as soon as they can, help them to walk and demonstrate how to use crutches properly.
• Help the family deal with the fracture and help the child understand what's happening.

Postscript

• Encourage the child to talk about the experience and express their feelings after the emergency is over; use this time to answer questions and clear up misconceptions (as would usually be done before treatment).

Different histories

Fractures can result from physical abuse and so health care professionals must be alert to the history, details and information given by caregivers in comparison with the child's injuries. Where there are concerns, the health professional must follow local safeguarding children procedures.

Juvenile rheumatoid arthritis

JRA is a chronic, autoimmune disease of the connective tissue. It's a group of conditions characterised by the presence of chronic synovial inflammation. Immunogenetic traits in children with JRA are different from those in adults with adult rheumatoid arthritis. These traits may be significant because of their effect on the formation of cellular antibodies, the immune system and consequent chronic inflammation.

What causes it

The exact cause of JRA is unknown. Some experts believe that tissue injury in a joint causes normal immunoglobulins within the joint to become antigenic. This tissue injury may be a result of infection, possibly viral. Researchers haven't pinpointed a specific infectious gene marker, or even identified the mechanism that provokes the systemic and local immune responses in children with JRA.

How it happens

Autoantibodies develop in response to injured joint tissue. These autoantibodies are known as rheumatoid factors. These factors then lodge in the joint's synovial fluid and cause inflammation. As the inflammatory process continues, the synovial membrane thickens, production of synovial fluid increases and cellular composition is altered. This process results in pain, swelling and limited mobility.

What to look for

There are three major presentations of JRA. Most children with JRA exhibit some joint swelling, warmth and morning stiffness. (See *Types of JRA*.)

What tests tell you

There's no diagnostic test for JRA. In early stages of the disease, only soft tissue swelling may be seen on X-ray. MRI of the involved joints may show joint damage.

When things happen quickly, encourage the child to express concerns and ask questions *after* the emergency is over

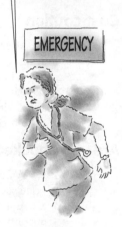

EMERGENCY

Types of JRA

There are three major types of juvenile rheumatoid arthritis (JRA), each with its own presentation.

Pauciarticular (oligoarthritis) disease

Pauciarticular disease is characterised by chronic arthritis in four or fewer joints. The large joints (knees, ankles, elbows) are most commonly affected. This presentation accounts for 50% of all JRA cases. The symptoms are typically mild with possibly little or no pain. Systemic features are uncommon but the eyes can be severely inflamed.

Polyarticular pattern

The polyarticular pattern of JRA most closely resembles the adult disease. Chronic pain and swelling occur in five or more joints, usually the knees, wrists, ankles, neck and elbows. Systemic features are usually less prominent, although a low-grade fever, fatigue and anaemia may be present. This process may wax and wane over the course of years. It accounts for approximately 30% of all cases and affects girls more commonly than boys.

Systemic JRA

In systemic JRA, an acute presentation of the disorder, a salmon-pink rash appears on the trunk and extremities, high fever occurs and anorexia and weight loss are common. Joint involvement occurs later in the disease process. Other areas of the body may be affected, including the heart, liver, lungs and blood. This type of presentation accounts for approximately 20% of all JRA cases and may be episodic. Remission of the systemic features may occur within 1 year.

Haematological tests may help confirm the diagnosis if clinical manifestations are present:
- Rheumatoid factor is positive in only 15% of cases.
- Leucocytes may be elevated, suggesting an inflammatory process.
- Erythrocyte sedimentation rate may be normal or elevated.
- Antinuclear antibodies may be present.

Complications
The prognosis for children with JRA is very good. It's a self-limiting disease, and 70% to 90% survive JRA without functional limitations. However, some complications do occur:
- In children with early-onset pauciarticular disease involving only one knee, there may be a significant difference in leg length.

Thrown another curve

- The incidence of scoliosis may be up to 10 times higher in children with JRA than in the general population.
- Cervical spine involvement and other skeletal abnormalities may develop in up to 70% of children with arthritis.
- Anaemia is a common feature of systemic and polyarticular arthritis.

The eyes have it

- Up to 30% of children with pauciarticular arthritis develop an inflammation of the iris and ciliary bodies of the eye (uveitis) which produces no symptoms but may cause blindness if left untreated.
- Children with JRA are at increased risk for iridocyclitis (inflammation of the iris and ciliary body in the eye).

How it's treated
Treatment of JRA aims to reduce disease activity, relieve symptoms and maintain function.

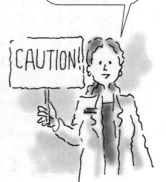

A child with JRA should be referred to an ophthalmologist who will check for signs of eye involvement.

Non-steroidal anti-inflammatory drugs (NSAIDs) first unless pain is worse.

NSAIDs are prescribed to decrease inflammation and relieve pain; aspirin (one of the rare occasions and must be prescribed by a consultant) may be given or another drug, such as naproxen or ibuprofen, may be used. If NSAIDs fail, then disease-modifying drugs (DMDs) are used and may include:
- Methotrexate, hydroxychloroquine, gold, penicillamine, sulphasalazine
- Immunosuppressants such as cyclosporin A, azathioprine, cyclophosphamide and chlorambucil
- Intravenous Gamma globulin
- Corticosteroids
- Etanercept (cytokine modulator).
  Occasionally, local corticosteroid injections or joint replacement is required.

Up and active

ROM and muscle strengthening exercises are ordered and carried out by a physiotherapist. Unless JRA is in the most acute stage, bed rest should be avoided. Involvement of the eye should be treated by an ophthalmologist.

What to do

The child and his parents will need help adjusting to the realities of a chronic disease. Parents may tend to be overprotective, and may need help to find the balance between allowing their child to live a normal life and protecting them from injury and complications.

In addition, follow these steps:
• Monitor the child for signs of joint limitation and pain.
• Teach the family about the disease process and how to monitor for complications.
• Help parents acquire the skills needed to parent a child with a chronic illness.

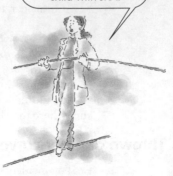

It's a balancing act. There's a fine line between protecting and overprotecting a child with JRA.

Helpful or harmful?

• Help family members distinguish between harmless interventions and those that are potentially harmful; some studies show that most children will try alternative medicines for JRA, including copper bracelets, acupuncture, herbs and other medicines and diet.
• During inflammatory exacerbations, administer NSAIDs or prescribed medication on a regular schedule.

Energy conservation

• Allow the child to rest frequently throughout the day to conserve energy for times when they must be mobile.
• Ensure the child receives regular slit-lamp examinations to enable early diagnosis and treatment of iridocyclitis.

Legg–Calvé–Perthes disease (often shorted to perthes)

Legg–Calvé–Perthes disease is an avascular necrosis of the femoral head. It may involve the entire femoral head or only a portion of it. There may be a widening and flattening of the femoral head. The disorder can appear at any time between 2 and 12 years, although it's most commonly seen between 4 and 8. Boys are five times more likely to be affected than girls. It usually affects only one hip. If both hips are symmetrically affected, an underlying systemic disorder should be considered.

What causes it

Necrosis of the bone is caused by diminished blood supply to the femoral head. It isn't known what causes the blood supply to be interrupted.

Epidemiologic studies show an increased association of Legg–Calvé–Perthes disease with such factors as low birth weight, older parental age at conception and lower socioeconomic status, to name a few. Short stature as well as delayed bone maturation for age also seem to be risk factors.

Other theories have focused on conditions that could directly impede blood flow to the femoral head. Disorders of coagulation, such as thrombophilia, may predispose a child to Legg–Calvé–Perthes disease.

How it happens

Legg–Calvé–Perthes disease has three distinct stages:

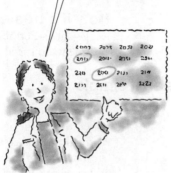

It's worth the wait. A few years of healing can result in completely normal bone in a child with Legg–Calvé–Perthes disease.

The avascular stage is characterised by the interference of the blood supply to the head of the femur; without an appropriate blood supply, death of the bone cells (osteocytes) and bone marrow cells occurs. This stage can last several months to 1 year.

During the revascularisation stage, vascular and connective tissue invade the dead bone in a process called creeping substitution; the necrotic tissue is replaced with living bone, although the bone isn't yet calcified.

In the final stage, also called the healing stage, ossification occurs; this process can take between 2 and 3 years to complete.

A job well done

The replacement of necrotic bone may be so complete and perfect that a completely normal bone results.

What to look for

Typically, children with Legg–Calvé–Perthes disease demonstrate a painless limp. Occasionally, pain is present and is made worse by activity. Pain is usually referred to the knee. Children may also complain of anterior thigh or groin pain.

What tests tell you

Symptoms may occasionally follow an injury, but studies usually show the disease was present before the injury.

X-rays correlate with the progression of the disease and the extent of the necrosis. There may be evidence of decreased bone mass and a smaller ossification centre. A subchondral fracture may be an early finding in the child with Legg–Calvé–Perthes disease. As the disease progresses, X-rays will show changes.

Complications

Osteochondritis dissecans occurs in less than 5% of children with Legg–Calvé–Perthes disease. In this disorder, a wedge-shaped necrotic area of bone and cartilage develops adjacent to the joint. It may break off and become lodged within the joint itself. The growth plate may be affected in severe disease.

Prognosis depends on the child's age, the extent of femoral head involvement, the disease's duration and ROM. Some long-term studies have suggested that osteoarthritis leading to the need for total hip replacement will commonly develop later in life.

How it's treated

Legg–Calvé–Perthes disease is a self-limiting disease with no known treatments to speed the return of blood to the femoral head.

Keep it simple

Treatment consists simply of protecting the joint. If the joint is deeply seated within the acetabulum and normal joint motion is maintained, then a reasonably good result can be expected.

The goal of treatment is to reduce hip irritability, restore normal ROM and prevent subluxation or dislocation. Surgical intervention is sometimes required.

Non-surgical intervention includes physiotherapy, traction and crutches. Casts and abduction bracing have been used in an attempt to hold the femoral head in place while the disease runs its course, but recent studies have shown no benefit from this type of treatment.

What to do

The child (and his parents) will need continuous emotional support. They should be encouraged to talk about their fears, anxiety and frustration. Explaining all procedures as well as the need for bed rest will help reduce anxiety.

In addition, follow these steps:
- Administer analgesics as ordered.
- Encourage parents to participate in their child's care.
- Stress the need for follow-up care to monitor rehabilitation.

Party at Tommy's bedside! RSVP

- Stress the need for home tutoring and socialisation to promote normal mental and emotional growth and development.
- Offer tips for making home management of the bedridden child easier; tell parents what different items might be needed, such as pyjamas and trousers in a size larger than usually worn (with the side seam opened and Velcro fasteners attached to close it), a bedpan, adhesive tape, sheepskin and, possibly, a hospital bed.
- Involving the community children's nursing team will assist the family to cope with managing the treatments at home.

When kids talk about hanging out, this isn't what they have in mind! Diversional activities keep boredom in check, and will help keep development on track.

It's hard to be a patient patient

• Remind the child and parents that, although recovery may be a long and frustrating process, this is a self-limiting disease and the child will ultimately recover.

Scoliosis

Scoliosis is a spinal deformity; it's defined as a lateral curvature of the spine that's greater than 10 degrees, and is always associated with some rotation of the involved vertebrae. Posterior curvature of the spine is known as kyphosis, and anterior curvature is known as lordosis. Although some curvature is normal, excessive curvature becomes pathologic. Scoliosis is classified as either non-structural (functional) or structural. (See *Looking at scoliosis*.)

Scoliosis can occur at any age, but idiopathic scoliosis is seen in greatest numbers in children after 8 years. Girls are four to five times more likely to be affected than boys, and the incidence is higher if another family member is affected. The deformity progresses during growth periods and stabilises when vertebral growth is complete.

What causes it

In non-structural scoliosis, the spine is structurally normal and the disorder never progresses to structural scoliosis. Non-structural scoliosis may be caused by poor posture, leg-length discrepancies, an irritated sciatic nerve, or an infectious process such as appendicitis. A very rare psychological scoliosis is known as hysterical scoliosis.

Not sure about structure

Structural scoliosis can be caused by neuromuscular disorders, such as cerebral palsy, poliomyelitis or muscular dystrophy. Birth defects, injuries, certain infections, tumours and metabolic factors are also identified causes. Connective tissue disorders and rheumatic disease may also cause structural abnormalities. The cause of idiopathic scoliosis, the most common type of structural scoliosis, is unknown.

How it happens

The spine is normally curved in order to maintain proper balance, with the muscles on either side of the spine supporting it. If a lateral curve has developed, a convex rotation of the spine and ribs will eventually cause the vertebrae to become rotated or wedge-shaped. Muscles become contracted and a compensatory curve develops so that the body can maintain balance and posture.

What to look for

Examination of the child usually begins with a general inspection of the back with the child in a standing position. Obvious asymmetries can be seen, including:

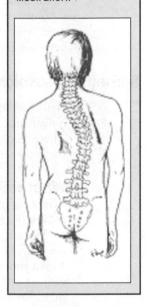

Looking at scoliosis

The spinal deformity that occurs in scoliosis is shown in this illustration.

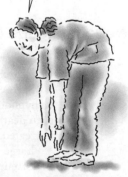

The signs of scoliosis are even more obvious when the child bends over.

- one shoulder higher than the other
- prominent scapula
- uneven waistline
- rib hump.

Over for obvious

As the child bends over, these asymmetries become even more obvious. The shoulder and hip levels become uneven. The head should normally align directly over the sacrum but, in persons with a spinal deformity, there may be deviation from the midline.

Something suspicious

Scoliosis classically produces no symptoms. If the child has pain, the scoliosis is likely due to some other disorder such as a bone or spinal cord tumour. These secondary causes must be ruled out. In cases of secondary scoliosis, the curvature will resolve when the underlying cause is treated.

What tests tell you

X-rays are used to evaluate the entire spine in the standing position, looking at both the anteroposterior and lateral planes.
- Measurement of skeletal maturity and shoulder and hip levels determines the degree of scoliosis.
- An abnormal forward bending test, in which the patient bends forward 90 degrees with the hands joined at the midline, demonstrates asymmetry of the shoulders and height of the ribs.
- Two types of measurement devices a level plane ruler, used for measurement while the patient is bending over, and a scoliosometer, designed to assess the angle of trunk rotation, are used only when management decisions will be affected, or to help reassure the child and family (both types of measurements are difficult to standardise).

Complications

Complications can sometimes lead to serious, debilitating, or even life-threatening sequelae.

Negotiating the curves

The severity of complications increases with the severity of the curvature:
- Severe curves can affect vital lung capacity, causing tachypnoea or even hypoxia; severe restrictive lung disease and even death from cor pulmonale may occur if scoliosis is left untreated.
- Large thoracic curves greater than 60 degrees are associated with a shortened life span.

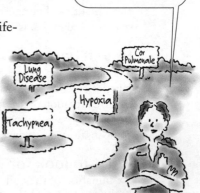

Severe curves can have severe consequences in a child with scoliosis.

- Large lumbar curvatures may lead to subluxation of the vertebrae and arthritic changes in the spine; disabling pain in adulthood may result because of these changes.
- Neurological sequelae and paralysis may be a complication if the vertebral column is manipulated during surgery.
- Infection is always a risk after surgery.

How it's treated

Treatment of scoliosis depends on the magnitude of the curve, skeletal maturity and the risk of progression. No treatment is necessary in children with functional scoliosis or in whom the curve is less than 20 degrees. Structural scoliosis is treated as early as possible in order to lessen or prevent progression. Stretching and strengthening the back muscles improve posture and maintain flexibility.

Brace yourself

Bracing is used in skeletally immature children with curves between 20 and 40 degrees. A silastic, thoracolumbosacral brace is moulded to the child and exerts gentle pressure on the spine. This brace is worn 23 hours per day until growth is complete, usually for several years. It's removed only for hygiene and skin care.

No confusion, it's spinal fusion

Spinal fusion surgery, rod placement and bone grafting may be required to correct curves greater than 45 degrees. Activities are restricted for several months until the fusion is solid.

What to do

It's essential to assess continually for compliance, as non-compliance with recommended treatment measures may be detrimental. In addition, follow these steps:
- Teach the prescribed treatment routines to the child and parents, and explain the consequences of not following these recommendations (to help ensure the best possible outcome).
- Emphasise activity restrictions; provide alternative exercises and activities that are beneficial.

Stealth brace

- Help the child find clothing that minimises the appearance of the brace to enhance their self-image; teach them to wear a light T-shirt underneath the brace and to place a smooth cloth over the chin pad (to minimise skin breakdown and promote skin integrity).

A strange new world

- For children requiring surgical correction, pre-operative teaching is essential. Prepare the child for the presence of various catheters, a special bed

(Stryker frame), and the use of certain body mechanics in order to restrict bending at the fusion site. (Peer support groups may be helpful when the child can return home.)

Quick quiz

1. Ortolani's test is performed to rule out:
    A. JRA.
    B. congenital talipes.
    C. DDH.
    D. osteogenesis imperfecta.

Answer: C. Ortolani's test is performed to reveal hip instability associated with DDH.

2. Why are children less prone to fractures than adults?
    A. Children have more calcium in their bones.
    B. Children have stronger bones.
    C. Adults have brittle bones.
    D. Children have more cartilaginous bones.

Answer: D. Because young children have a more cartilaginous skeleton, they may be less prone to fractures than adults.

3. A nurse is caring for an infant with DDH. When teaching the parents to care for this child, the nurse should tell them:
    A. to have the child wear the Pavlik harness only when out of bed.
    B. to apply three nappies to the child to provide abduction to the hip.
    C. that immunisations will be delayed until the Pavlik harness is removed.
    D. that when the hips are stabilised, after about 2 or 3 weeks, the Pavlik harness can be removed for bathing purposes; otherwise, it should remain in place at all times.

Answer: D. The harness should be in place as much as possible to ensure proper joint alignment with the head of the femur in the acetabulum.

4. A child who's wearing a cast develops an itch under the cast. What should the nurse do to help relieve the itch?
    A. Use sterile applicators to scratch the itch.
    B. Apply cool air under the cast with a blow-dryer.
    C. Apply cool water under the cast.
    D. Apply hydrocortisone cream.

Answer: B. Itching underneath a cast can be relieved by directing a blow-dryer on the cool setting towards the itchy area.

5. How many hours per day should a child wear a brace for treatment of scoliosis?

    A. 8
    B. 12
    C. 23
    D. 24

Answer: C. A brace for the treatment of scoliosis should be worn 23 hours per day. The brace may be removed for 1 hour per day for bathing and hygiene purposes.

Scoring

⭐⭐⭐   If you answered all five items correctly, hip-hooray! You've earned the right to flex your muscles.

⭐⭐   If you answered four items correctly, fine work! Now you're ready to bone up for the next quiz.

⭐   If you answered fewer than four items correctly, don't let it rattle your bones! There are still four quizzes in your future – no bones about it.

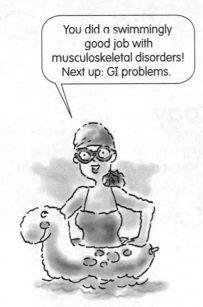

You did a swimmingly good job with musculoskeletal disorders! Next up: GI problems.

Gastrointestinal (12) problems

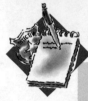

Just the facts

In this chapter, you'll learn:

♦ anatomy and physiology of the GI system
♦ diagnostic tests for children with GI disorders
♦ treatments and procedures used for children with GI disorders
♦ GI disorders that affect infants and children.

Anatomy and physiology

The functions of the GI tract enable ingestion and propulsion of food, digestion and absorption of food and nutrients needed by the body, and elimination of waste products.

Structures of the GI system

The GI system consists of two major components:

alimentary canal

accessory organs of digestion.

It's alimentary, my dear Watson

The alimentary canal of the GI tract consists of a hollow, muscular tube that begins in the mouth and ends at the anus. It includes the:
- oral cavity
- pharynx
- oesophagus

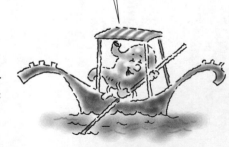

If neighbours make the neighbourhood, the alimentary canal is the best! To my north is Mr. Oesophagus, and to my south are the Intestines.

- stomach
- small intestine
- large intestine.

Accessories make the system

Accessory glands and organs that aid GI function include the:
- salivary glands
- liver
- biliary duct system (gallbladder and bile ducts)
- pancreas.

Digestion

Digestion starts in the oral cavity, where chewing (mastication), salivation (the beginning of starch digestion), and swallowing (deglutition) take place. (See *The growing GI system*.)

Growing pains

The growing GI system

Here are some highlights of the developing GI system during the first few years of life.

Salivary assistance

- Saliva production begins at age 4 months and aids in the process of digestion.
- The sucking and extrusion reflex (a reflex that protects the infant from food substances his system is too immature to digest) persists until ages 3 to 4 months.

Stomach

- The stomach capacity of the neonate is 30 to 60 ml, and gradually increases to 200 to 300 ml by 12 months.
- Up until 4 to 8 weeks, the neonatal abdomen is larger than the chest and the musculature is poorly developed.
- Spit-ups are frequent in the neonate because of the immature muscle tone of the lower oesophageal sphincter and the low volume capacity of the stomach.
- Peristalsis occurs within 2½ to 3 hours in the neonate and extends to 3 to 6 hours in older infants and children.
- Digestive enzymes are deficient until at least the age of 4 to 6 months; wind, diarrhoea, sensitisation for food allergies and microscopic haemorrhages can develop if solid foods are introduced before this time.

Intestinal

- From 1 to 3 years, the composition of intestinal flora becomes more adult-like and stomach acidity increases, reducing the number of GI infections.
- Exposure to breast milk increases intestinal flora early on and provides some protection against viruses and pathological flora.
- Increased myelination of nerves to the anal sphincter allows for physiologic control of bowel function, usually at about age 2; psychological readiness may occur at a later age.

Liver

- The liver is immature at birth, resulting in inefficient detoxifying of substances and medications; medication dosages may need to be adjusted.
- The liver's slow development of glycogen storage capacity makes the infant prone to hypoglycemia.
- Infants are more prone to dehydration and fluid and electrolyte imbalances due to greater body surface area, high rate of metabolism, and immature kidney function.

The rise and fall of hormones

Hunger is controlled by the lateral hypothalamus in the brain. A fall in blood nutrients, a rise or fall in hormones governing metabolism, hunger contractions from the stomach, and emotional input signal the hypothalamus to stimulate hunger. Fullness of the stomach, blood levels of nutrients and hormones, and emotions or habits stimulate the satiety centre in the ventromedial area of the hypothalamus to decrease hunger.

The tasteful tongue

The tongue provides the sense of taste and is the strongest muscle in the body. Saliva secreted from the salivary glands moistens the mouth and lubricates the food bolus to ease swallowing.

Look out stomach, here it comes!

When a person swallows a food bolus:

The upper oesophageal sphincter relaxes, allowing food to enter the oesophagus.

The epiglottis closes with swallowing to prevent food from being aspirated into the trachea.

As food moves through the oesophagus, glands in the oesophageal mucosal layer secrete mucus, which lubricates the food and protects the oesophageal mucosal layer from being damaged by poorly chewed foods. (See *Choking hazards*.)

Lower oesophageal contractions (called peristalsis) gradually push the food down the oesophagus and through the lower oesophageal sphincter into the stomach.

Stomach

Until the child is approximately 2 years, the stomach is round. It will gradually elongate and take the adult shape and position in the abdomen by 7 years of age.

The stomach lies in the left upper quadrant of the abdomen and is made up of three parts:

The fundus is an enlarged portion above and to the left of the oesophageal opening in the stomach; the cardiac sphincter is at the opening of the oesophagus to the stomach.

The body is the middle portion of the stomach.

The pylorus is the lower portion of the stomach, lying near the junction of the stomach and the duodenum. The pyloric sphincter is at the opening of the stomach to the duodenum.

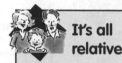

It's all relative

Choking hazards

Foods that are round and less than 1¼" (3.2 cm) in diameter can obstruct the airway of a child when swallowed whole. Teach parents to cut foods into small pieces to prevent obstruction of the airway. Common foods that may cause choking include:

- sausages
- nuts
- popcorn
- marshmallows
- grapes
- hard sweets
- fruits with stones.

A gastric response

The secretory cells in the lining of the stomach are believed to be functional at birth. The lining of the stomach secretes gastrin in response to stomach wall distension. In turn, gastrin stimulates the release of highly acidic digestive secretions consisting mainly of pepsin, hydrochloric acid, intrinsic factor, and proteolytic enzymes. Limited amounts of water, alcohol, and some drugs are absorbed in the stomach.

Triple overtime

The stomach's three functions are to store food, mix food with gastric juices via peristaltic contractions, and slowly distribute this food (now called chyme) into the small intestine through the pyloric opening for further digestion and absorption.

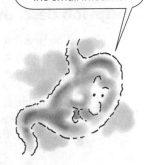

There's no such thing as a day off when you store the food, mix it with gastric juices, and send the chyme into the small intestine.

Small intestine

Nearly all digestion and absorption takes place in the small intestine. The small intestine lies coiled in the abdomen and consists of three major sections:

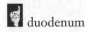 duodenum

jejunum

ileum.

Contractions and secretions

Peristaltic contractions and various digestive secretions break down carbohydrates, proteins and fats, enabling the intestinal mucosa to absorb these nutrients, along with water and electrolytes. Secretin and cholecystokinin are the hormones that affect intestinal secretions and gastric motility.

Distribution centre

The surface area of the small intestine is increased by millions of villi in the mucous membrane lining. Digested food is absorbed through the mucosal walls and into the blood for distribution throughout the body. Failure to feed, malnutrition, ischemia, and infections affect the small intestine's ability to absorb nutrients, resulting in growth delays.

Large intestine

The ileocecal valve is the sphincter between the ileum of the small intestine and the caecum of the large intestine. It prevents secretions from returning to the ileum. By the time chyme passes through the small intestine and enters the ascending colon of the large intestine, it has been reduced to mostly indigestible substances.

Downward spiral

From the ascending colon, chyme passes through the transverse colon and descending colon to the rectum, and finally into the anal canal, where it's expelled. The anal sphincter voluntarily controls defecation except in infants and patients with spinal cord injuries.

A large job description

The large intestine doesn't produce hormones or digestive enzymes; it is, however, the site of water and sodium absorption. The large intestine also harbours bacteria, such as *Escherichia coli* and *Enterobacter aerogenes*, which help synthesise vitamin K and break down cellulose into usable carbohydrates. The mucosa does produce alkaline secretions that lubricate the intestinal wall as chyme pushes through and protect the mucosa from acidic bacterial actions.

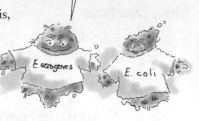

We aren't always the bad guys. As residents of the large intestine, we help synthesise vitamin K and break down cellulose.

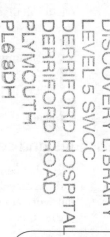

Accessory glands and organs

Allied with the GI tract are the liver, biliary duct system and pancreas, which contribute the hormones, enzymes and bile that are vital to digestion.

Liver

The liver is located in the right upper quadrant (RUQ) of the abdomen and is the body's largest gland. It plays an important role in carbohydrate metabolism, detoxifies various endogenous and exogenous toxins in plasma, and synthesises plasma proteins, non-essential amino acids and vitamin A.

Essential storage

The liver also stores essential nutrients, such as iron and vitamins K, D and B12. It secretes bile and removes ammonia from body fluids, converting it to urea for excretion in urine.

Biliary duct system

Bile is a greenish fluid that aids the small intestine to emulsify and absorb fats and fat-soluble vitamins. Bile exits through bile ducts that merge into the right and left hepatic ducts to form the common hepatic duct. This common duct joins the cystic duct from the gallbladder to form the common bile duct to the duodenum.

Gallbladder

The gallbladder, located beneath the liver, stores and concentrates bile produced by the liver. Secretion of the hormone cholecystokinin causes the gallbladder to contract and relax the ampulla of Vater, releasing bile into the common bile duct for delivery to the duodenum.

The stomach gets all the credit, but digestion would be a disaster without the accessory glands and organs!

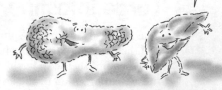

Pancreas

The pancreas is a large gland located behind the stomach and attached to the duodenum. The pancreas performs exocrine and endocrine functions. Its exocrine function involves cells that secrete digestive enzymes, bicarbonate and hormones into the small intestine to aid in digestion.

Alpha beta Langerhans

The endocrine function of the pancreas involves the islets of Langerhans, which house alpha and beta cells. Alpha cells secrete glucagon, which stimulates glycogenolysis in the liver. Beta cells secrete insulin to promote carbohydrate metabolism.

Diagnostic tests

Tests used to diagnose GI disorders include barium enema, barium swallow, endoscopic retrograde cholangiopancreatography (ERCP), endoscopy and stool specimen testing.

Barium enema

A barium enema, also called a lower GI series, allows X-ray visualisation of the colon. Barium is dripped into the rectum by gravity, and a series of X-rays is taken as the barium passes through the lower GI tract.

Nursing considerations

Explain the procedure to the child and parents. Prepare the child for insertion of the barium, and explain that they may be slightly uncomfortable when changing positions on the X-ray table. Also explain that the child will have to wait until the test is over to go to the toilet, and that bowel movements may look whitish until the barium has passed through his system.

• Sometimes, the child will be on a liquid diet for 24 hours before the test.

An interesting way to start the day

• Bowel preparations vary with amongst different units but in many case all that is needed for is for the child to avoid food with fibre the day before and then just have fluids from the night before.

• In some cases enemas are required the night before the test, the morning of the test, or both but this should be avoided where possible. (Prepare the child for the enema and provide as much privacy as possible.)

• Tell the child that X-rays will be taken on a special table and that they must try to lie still (even though they'll feel like going to the toilet).

• Cover the genital area with a lead apron during the X-rays.

Exit the barium

- Hydrate the child well with electrolyte-containing fluids after the procedure to prevent dehydration and to help expel the barium to prevent barium impaction and constipation.

Barium swallow

A barium or diatrizoate meglumine (Gastrografin) swallow, also called an upper GI series, provides imaging of the upper GI tract. It's used primarily to examine the oesophagus.

Follow the swallow

A series of X-rays is taken while the swallowed barium or Gastrografin moves into the oesophagus, stomach and duodenum, to reveal abnormalities. The barium outlines the stomach walls and delineates ulcer craters and filling defects. Gastrografin and barium facilitate imaging through X-rays, but Gastrografin is less toxic if it escapes from the GI tract.

Seeking the ileocaecal valve

A small bowel series is an extension of the upper GI series; additional imaging is done as the barium or Gastrografin flows farther down the GI tract, through the small intestine to the ileocaecal valve.

Nursing considerations

- Explain the procedure to the child and parents. Tell the child that they'll need to take big swallows of a thick drink that looks like a milkshake (but doesn't taste as nice so flavourings are often added!). Explain that pictures will be taken while they're drinking and afterward, and that they'll need to stay still during the X-rays.
- Depending on local policy, the child should not have breakfast on the day of the test but can be given some clear fluids up until a few hours before.
- After the test, monitor bowel movements for excretion of barium and monitor GI function.

Endoscopic retrograde cholangiopancreatography

In ERCP, a contrast medium is injected into the duodenal papilla to allow radiographic examination of the pancreatic ducts and hepatobiliary tree.

Nursing considerations

As a general anaesthetic is given obtain written, informed consent after explaining the procedure to the child and parents. In addition:
- check the child's history for allergies to cholinergics and iodine.

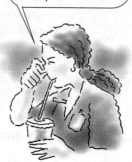

Barium preparations are disguised as milkshakes but they taste more like chalk! They're easier to swallow when they're ice cold.

It's all over

After the procedure:
• monitor the child's gag reflex (The child remains on NBM until his gag reflex returns.)
• protect the child from aspiration of mucus by positioning on their side
• monitor the child for urine retention.

Endoscopy

Endoscopy allows visualisation of the GI system (and, when needed, biopsy of tissue) with a fibre-optic scope.

The direct approach

Fibre-optic testing allows direct visualisation of the GI tract.
    Different types of fibre-optic testing are used to examine different portions of the GI tract:
• Gastroscopy allows visual inspection of the oesophagus, stomach and duodenum.
• Colonoscopy allows direct visualisation of the descending, transverse and ascending colon.
• Proctosigmoidoscopy allows inspection of the anus, rectum and distal sigmoid colon.

Nursing considerations

• Explain the procedure to the child and parents, and make sure that written, informed consent has been obtained.
• Prepare the child for sedation by explaining that it will make them sleepy and stop anything from hurting during the procedure.
• A mild sedative may be administered before the examination; prepare the child for insertion of an IV cannula for sedation during this procedure.
• The child may be kept NBM beginning at midnight before the test for an upper GI series.
• The child may be placed on a liquid diet for 24 hours before the examination or require enemas and laxatives until the bowel is clear for a lower GI series.
• After the procedure, assess vital signs for dyspnoea and fever with a decrease in blood pressure and an increase in pulse, indicating the possibility of bleeding from perforation.

Stool specimen

Stool specimens are obtained to examine the stool for suspected GI bleeding, infection or malabsorption. Tests include testing for occult (hidden) blood and microscopic tests for ova, parasites and fat.

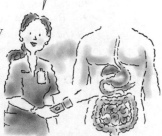

It's hard to hide from endoscopy! A fibre-optic scope can 'shine a light' on the entire GI system.

Nursing considerations

Nursing interventions focus on proper collection and handling of the specimen.
• Obtain the specimen in the correct container (the container may need to be sterile or contain a preservative).
• Be aware that the specimen may need to be transported to the laboratory immediately or placed in the refrigerator.
• For infants, stool specimens may be obtained from the nappy. However, apply a urine bag to prevent urine from contaminating the stool.

Treatments and procedures

Treatments and procedures for children with GI disorders include alternative feeding methods, total parenteral nutrition (TPN), GI intubation and ostomy creation.

Alternative feeding methods

Children who are unable to take nutrients by mouth (e.g. premature neonates with a poor sucking reflex, children who can't take in enough calories or children with disorders of the mouth and oesophagus, such as atresia and fistulas) are fed by alternative feeding methods. These methods include nasogastric (NG) or orogastric (OG) feeding, duodenum and jejunum gavage, gastrostomy or jejunostomy feeding. These feeds may be administered intermittently or continuously.

Nursing considerations

Explain to the child and parents why the alternative feeding method is needed, and prepare the child for insertion of the feeding tube. For the majority of children, the insertion of a tube is an unpleasant and uncomfortable experience and the extent to which they can assist will depend on age and cognitive development.

Nasogastric and orogastric feeds

In NG and OG feeds, a tube is inserted into the stomach by way of one of the nares (NG) or the mouth (OG). Follow these steps:
• To determine the correct length of the feeding tube, measure from the tip of the child's nose to his ear and add to that amount the length from his ear to his xiphoid process.

Cold coil in a cup

• Lubricate the tube with sterile water administration.
• Facilitate insertion of the NG tube by having the child take large swallows of water as the tube is being inserted; allow the child to practice first.

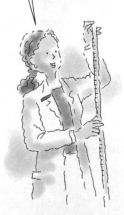

How long should it be? Do the maths! The tip of the child's nose to the ear + the ear to the xiphoid process = the tube length.

- When thc feeding tube is secured, check placement immediately, at the start of intermittent feeds, and at least every 4 hours thereafter.
- The only safe way of checking the placement is by aspirating and then testing with PH paper. It should be acidic (5.5 or less). However, radiographic confirmation of tube placement may also be undertaken but aspiration testing should still take place.
- The Woosh test, where air is inserted whilst listening to the abdomen, should not be used as it is potentially dangerous.

Recycle the residual

- Check the residual amount of formula by aspirating stomach contents into a syringe. Record the amount of residual formula and the colour, odour and consistency of the gastric contents before re-feeding the contents.
- Administer feeding by gravity or feeding pump.

Clear the clogs

- Irrigate the feeding tube with 10 ml of sterile water after each feeding to prevent stagnant formula from clogging the tube.
- Record the total amount of formula administered and how well it was tolerated. Observe for signs of aspiration and intolerance, including low oxygen saturation, difficulty breathing, increased crying or discomfort and vomiting.

Pinch and position

- If the feeding tube is to be removed after feeding, pinch the tube while withdrawing it to prevent aspirating fluid left in the tube.
- Position the child with his head elevated during the feeding and for 1 hour afterward to prevent aspiration.

Sucking for satiation

- When feeding infants by NG or OG tube, non-nutritive sucking is essential for oral stimulation. It helps the infant to relate a full stomach with oral sucking and fulfils the developmental need to suck.

Duodenum and jejunum gavage feeds
Duodenum and jejunum gavage feeds are administered with indwelling feeding tubes in the duodenum or jejunum.

Feeds are administered as they are with NG and OG feeds; however, the residual gastric contents and tube placement don't need to be checked. Duodenum and jejunum feeding tubes aren't removed after each feeding.

Gastrostomy and jejunostomy feeds
Gastrostomy and jejunostomy feeds are administered via a surgically placed feeding tube. The tube has one exit site on the abdomen but is composed of two separate chambers, each with a unique entry port. One side of the tube

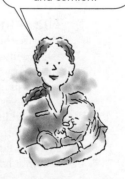

An infant who's receiving tube feeding still needs to suck. It provides stimulation and comfort.

ends in the stomach and is typically used for medication administration. The other side of the tube ends in the jejunum and is typically used for formula administration. Two types of gastrostomies are used: 'PEG' (percutaneous endoscopic gastrostomy) and the 'button' device.

It wouldn't work in outer space

In gastrostomy and jejunostomy feeds:
•   Boluses of formula or water are administered by gravity or by feeding pump.
•   The feeding tube must be flushed with sterile water after each feeding to prevent clogs.
•   The child should be positioned with his head elevated at a 30-degree angle after feeding to prevent aspiration and encourage gastric emptying.
•   Long-term gastrostomy tubes have a button closure that allows for the removal of the gastrostomy tube between feeds.
•   As with NG or OG tubes, infants fed by gastrostomy tube should engage in non-nutritive sucking for oral stimulation. It helps the infant to relate a full stomach with oral sucking and fulfils the developmental need to suck.

Total parenteral nutrition

TPN provides nutrients intravenously for infants and children who aren't able to take GI feeds, if GI feeds can't provide enough nutrition, or if feeding is needed long-term.

Concentrate on TPN

TPN is a highly concentrated solution of protein, glucose, vitamins and minerals. It's infused through IV tubing with a special filter to remove particulate matter and microorganisms. Low glucose solutions may be administered through a peripheral IV line. High glucose solutions are administered through central IV lines. Some medications, such as heparin and ranitidine (Zantac), may be added to the TPN solution and, therefore, shouldn't be administered separately.

TPN is typically administered with an intralipid infusion that provides necessary lipids and calories.

Nursing considerations

Prepare the child for insertion of the peripheral or central line. It can be frightening to a child (and their parents) if a line is inserted in the neck or shoulder area. Using a doll to demonstrate may help the child understand what will happen.

Asepsis is crucial when putting up or taking down TPN solution.

In addition, follow these steps:
•   Monitor the infusion rate via the IV pump. Cycling TPN, if ordered, involves tapering the drip rate at the start and end of the infusion, which commonly requires hourly rate changes.

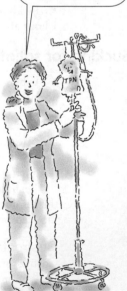

Parents may need reassurance that all the nutrition their child needs is in the TPN solution.

Infection inspection

- Assess the insertion site for signs of infection and infiltration because TPN can cause significant tissue damage.
- Bags of TPN should be changed every 24 hours; tubing should be changed according to your Trust's policy. The medical staff in consultation with dieticians and pharmacists will prescribe changes to the contents of the TPN solution based on the child's daily laboratory values. Inspect the bag of TPN; don't hang it if the solution appears cloudy or if there are precipitates visible (if so, return it to the pharmacy).

Not too much, not too little

- Electrolytes should be monitored for excesses and deficits, particularly hyperkalaemia and hypophosphataemia.
- Monitor the child's blood glucose for hyperglycaemia and administer insulin as prescribed.
- Reassure the parents that the TPN will provide all the nutrition the child needs.

GI intubation

GI intubation is the insertion of an NG tube for diagnostic and therapeutic purposes. It's used to:
- empty the stomach and intestine
- aid in diagnosis and treatment of stomach and upper GI tract disorders
- decompress obstructed areas
- detect and treat GI bleeding
- administer medications or feeds.

Nursing considerations

Prepare the child for insertion of the NG tube with a simple, age-appropriate explanation. Because many children panic at the sight of the tube, it's important to maintain a calm and reassuring manner and provide emotional support.

In addition, follow these steps:
- When inserting the tube, instruct the child to take swallows of water to ease insertion, which also gives the child a job to do and provides a degree of distraction.

What goes in must come out

- Maintain accurate intake and output records.
- Record the amount, colour, odour and consistency of gastric drainage every 4 hours.
- When irrigating the tube, note the amount of normal saline solution instilled and aspirated.

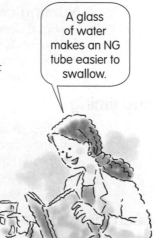

A glass of water makes an NG tube easier to swallow.

- Check for fluid and electrolyte imbalances.
- Provide good oral and nasal care. Make sure the tube is secure and doesn't put pressure on the nostrils.

Anchors away

- To support the tube's weight and prevent its accidental removal, anchor the tube to the child's clothing.
- After removing the tube from a child with GI bleeding, watch for signs and symptoms of recurrent bleeding.

Ostomy

An ostomy is an opening in the intestines with the intestinal wall drawn to the abdomen. A stoma is created to allow passage of intestinal contents. An ostomy can be permanent or temporary, depending on the reason for the ostomy and how much of the intestine has been removed.

Correct the defect

An ostomy is created to correct an anatomical defect, relieve an obstruction or permit treatment of an infection or injury to the intestinal tract. The most common reasons for an ostomy in infants and children are imperforate anus, necrotising enterocolitis, Hirschsprung's disease and inflammatory bowel diseases.

Location, location, location

An ileostomy is placed in the ileum portion of the small intestine. A colostomy is placed in the large intestine and may be ascending, transverse or descending, depending on where it's placed.

Nursing considerations

Explain the procedure in simple, age-appropriate terms, preparing the child and parents for all aspects of the surgery. Prepare the child and parents for the post-operative period; specifically, what the child will see on their body and how it might feel.

Bad timing

For older children and young people, who are already concerned with appearance and acceptance by their peers, concerns about body image and sexuality are likely. Encourage them to express these concerns and ask questions. (A same-gender nurse may be easier for the child to talk with.)

Been there, done that

If possible, introduce the child to a peer who has had the procedure and is handling it well. Refer the child to other

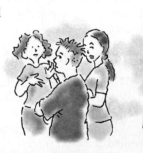

I want to be just like my friends, and having an ostomy makes me feel different. It helps to talk about it, and to have my questions answered.

health care professionals who can help them deal with body image issues. Also note the following:

- Mucous secretions begin within 48 hours after surgery.
- Faecal drainage begins within 72 hours after surgery.
- Oedema of the stoma is present for 2 to 3 weeks after placement.

A wash and a pat-dry

- When changing the stoma appliance (as needed), record the amount, character, colour and odour of the drainage; wash the peristomal area with warm water and gauze, rinse, pat dry, apply adhesive material (skin sealant and stoma paste) and reapply the drainage bag.
- Instruct the child and parents in care of the ostomy.
- If the skin is irritated, apply a protective ointment before applying the appliance.
- An infant's stoma may be left unpouched with a protective wafer around the stoma.

Pouch protector

- In young children, protect the pouch from being pulled off by using one-piece shirt-and-trouser outfits.
- To control odour in the appliance, use deodorant drops as advised.
- A low-residue diet may be required; avoid gas-producing foods or foods with strong odours.

Pass the salt

- With an ileostomy, sodium levels should be monitored and supplements prescribed as necessary.
- Protect the skin around the stoma from enzymes in liquid stool by using a skin protectant or by making sure that the opening to the wafer is cut close to the sides of the stoma.
- Have lots of fluid to replace that lost through the ileostomy.

GI disorders

GI disorders that may affect children include appendicitis, coeliac disease, cleft lip and palate, Crohn's disease, hepatitis, Hirschsprung's disease, intussusception, pyloric stenosis, tracheoesophageal fistula and oesophageal atresia, ulcerative colitis and volvulus.

Appendicitis

Appendicitis is an inflammation and obstruction of the blind sac (vermiform appendix) at the end of the caecum. It's the most common major surgical disease in school-age children and its peak incidence occurs in children

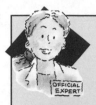

Advice from the experts

Abdomen assessment tips

Keep these tips in mind when assessing a child's abdomen:

- Wash and warm your hands before beginning the assessment.
- Note guarding of the abdomen and the child's ability to move around on the examination table.
- Flex the child's knees to decrease muscle tightening in the abdomen.
- Have child use deep breathing or distraction during the examination; a parent can help divert the child's attention.
- Have the child 'help' with the examination. Place your hand over the child's hand on the abdomen and extend your fingers beyond the child's fingers to decrease ticklishness of palpating the abdomen.
- Before palpation, auscultate the abdomen as palpation can produce erratic bowel sounds; lightly palpate tender areas last.

between 10 and 12 years. Although the appendix has no known function, it does regularly fill and empty itself with food.

What causes it

The appendiceal lumen becomes obstructed with faecal matter, calculi, tumours or strictures from trauma or infection due to bacteria, viruses or parasites.

How it happens

The obstruction of the appendiceal lumen sets off an inflammatory process that can lead to infection, thrombosis, necrosis and perforation. If the appendix ruptures or perforates, the infected contents spill into the abdominal cavity, causing peritonitis.

What to look for

At first, mid-abdominal cramps and tenderness are diffuse; eventually, they localise in the right lower quadrant (RLQ) at McBurney's point. The child will guard against anyone trying to examine their abdomen. (See *Abdomen assessment tips*.)

They may experience nausea and vomiting, and have a low-grade fever. Later complaints include lethargy, irritability, constipation and, rarely, diarrhoea.

Much ado about the RLQ

Auscultation reveals normal bowel sounds. As the inflammation increases, constant pain is noted in the RLQ with rebound tenderness; the pain is exacerbated by coughing and deep breathing.

Calm before the storm

If peritonitis occurs, abdominal distension and rigidity progress. Sudden cessation of abdominal pain signals perforation or infarction.

When the pain from appendicitis stops suddenly, it's the calm before the storm of perforation, or infarction, that is.

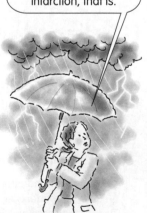

What tests tell you

Diagnosis of appendicitis is based on physical findings and characteristic clinical symptoms. A moderately elevated white blood cell (WBC) count with increased numbers of immature cells supports the diagnosis. Abdominal ultrasound may also be performed although the appendix can hide!

Complications

The most common complication of appendicitis is peritonitis from appendix rupture, which is a clinical emergency. Signs and symptoms of peritonitis include fever, abdominal distension and rigidity, sudden relief of pain, decreased bowel sounds, nausea and vomiting. Other possible complications include ischemic bowel and post-operative wound infection.

How it's treated

Appendectomy is the only effective treatment of appendicitis. Laparoscopic appendectomy decreases recovery time and hospital stay. If peritonitis develops, treatment involves GI intubation, parenteral replacement of fluids and electrolytes and administration of antibiotics.

What to do

Because an appendectomy is usually performed on an emergency basis, there may not be time to formally prepare the child for surgery.

Seize the day

Seize the opportunities that nursing care provides (bedside care, transporting the child, administering medications) to provide brief explanations and answer the child's questions. At the very least, tell the child that they'll be given a special medicine and won't feel anything during surgery.

Tell them where they'll be when waking up and when they'll see their parents. Tell the child what to expect when they wake (IV line, NG tube, level of discomfort and what will be done to make them feel better). In addition, follow these steps:
• Allow the child to find a position to decrease pain.
• Administer IV fluids to prevent dehydration, and keep the child NBM until after surgery is performed.
• Never apply heat to the right lower abdomen; this may cause the appendix to rupture.
• Although analgesia may mask some of the symptoms the child should be kept as pain-free as possible.

Post-operative care

• Be aware that the child with a ruptured appendix may have a drain and an NG tube attached to low intermittent suction.
• Keep the incision site clean and dry; change dressings when soiled.

A malodorous sign

- Document the return of bowel sounds, the passing of flatus and bowel movements – all signs of peristalsis.
- Administer antibiotics and pain medication as prescribed.

Infection detection

- Instruct the parents in care of the wound and the signs and symptoms of infection.

Coeliac disease

Coeliac disease is an inborn error of metabolism characterised by poor food absorption and intolerance of gluten (a protein found in grains, such as wheat, rye, oats and barley). The disease usually generally becomes apparent between 6 and 18 months of age, after gluten-containing foods are introduced into the diet.

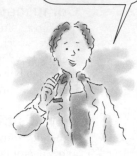

To the child with coeliac disease, gluten is the enemy. The child is born with an intolerance of the protein.

What causes it

This relatively uncommon disorder probably results from environmental factors and a genetic predisposition, but the exact mechanism is unknown. Two theories prevail:

The first theory suggests that the disease involves an abnormal immune response.

The second theory proposes that an intramucosal enzyme defect produces an inability to digest gluten.

How it happens

A decrease in the amount and activity of enzymes in the intestinal mucosal cells results in damage to those cells when exposed to gluten. This damage causes the villi of the proximal small intestine to atrophy and decreases intestinal absorption.

Inspection of a child with coeliac disease may reveal malnutrition.

What to look for

Symptoms vary but typically include recurrent attacks of diarrhoea, steatorrhoea (fatty, foul-smelling stools), abdominal pain and distension, vomiting, anorexia, irritability and coagulation difficulties from the malabsorption of fat-soluble vitamins. Inspection reveals signs of generalised malnutrition and failure to thrive, such as a potbelly or muscle-wasting.

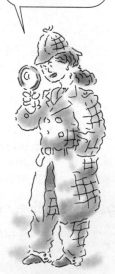

What tests tell you

- Histological changes seen on small-bowel biopsy specimens confirm the diagnosis.
- A glucose tolerance test shows poor glucose absorption.

- Serum laboratory tests indicate decreases in levels of albumin, calcium, sodium, potassium, cholesterol and phospholipids.
- Haemoglobin level, haematocrit, WBC counts and platelet counts may also be decreased.
- Immunological assay screen (immunoglobulin [Ig] A and IgG antibodies) is positive for coeliac disease.
- Stool specimens reveal a high fat content.

Complications

If not detected and properly treated, coeliac disease can be fatal because children become malnourished and debilitated. Complications include anaemia, bleeding disorders, small-bowel ulcerations, intestinal lymphoma and lactose intolerance.

How it's treated

Lifelong elimination of gluten from the child's diet is essential. A high-protein, low-fat, high-calorie diet that includes corn and rice products, soy and potato flour, breast milk or soy-based formula and all fresh fruits is required. Supportive treatment includes folic acid and iron supplements and administration of vitamins A and D in water-soluble forms.

What to do

Because of the need for lifelong adherence to the diet, the child and parents should be referred to a dietician who can help them make informed choices and plan a nutritious diet. (See *Teaching points for coeliac disease*.)

Cleft lip and palate

A cleft lip and palate occur when the bone and tissue of the upper jaw and palate fail to fuse completely at the midline in the first trimester of pregnancy. They may occur separately or together. Cleft deformities usually occur unilaterally or bilaterally, but rarely midline. Only the lip may be involved or the defect may extend into the upper jaw and nasal cavity. (See *A look at cleft lip and cleft palate*, page 422.)

What causes it

Cleft lip or palate most commonly occurs as an isolated birth defect. It may also occur as part of a chromosomal abnormality or after prenatal exposure to teratogens, such as anticonvulsant medications and alcohol.

How it happens

Defects originate in the second month of pregnancy, when the front and sides of the face and the palate shelves fuse imperfectly.

What to look for

Cleft lip can range from a simple notch on the upper lip to a complete cleft from the lip edge to the floor of the nostril. A cleft palate that occurs alone

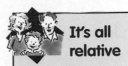

It's all relative

Teaching points for coeliac disease

Nursing interventions for a child with coeliac disease focus primarily on educating the parents about caring for the child at home, with an emphasis on dietary needs:

- Eliminate gluten from the diet.
- Provide a diet that includes corn and rice products, soy and potato flour and fresh fruits and vegetables; for the infant, give breast milk or soy-based formula.
- Replace vitamins and calories; give small, frequent meals.
- Monitor for steatorrhoea; its disappearance is a good indicator that the child's ability to absorb nutrients is improving.
- Read nutrition labels for sources of gluten.

A look at cleft lip and cleft palate

These illustrations show the four variations in cleft lip and cleft palate.

Notch with vermilion border **Unilateral cleft lip and cleft palate** **Bilateral cleft lip and cleft palate** **Cleft palate**

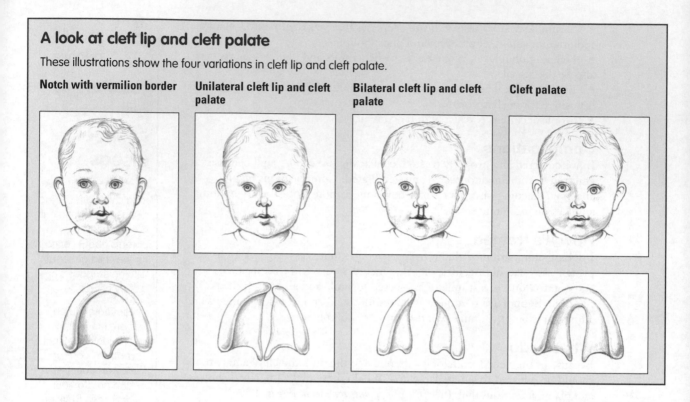

(without cleft lip) may be partial or complete, involving only the soft palate or extending from the soft palate completely through the hard palate.

What tests tell you

Prenatal ultrasonography where performed may detect two-thirds of occurrences. A typical clinical picture confirms the diagnosis. Cleft lip with or without cleft palate is obvious at birth. Cleft palate without cleft lip may not be detected until a mouth examination is done or until feeding difficulties develop.

Possible effects of the cleft

The effects of a simple cleft lip are largely cosmetic. Speech difficulties and failure to thrive (due to inadequate oral intake) are possible complications of unrepaired cleft palates. In addition, dentition problems, nasal defects, increased episodes of otitis media, hearing defects and appearance are concerns. The infant is also at increased risk for aspiration and upper respiratory infections. Parents' feelings of shock, guilt and grief may interfere with parent–child bonding.

How it's treated

Cheiloplasty (cleft lip surgery) is performed between 3 and 4 months; it unites the lip and gum edges. It's performed in anticipation of tooth eruption,

Advice from the experts

Preoperative cleft lip and cleft palate care

Nursing interventions before cleft lip or cleft palate repair (usually performed at 3 to 4 months of age) will help to ensure an optimal outcome.

Cleft lip

- Feed the infant slowly and in an upright position to decrease the risk of aspiration.
- Wind the infant frequently during feeding to eliminate swallowed air and decrease the risk of vomiting.
- Use gavage feedings if oral feedings are unsuccessful.
- Give a small amount of water after feedings to prevent milk from accumulating and becoming a medium for bacterial growth.
- Give small, frequent feeds to promote adequate nutrition and prevent tiring.

- Hold the infant while feeding, and promote sucking between meals; sucking is important for speech development.

Cleft palate

- It is advised that the infant is weaned from the bottle or breast before cleft palate surgery and should be able to drink from a cup.
- Teach the parents that the infant is susceptible to pathogens and otitis media from the altered position of the eustachian tubes.

providing a route for adequate nutrition and sucking. (See *Preoperative cleft lip and cleft palate care*.)

An early start

Palatoplasty (cleft palate repair surgery) is performed between 6 and 18 months, before speech patterns develop. The infant must be free from ear and respiratory infections before surgery.

A group effort

Long-term, team-oriented care aims to address speech defects, dental and orthopaedic problems, nasal defects and possible alterations in hearing.

What to do

Parents may experience grief over the 'perfect' child they had hoped for and expected. Those feelings may, in turn, cause feelings of guilt. Referral to a specialist nurse or a cleft lip and palate support group may be helpful in working through these feelings so appropriate parent–child bonding can take place.

In addition, follow these steps:
- To help determine an effective feeding method, assess the quality of the infant's sucking by determining if they can form an airtight seal around a finger or nipple that's placed in their mouth; special nipples are available for infants with cleft lip or palate.

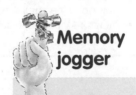

Memory jogger

When feeding an infant with cleft lip or cleft palate, remember the mnemonic ESSR:

E – *Elevate* the head during feeding and use an *Enlarged* nipple.
S – *Stimulate* the sucking reflex.
S – Wait for the child to *Swallow* to prevent choking.
R – Allow for a *Rest* period after each swallow.

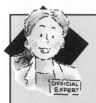

Advice from the experts

Post-operative cleft lip and cleft palate care

Many nursing interventions are needed after the surgical repair of a cleft lip or cleft palate.

Cleft lip

- Maintain a patent airway; oedema or narrowing of a previously large airway may make the infant appear to be in distress.
- Observe for cyanosis to detect signs of respiratory compromise as the infant begins to breathe through their nose.
- Maintain an intact suture line by keeping the infant's hands away from their mouth.
- Clean the suture line after feeds.
- Anticipate the infant's needs; this will help prevent crying.
- Give extra care and support because the infant's emotional needs can't be met by sucking.
- When feeds resume, use a syringe with tubing to administer foods at the side of the mouth to prevent trauma to the suture line.
- Monitor for pain and administer analgesia as prescribed.

Cleft palate

- Position the infant on their abdomen or side to maintain a patent airway.
- Assess for signs of altered oxygenation to promote good respiration.
- Use a cup for feeding to prevent injury to the suture line; don't use a nipple or pacifier.
- Keep hard or pointed objects away from the infant's mouth to prevent trauma on the suture line.
- Use elbow restraints to keep the child's hands out of his mouth; remove one restraint at a time.
- Provide soft toys to prevent injury.
- Distract or hold the infant to try to keep his tongue away from the roof of his mouth.
- Start the infant on clear liquids and progress to a soft diet.
- Rinse the suture line by giving the infant a sip of boiled and cooled water after each feed to prevent infection.
- Follow local guidelines for specific post-operative management

---

- Monitor vital signs and intake and output to determine fluid volume status.
- Prepare the child and parents for surgical repair of the defect.
- Monitor for complications and prepare the family to take over the follow-up care post-operatively. (See *Post-operative cleft lip and cleft palate care*.)

Crohn's disease

Crohn's disease is a chronic inflammation and ulceration of the GI tract anywhere from the mouth to the anus, usually involving the terminal ileum. The disease extends through all layers of the intestinal wall and may involve regional lymph nodes and the mesentery.

What causes it

Although the exact cause is unknown, possible causes include allergies and other immune disorders and infection (although no infecting organism has been identified). Genetic factors may also play a role.

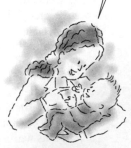

A special feeding nipple may be needed for the infant with cleft lip or palate.

How it happens

An inflammatory response causes mucosal ulcers to grow in size and depth in the mucosal wall of the GI tract. Fibrosis and stiffening of the mucosal wall can occur. Fistulas can develop between bowel loops or adjoining organs. Healing lesions develop scar tissue, leading to strictures.

What to look for

The child may report a gradual onset of symptoms, marked by periods of remission and exacerbation:
• Acute symptoms include steady, colicky pain in the RLQ (cramping); diarrhoea and flatulence; fever and bloody stool.
• Chronic symptoms, which are more typical of the disease, are more persistent and less severe. These symptoms include diarrhoea (four to six stools per day), pain in the RLQ, excess fat in stool, weight loss, weakness and fatigue, cramping and abdominal distension.

What tests tell you

Laboratory test findings indicate an increased WBC count and erythrocyte sedimentation rate (ESR). Other findings include hypokalaemia, hypocalcaemia, hypomagnesaemia and decreased haemoglobin level.

A string thing

Barium enema shows segments of stricture separated by normal bowel ('string sign'). Sigmoidoscopy and colonoscopy show patchy areas of inflammation. A biopsy is required for definitive diagnosis. Laboratory analysis to detect occult blood in stool is usually positive.

Complications

Complications of Crohn's disease include intestinal obstruction, fistula formation between the small bowel and bladder, perianal and perirectal abscesses and fistulas, intra-abdominal abscesses, bowel perforation, growth retardation and toxic megacolon.

A toxic outcome

Toxic megacolon is an acute dilation of the colon secondary to severe inflammation of bowel mucosa. Signs and symptoms are spiking fever, acute abdominal pain and abdominal distension. The bowel mucosa shreds, leading to haemorrhage and peritonitis, and may cause death.

How it's treated

The inflammatory response is controlled by the administration of corticosteroids, aminosalicylates, anti-infectives and immunosuppressive agents.

Give the bowel a rest

Effective treatment requires nutritional support with high-protein, high-calorie, low-fibre foods and supplements with iron, folic acid and vitamins.

Enteral formulas may be used as supplements. TPN may be administered to give the bowel a rest for healing.

A temporary fix

Surgical treatment may involve a bowel resection for obstructions or fistulas or a total colectomy with ileostomy if the bowel perforates or toxic megacolon occurs. Surgery doesn't cure Crohn's disease but relieves symptoms temporarily until the next exacerbation.

What to do

The child with Crohn's disease may need multiple hospitalisations.

Child interrupted

Do everything possible to 'normalise' the child's life during hospital stays. Maintain routines to the extent possible. Encourage the child to keep up with schoolwork, provide age-appropriate activities and diversions to maintain development and alleviate boredom and encourage his family and friends to spend as much time as possible with the child.

In addition, follow these steps:
• Administer analgesics and antispasmodics to decrease abdominal pain, and corticosteroids to decrease bowel inflammation.
• Withhold food and fluids, using parenteral nutrition in place of feeding to rest the bowel.

Keep it at bay

• Teach proper nutritional support to the child and parents, including the need for small, frequent meals that are high-protein, high-calorie and low-fibre; the use of multivitamin and iron supplements; and the need for bland foods when the child has mouth ulcers.
• Encourage medication compliance even while the child is in remission.
• Promote stress reduction through relaxation and distraction, and promote enhanced self-image and self-esteem; encourage participation in support groups.

Hepatitis

Hepatitis is a communicable, inflammatory condition of the liver; it can be acute or chronic. Hepatitis can be caused by several viruses, and the incubation period differs depending on the type of virus that causes it. Such disease processes as cancer and liver abscesses may also cause hepatitis. Neonatal hepatitis can occur in an infant born to a hepatitis B virus (HBV) – positive mother.

What causes it

There are several different viruses that cause hepatitis.

ABCs (and D's) of hepatitis

Hepatitis A virus (HAV) is the most common type in children and is transmitted by person-to-person contact (faecal-oral route) or through the ingestion of contaminated food, milk or water.

HBV is transmitted by direct contact with contaminated blood, secretions and faeces, most commonly through perinatal exposure from a HBV – positive mother.

Hepatitis C virus (HCV) is transmitted by exposure to blood or blood products, IV or intranasal drug use, and sexual contact, and may also be transmitted perinatally. HCV is most commonly transmitted through transfused blood from asymptomatic donors.

Hepatitis D virus (HDV) occurs only in children who also have HBV and is transmitted by intimate contact with a person who also has HBV.

The E and the G

Hepatitis E virus (HEV), not usually reported in children in the UK, is transmitted by inadequate hand washing or contaminated food and water. HEV is seen in countries with poor sanitation as the virus is found in stool. Hepatitis G virus (HGV) is a newly recognised virus also not reported in children. HGV is transmitted by blood transfusion, organ transplantation, IV drug abuse and sexual contact.

How it happens

Exposure to the virus or causative agent causes an inflammatory reaction in the liver. Lesions develop and cause necrosis of hepatic cells and scarring. Blood flow becomes obstructed, causing engorgement and hepatomegaly. Bile ducts become obstructed and bile accumulates in the blood, causing jaundice.

In mild forms of hepatitis, the liver cells regenerate and the patient recovers. In severe forms of hepatitis, the liver becomes necrotic and death occurs.

What to look for

Assessment findings are similar for the different types of hepatitis. Typically, signs and symptoms progress in several stages.

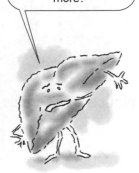

Hepatitis does a real number on me – inflammation, lesions, necrosis, scarring, hepatomegaly and jaundice. Need I say more?

Tired and irritable

In the prodromal stage, the child complains of fatigue, anorexia, mild weight loss, malaise, irritability, headache, weakness, photophobia and nausea with vomiting. Assessment reveals fever, the onset of clinical jaundice, dark-coloured urine and clay-coloured stools. Children younger than age 2 years are commonly asymptomatic with HAV.

Itchy and uncomfortable

During the clinical jaundice stage, the child has itching, abdominal pain, indigestion, skin rashes and hives. Palpation reveals RUQ discomfort and an enlarged, tender liver.

What tests tell you

Elevated liver enzymes (aspartate aminotransferase, alanine aminotransferase, alkaline phosphatase) are revealed in the prodromal stage. ESR and bilirubin levels are elevated, and prothrombin time is elongated.

A view from the side

A hepatitis profile, which identifies antibodies specific to the causative virus, establishes the type of viral hepatitis. A liver biopsy is performed if chronic hepatitis is suspected.

Complications

Complications of hepatitis include cirrhosis, liver cancer, chronic hepatitis, pancreatitis, myocarditis, pneumonia, aplastic anaemia and life-threatening fulminant hepatitis.

No turning back

Fulminant hepatitis causes unremitting liver failure with encephalopathy, which progresses to coma and usually leads to death within 2 weeks. Signs and symptoms of fulminant hepatitis include:

- vomiting
- anorexia
- jaundice
- ascites
- GI bleeding
- abdominal pain
- lethargy
- progressing disorientation
- coma.

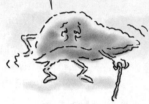

Fulminant hepatitis is too much for me. All that's left is failure without remission.

Notice of necrosis

A decrease in hepatomegaly is an ominous sign of tissue necrosis. Children with HBV have a much greater chance of becoming chronic carriers than adults, and of developing cirrhosis and liver cancer.

How it's treated

Treatment of hepatitis is supportive and focuses on rest, comfort and good nutrition. Antihistamines are administered to decrease the inflammatory process and relieve itching from the rash.

Hepatitis prevention

Immunoglobulin is administered within 2 weeks of exposure to HAV or HBV to prevent the disease. The neonate born to an HBV – positive mother should receive the HBV vaccine and hepatitis B immunoglobulin within 12 hours of birth. Additional doses of the hepatitis B vaccine should be administered at 1 and 6 months.

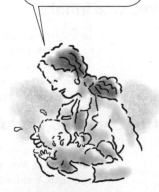

A few needle sticks is a small price to pay. HAV vaccine is recommended where the disease is prevalent, and HBV vaccination is recommended for all neonates.

What to do

Hepatitis is a frightening diagnosis for parents. Provide reassurance and assist parents in getting their questions answered. Prepare the child for blood taking and IV line insertions. In addition, follow these steps:
• Promote comfort to decrease abdominal discomfort.

A little here, a little there

• Provide small, frequent meals and snacks to support nutrition.
• Administer anti-emetics to decrease nausea and antihistamines to decrease itching; avoid paracetamol and other drugs metabolised by the liver.
• Limit activity to promote rest.

Back to school

• Educate the parents about the disease.
• Teach the parents about preventive measures, such as immunisations, good hand-washing habits and proper disposal of nappies; explain the need to avoid sharing contaminated items.
• Instruct the parents to seek appropriate advice before administering medications or over-the-counter products (because of impaired liver function).
• Instruct parents to watch for signs and symptoms that indicate worsening of hepatitis, leading to fulminant hepatitis.

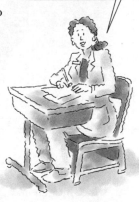

When a child has hepatitis, it's the parents who need an education – on everything from hand washing to recognising signs of worsening disease.

Hirschsprung's disease

Hirschsprung's disease is the absence of parasympathetic ganglionic cells in a segment of the colon, usually at the distal end of the large intestine. The lack of nerve innervation causes an absence of, or alteration in, peristalsis in the affected part of the colon. (See *A look at Hirschsprung's disease*, page 430.)

What causes it

Hirschsprung's disease is believed to be the result of a congenital, usually familial, defect. The disease may coexist with other congenital anomalies, particularly Down's syndrome and anomalies of the urinary tract.

How it happens

As stool enters the affected part, it remains there until additional stool pushes it through. The affected part of the colon dilates; a mechanical obstruction may result.

What to look for

In a neonate, history commonly reveals a failure to pass meconium and stool within the first 24 to 48 hours after birth. On inspection, the infant may have abdominal distension and easily palpable stool masses. When stool does pass through, it's liquid or ribbon-like.

A look at Hirschsprung's disease

Hirschsprung's disease is a congenital disorder of the large intestine characterised by the absence or marked reduction in parasympathetic ganglion cells in the colorectal wall.

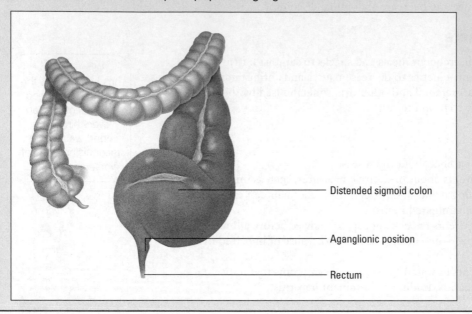

Distended sigmoid colon

Aganglionic position

Rectum

Suspicious stain

Children may experience bile-stained or faecal vomiting, irritability, lethargy and weight loss. They may exhibit signs of dehydration, including pallor, dry mucous membranes and sunken eyes.

What tests tell you
- Rectal biopsy provides definitive diagnosis by showing the absence of ganglion cells.
- Suction aspiration, using a small tube inserted into the rectum, also determines the absence of ganglion cells.
- Full-thickness surgical biopsy under general anaesthesia may be performed if findings from suction aspiration are inconclusive.
- Rectal manometry reveals failure of the internal anal sphincter to relax and contract.
- Abdominal X-rays show distension of the colon.

Complications
Disease progression causes the most complications, including severe diarrhoea, bowel perforation, sepsis, incontinence, stricture formation, enterocolitis and hypovolemic shock.

In infants, the main cause of death is enterocolitis (when not treated), caused by faecal stagnation that leads to bacterial overgrowth, production of bacterial toxins, intestinal irritation, profuse diarrhoea, hypovolemic shock and perforation.

How it's treated

Surgery is the treatment of choice in these children and should be performed as soon as the child's fluid and electrolyte imbalances are stabilised.

Out with the bad

Laparoscopic surgery involves pulling the ganglionic segment of bowel through the anus to remove the affected portion. Surgery is usually delayed until the infant is at least 10 months old. If a total obstruction is present, a temporary colostomy or ileostomy may be necessary to decompress the colon. Next, a second operation is performed to remove the affected segment of bowel and close the ostomy.

What to do

The infant's parents will need a great deal of emotional support. Prepare them for each procedure, including surgery, by offering thorough explanations and making sure that their questions are answered. Encourage them to express their feelings and concerns, and encourage their participation in the infant's care to the extent possible.

Pre-operative care
• Administer IV fluids to maintain fluid and electrolyte balance and prevent dehydration and shock.
• Maintain NBM status and insert an NG tube for gastric decompression.

Forced evacuation

• Administer isotonic enemas (normal saline solution or mineral oil) to evacuate the bowels.
• Administer antibiotics (and an antibiotic enema) as ordered.

Post-operative care
After colostomy or ileostomy, follow these steps:
• Monitor fluid intake and output; an ileostomy is especially likely to cause excessive electrolyte loss.
• Keep the area around the stoma clean and dry; use colostomy or ileostomy appliances to collect drainage.
• Monitor for return of bowel sounds to begin diet.
  After corrective surgery, follow these steps:
• Keep the wound clean and dry to prevent infection.
• Don't use a rectal thermometer or suppositories.

Bowel sounds = dinner bell

• Begin oral feeds when active bowel sounds begin and NG drainage decreases.

- Educate the parents about care of sutures.
- Teach the parents how to recognise the beginning signs of constipation, such as straining during defecation and a distended abdomen, fluid loss and dehydration (decreased urine output, sunken eyes, poor skin turgor), enterocolitis (vomiting, diarrhoea, fever, lethargy, sudden marked abdominal distension) and strictures (abdominal distension, constipation, vomiting).

Expert advice

- Before discharge a stoma care nurse specialist will provide the parents with valuable tips on colostomy or ileostomy care.
- Teach the parents which foods increase the number of stools (raisins, prunes, plums) and tell them to avoid offering these foods. (Reassure them that their child will, in time, probably gain sphincter control and eat a normal diet.)

Patience is a virtue

- Caution the parents that complete continence of stool can take years to develop, and that constipation may occur.

Intussusception

Intussusception is a telescoping of a bowel segment into itself, the most common site being the ileocaecal valve. It usually occurs at about 6 months, but can occur in children up to 3 years of age and, rarely, in older children. It's three times more likely to occur in males than in females, and is more likely to occur in children with cystic fibrosis.

Intussusception can be fatal, especially if treatment is delayed for more than 24 hours. (See *Understanding intussusception*.)

What causes it

The cause of intussusception is unknown in most cases. It may result from polyps, hyperactive peristalsis or an abnormal bowel lining. It may also be linked to viral infections because seasonal peaks are noted (spring and summer).

How it happens

When a bowel segment invaginates, peristalsis propels it along the bowel, pulling more bowel along with it. Invagination causes inflammation and swelling at the affected site. Oedema eventually causes obstruction and necrosis from occlusion of the blood supply to the bowel.

What to look for

The medical history may reveal intermittent attacks of colicky pain characterised by screaming, drawing knees to the chest, sweating and grunting. Parents report vomit containing bile or faecal material, which can lead to dehydration, fluid and electrolyte imbalance and metabolic alkalosis.

Understanding intussusception

In intussusception, a bowel section invaginates and is propelled along by peristalsis, pulling in more bowel. In this illustration, a portion of the caecum invaginates and is propelled into the large intestine. Intussusception typically produces oedema, haemorrhage from venous engorgement, incarceration and obstruction.

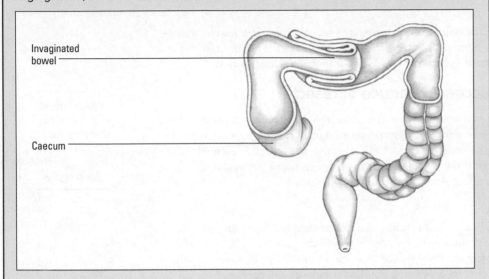

Invaginated bowel

Caecum

They also describe the passage of 'redcurrant jelly-like' stool containing mucus and blood.

Tender to the touch

Inspection and palpation may reveal a distended and tender abdomen with a palpable, sausage-shaped abdominal mass. Other clinical signs include fever, increased pulse, shallow respirations and decreased blood pressure (shock-like state).

What tests tell you
• Abdominal X-rays show a soft tissue mass and signs of complete or partial obstruction.
• Barium enema confirms colonic intussusception when it shows the characteristic coiled spring sign.

Complications
Without proper treatment, strangulation of the intestine may occur, with gangrene, shock, perforation and peritonitis. These complications can be fatal.

How it's treated

An NG tube is inserted to decompress the intestine and minimise vomiting. Ten per cent of children with intussusception may have spontaneous reduction in the bowel. Therapy may include hydrostatic reduction or surgery.

Forceful introduction

During hydrostatic reduction, air pressure or a solution of barium or water-soluble contrast medium is introduced into the rectum. The force from the fluid or air moves invaginated bowel back into its original position.

If at first you don't succeed … reduce or resect

Surgery is indicated when hydrostatic reduction fails, intussusception recurs, or signs of shock or peritonitis are present. Manual reduction is attempted first by pulling the intussusception back through the bowel. If manual reduction fails, or if the bowel segment is gangrenous or strangulated, resection of the affected bowel segment is performed.

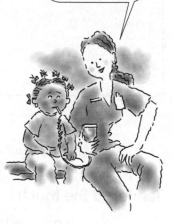

When time is of the essence, use care-giving opportunities to prepare the child for surgery.

What to do

Intussusception is a painful condition; onset of symptoms may be sudden and severe. The child may be inconsolable and the parents are likely to be terrified and distressed from seeing their infant or toddler in so much pain. Provide the parents with as much emotional support and reassurance as possible.

Explain on the go

Because intussusception is treated as an emergency, use care-giving opportunities (during bedside care, medication administration, transport to testing areas) to provide as much explanation as possible about tests and procedures, and make sure the parents' questions are answered.

Music to soothe

To the extent possible, allow the parents to remain with their child providing comfort and support.

Better days ahead

For the child who's old enough to understand, provide simple explanations as procedures are being performed, and reassure them that you're there to help and they'll feel better soon.
• Prepare for enema insertion (barium or water-soluble contrast medium) to confirm the diagnosis and reduce the invagination by hydrostatic pressure.
• Monitor vital signs; a change in temperature may indicate sepsis.
• Monitor intake and output to prevent dehydration and administer IV fluids as ordered.

- Monitor NG tube output and replace volume lost, as ordered.
- Administer pain medication as ordered.
- For the child who has undergone hydrostatic reduction, monitor for the passage of stool (and barium, if used) to determine the need for surgery.

Post-operative care

After surgery, encourage the parents to stay with the child as much as possible. In addition, follow these steps:

- Administer antibiotics as prescribed to prevent infection.
- Monitor the incision site for signs of infection, such as inflammation, drainage and suture separation.
- Monitor for the return of bowel sounds to allow advancement of the diet.
- Continue to offer emotional support and encouragement to the parents.

Pyloric stenosis

Pyloric stenosis is hyperplasia (increased mass) and hypertrophy (increased size) of the circular muscle at the pylorus, the lower opening of the stomach leading to the duodenum. The increased mass and size of the muscle narrows the pyloric canal, preventing the stomach from emptying normally. Pyloric obstruction leads to vomiting and gastritis from prolonged filling of the stomach. It's most commonly seen in boys between ages 1 and 6 months.

What causes it

The exact cause of pyloric stenosis is unknown. It isn't an inherited disorder but may be associated with malrotation, oesophageal atresia and anorectal malformations.

How it happens

Spasms of the pylorus muscle cause the narrowing of the passageway between the stomach and duodenum. Swelling and inflammation further reduce the size of the lumen and could result in complete obstruction. Normal emptying of the stomach is prevented, resulting in vomiting and gastritis.

What to look for

Palpation reveals an olive-shaped bulge below the right costal margin and a distended upper abdomen.

Waving and projecting

The child experiences projectile vomiting during or shortly after feeds. The vomiting is preceded by reverse peristaltic waves (left to right) but not by nausea. Vomitus isn't bile-stained but may be blood-stained due to gastritis.

Stand back

Projectile means the vomit can come out like a projectile so be prepared if the child is being fed.

Déjà lunch

The child will resume eating after vomiting and exhibits poor weight gain. Symptoms of malnutrition and dehydration are present despite the child's apparent adequate intake of food.

What tests tell you
- Vomit may be positive for blood.
- Blood chemistry reveals hypocalcaemia, hyponatraemia, hypokalaemia and hypochloraemia.
- Arterial blood gas analysis may reveal metabolic alkalosis.
- Abdominal ultrasound and endoscopy reveal a hypertrophied sphincter.
- An upper GI series reveals delayed gastric emptying.

Complications

Complications of pyloric stenosis include malnutrition, dehydration, infection and metabolic alkalosis.

How it's treated

The child remains on NBM before surgery. IV fluids are administered to correct fluid and electrolyte imbalances and prevent dehydration, and an NG tube is inserted and kept open for gastric decompression. Surgical intervention consists of a pyloromyotomy performed by laparoscopy.

What to do

Provide the parents, who are usually very frightened, with an explanation of all tests, procedures and surgery. Make sure their questions are answered. In addition, follow these steps:
- Monitor vital signs and intake and output to assess renal function and check for dehydration.
- Record the amount of vomit as well as its frequency, characteristics and relation to feeds.
- Perform daily weight measurements on the same scale to assess growth.
- Assess abdominal and cardiovascular status to detect early signs of compromise.
- Position the child, preferably on the right side, to prevent aspiration of vomit.

Post-operative care
- Monitor IV fluids and infusions
- Feed the child small amounts of oral electrolyte solution; then increase the amount and concentration of food until normal feeding is achieved.

No need to say 'excuse me'

- Wind the child frequently during feeding.
- Provide a pacifier to maintain comfort and satisfy the infant's sucking reflex.

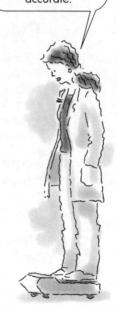

Using the same scale every day ensures that weight measurements for a child with pyloric stenosis will be accurate.

- Monitor intake and output.
- Keep the incision area clean to prevent infection; clean with soap and water and keep the nappy's contents away from the incision.

Going with the flow

- Position the child on his right side, allowing gravity to help the flow of fluid through the pyloric valve; elevate the child's head after feeding.
- Administer analgesics around the clock for pain management.
- Teach the parents wound site care, and monitor for signs and symptoms of infection and dehydration.

Tracheoesophageal fistula and oesophageal atresia

Tracheoesophageal fistula and oesophageal atresia are among the most serious congenital anomalies in neonates. They may develop separately but usually occur together. There's a higher incidence with prematurity and maternal polyhydramnios.

An unhealthy relationship

In tracheoesophageal fistula, an abnormal connection develops between the trachea and the oesophagus. In oesophageal atresia, the oesophagus is closed off at some point, and food can't enter the stomach through the oesophagus.

Combo conditions

These conditions may occur in several combinations and may be associated with other anomalies of the heart, anorectal area or genitourinary system. (See *Types of tracheoesophageal anomalies,* page 438.)

What causes it

These conditions are a result of the failure of the embryonic oesophagus and trachea to develop and separate correctly.

How it happens

In the foetus, there's a defective separation of the foregut into the trachea and oesophagus at about 4 to 5 weeks' gestation. The oesophagus fails to meet the stomach and ends in a blind pouch.

What to look for

At delivery, the neonate has frothy saliva in the mouth, and choking and coughing due to excessive secretions. During feeding the neonate experiences sudden coughing and gagging and shows signs of feeds coming out of nose and mouth. They may stop breathing and become cyanotic as the feed is aspirated into the lungs.

Types of tracheoesophageal anomalies

Congenital malformations of the oesophagus occur in about 1 in 3,000 live births. The American Academy of Pediatrics classifies the anatomic variations in tracheoesophageal anomalies according to type.

Type A	**Type B**	**Type C**	**Type D**	**Type E (or H-type)**
Oesophageal atresia without fistula (7.7%)	Oesophageal atresia with oesophageal fistula to the proximal segment (0.8%)	Oesophageal atresia with fistula to the distal segment (86.5%)	Oesophageal atresia with fistula to both segments (0.7%)	Tracheoesophageal fistula without atresia (4.2%)

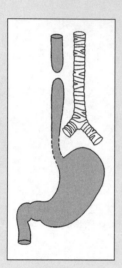 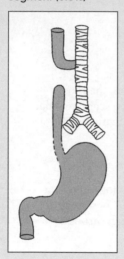 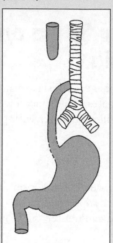 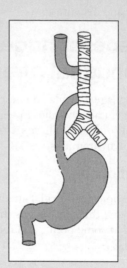 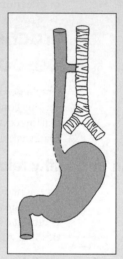

Belly full of air

Stomach distension occurs when air from the trachea enters the oesophagus or the stomach directly (through a fistula). Aspiration pneumonia occurs when the oesophagus joins the trachea and food regurgitates through the fistula into the lungs.

What tests tell you

A radiopaque catheter is inserted into the oesophagus, and an X-ray is taken to see where the catheter goes or what obstruction it hits. Bronchoscopy is performed to visualise the fistula between the trachea and oesophagus. Chest X-ray shows pneumonia and a dilated, air-filled upper oesophageal pouch.

Complications

Complications include leaking at the anastomosis site, strictures, gastroesophageal reflux, feeding difficulties and tracheomalacia (weakness of the tracheal wall, allowing the trachea to collapse).

How it's treated

Tracheoesophageal fistula and oesophageal atresia require surgical correction and are usually surgical emergencies. (Insertion of an NG tube is impossible in a neonate with oesophageal atresia).

A pump in the pouch

A sump pump may be inserted in the oesophageal pouch to remove accumulated secretions, reducing the risk of aspiration. A gastrostomy tube may be placed to decompress the stomach. The neonate's respiratory status must be closely monitored to maintain a patent airway. IV fluids are administered to prevent dehydration, and the neonate is kept NBM.

Ligate and lengthen

Surgical correction is performed to close fistulas and anastomose the oesophagus to the stomach. Oesophageal lengthening may be needed if the oesophagus is too short to join the stomach. A chest tube may be inserted to drain intra-pleural fluid and air. Antibiotics are administered to treat aspiration pneumonia.

What to do

Explain all procedures to the parents, make sure their questions are answered and provide support and reassurance. Allow them to spend as much time as possible with their child. In addition:
• suction excessive secretions from the mouth and pharynx frequently, and elevate the neonate's head to prevent aspiration
• keep the child NBM and begin IV fluids
• don't allow the infant to suck on a pacifier; this increases saliva secretions.

Post-operative care

After surgery, involve the parents in the child's care to help comfort both them and their child, reassure the parents and prepare them for caring for the child at home. In addition, follow these steps:
• An NG or OG tube is attached to low-suction or gravity drainage; document the amount and character of the drainage at least every 4 hours.
• Gastrostomy feeds may be given until the oesophagus heals.

Assess for distress

• Monitor for signs of respiratory distress.
• Monitor chest tube drainage and care of the chest tube site.
• Begin oral feeds with sterile water and advance to normal feeds as tolerated.

Sucking permitted

• Encourage sucking on a pacifier to prevent oral aversion.

The parents of a child who needs emergency surgery will look to the nurse to provide support and answer their questions.

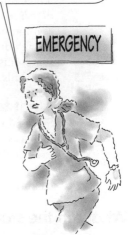

- Educate the parents on proper oral or gastrostomy feeding, signs of respiratory distress and signs of oesophageal constriction (such as drooling, difficulty swallowing, or regurgitating undigested food).

Ulcerative colitis

Ulcerative colitis is a chronic, recurrent inflammation of the colon and rectal mucosa with varying degrees of ulceration, bleeding and oedema. It usually begins in the rectum and sigmoid colon and may extend upward into the entire colon.

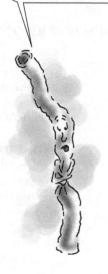

Vasoconstriction starts a painful chain of events – ruptures, ulcers, strictures and obstructions.

What causes it

Although the aetiology of ulcerative colitis is unknown, it may be related to an abnormal immune response in the GI tract, possibly associated with genetic factors. It's more prevalent among specific ethnic groups particularly people of Jewish heritage.

How it happens

Vasoconstriction initiates an immune response, producing ruptured capillary walls. The swollen bowel then develops ulcers. Healing ulcers can develop scar tissue, which results in strictures and obstructions.

What to look for

The hallmark sign of ulcerative colitis is frequent attacks of watery, bloody diarrhoea (in many cases containing pus and mucus) interspersed with asymptomatic remissions. However, one of the earliest signs may be faltering growth due to poor nutritional intake resulting from anorexia. Other symptoms include urgency with defecation, abdominal pain, cramping, fever and chills.

What tests tell you

Sigmoidoscopy confirms rectal involvement in most cases by showing increased mucosal friability, decreased mucosal detail and thick inflammatory exudate. Colonoscopy may be used to determine the extent of the disease and look for evidence of inflammation. A biopsy performed during the colonoscopy can help confirm the diagnosis.

What's in the stool?

Barium enema is used to evaluate the extent of the disease and detect complications. Stool specimen analysis reveals blood, pus and mucus, but no pathogenic organisms. Other laboratory tests reveal an elevated WBC count, an elevated ESR and decreased haemoglobin level and haematocrit.

Complications

Ulcerative colitis can lead to a variety of complications, depending on the severity and site of inflammation. Nutritional deficiencies are the most common complications, but the disease can also lead to perineal sepsis with anal fissure, anal fistula, perirectal abscess, haemorrhage, iron deficiency anaemia, coagulation defects and toxic megacolon. There's also an increased risk of colorectal cancer.

How it's treated

The goals of treatment are to control inflammation, replace nutritional losses and blood volume and prevent complications.

Down with inflammation!

Medical treatment begins with the administration of corticosteroids or other anti-inflammatory agent, such as aminosalicylates, to decrease inflammation. Supportive treatment includes dietary therapy and bed rest.
• Parenteral nutrition is used for children awaiting surgery or showing signs of dehydration, and is intended to give the bowel a chance to rest.
• A low-residue diet may be ordered for the child with mild signs and symptoms.
• Blood transfusions or iron supplements may be needed to correct anaemia.
• Surgery, the treatment of last resort, is performed if the child has toxic megacolon. (The most common surgical procedure is total proctocolectomy with ileostomy, which may cure the disease.)

What to do

Nursing care focuses on teaching the parents about diet, medication and stress reduction:
• Encourage small, frequent meals of a diet low in bran and fibre-rich foods. (See *Nutrition by culture*, page 442)
• Stress the importance of compliance with the medication regimen.
• Promote stress reduction through relaxation and distraction.
• Promote enhanced self-image and self-esteem.
• Instruct in ostomy care, if applicable.

Volvulus

Volvulus is a condition in which the bowel twists around itself at least 180 degrees. This results in vessel compression and ischemia

What causes it

The twisting in volvulus may result from an anomaly of rotation, an ingested foreign body or an adhesion. In some cases, the cause is unknown.

How it happens

A prolapsed portion of mesentery causes the bowel to become twisted. The twisted bowel is obstructed, leading to bowel distension and decreased absorption of water and electrolytes. Vomiting also occurs due to the

Cultured know how

Nutrition by culture

Nutrition varies among cultures and religions because dietary practices differ. Children need a well-balanced diet for growth and development, especially children on specific diets. The nurse and dietician should do a comprehensive nutritional assessment, and teach proper nutrition practices to enhance growth and development in children while respecting the cultural practices and beliefs of the family. Here are some tips on special cultural diet restrictions and characteristics:

- If the child is a vegetarian, the nurse should know proper protein foods to substitute for the lack of meat in the diet.
- Some Jewish children eat kosher meats that are typically high in sodium, which may be a problem in certain disease processes.
- In many cultures, use of herbal preparations in their diets and as medicinal treatments is common. The nurse should be aware of the types of preparations the child is eating or taking.

obstruction. A decreased blood supply to the affected bowel leads to necrosis. (See *What happens in volvulus*.)

What to look for
The child complains of severe abdominal pain and has bilious vomiting, which increases after feeding. Inspection reveals a distended abdomen with absent bowel sounds. The parents may report the passage of bloody stool.

What tests tell you
Abdominal X-rays show multiple distended bowel loops and a large bowel without gas. An upper GI series and barium enema help confirm the diagnosis. Blood chemistry indicates hyperkalaemia and hypocalcaemia.

Complications
Without immediate treatment, volvulus can lead to strangulation of the twisted bowel loop, ischemia infarction, perforation and fatal peritonitis.

Chain of events

Short gut syndrome may develop after surgical correction if an extensive area of bowel is removed. This syndrome results in decreased absorptive surface area which, in turn, leads to decreased absorption of nutrients.

How it's treated
If the bowel is distended but viable, surgery consists of detorsion (untwisting). If the bowel is necrotic, surgery includes resection and anastomosis. Prolonged TPN and IV administration of antibiotics are usually necessary.

Hirschsprung's disease

Also called *congenital megacolon* or *congenital aganglionic megacolon*, this congenital disorder of the large intestine is characterised by absence or marked reduction of parasympathetic ganglionic cells in the colorectal wall.

The resulting impaired intestinal mobility causes severe intractable constipation. Colonic obstruction then occurs, dilating the bowel and occluding the surrounding blood and lymphatic vessels.

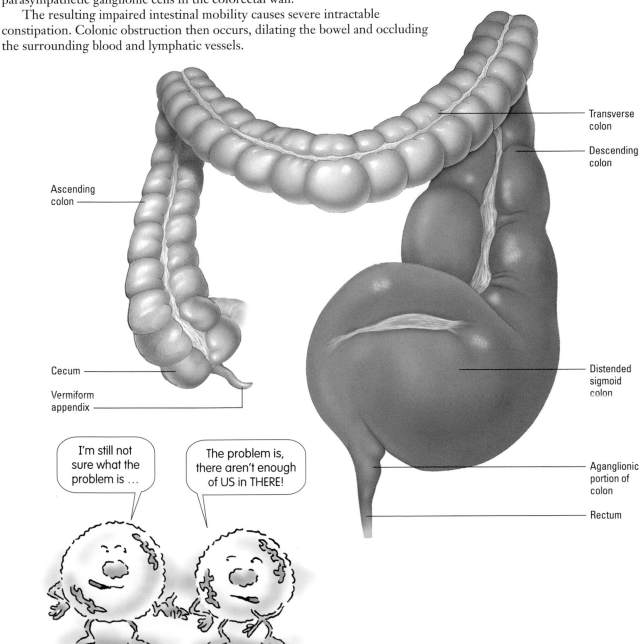

Acne

Acne is a chronic inflammatory disease of the sebaceous glands, associated with a high, rate of sebum production. When sebum blocks a hair follicle, one of two types of acne occurs.

In *inflammatory acne*, bacteria grow in the blocked follicle and lead to inflammation and eventual rupture of the follicle. In *non-inflammatory acne*, the follicle remains dilated by accumulating secretions but doesn't rupture.

Acne develops in 80% to 90% of adolescents or young adults, primarily between ages 15 and 18; however, the lesions can appear as early as age 8 years.

How acne develops

Excessive sebum production

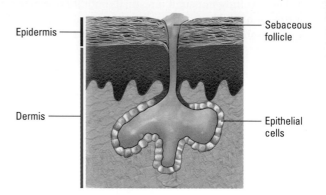

Epidermis

Dermis

Sebaceous follicle

Epithelial cells

Increased shedding of epithelial cells

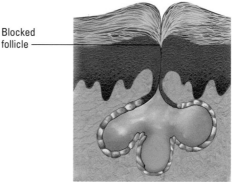

Blocked follicle

Inflammatory response in follicle

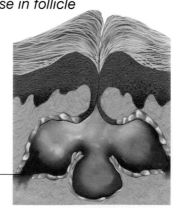

Ruptured follicle

When those sebaceous glands get inflamed, it's not a pretty sight!

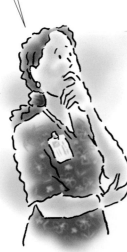

Comedones of acne

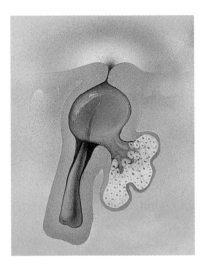

Closed comedo (whitehead)
A closed comedo doesn't protrude from the follicle and is covered by the epidermis.

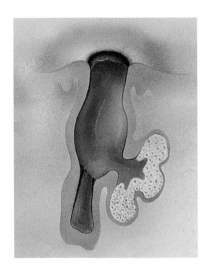

Open comedo (blackhead)
An open comedo protrudes from the follicle and isn't covered by the epidermis.
   Melanin or pigment of the follicle causes the black color.

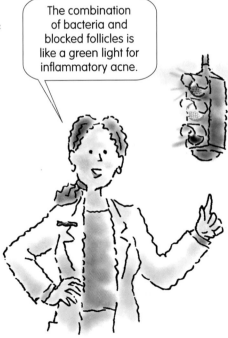

Rheumatic heart disease

Rheumatic fever is an inflammatory disease of childhood; it develops after an infection of the upper respiratory tract with group A beta-hemolytic streptococci. It mainly involves the heart, joints, central nervous system, skin and subcutaneous tissues.

The antigens of group A streptococci bind to receptors in the heart, muscle, brain and synovial joints, causing an autoimmune response. Because of a similarity between the antigens of the streptococcus bacteria and the antigens of the body's own cells, antibodies may attack healthy body cells by mistake.

Rheumatic heart disease refers to the cardiac manifestations of rheumatic fever and includes pancarditis (myocarditis, pericarditis, and endocarditis) during the early acute phase and chronic valvular disease later.

Just hearing *rheumatic heart disease* makes me shudder!

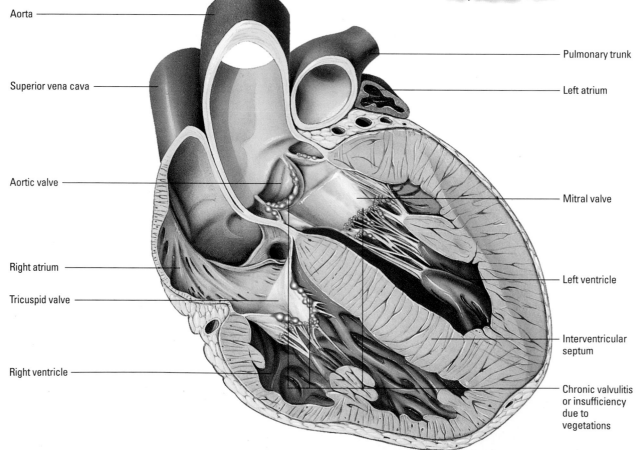

Aorta

Superior vena cava

Aortic valve

Right atrium

Tricuspid valve

Right ventricle

Pulmonary trunk

Left atrium

Mitral valve

Left ventricle

Interventricular septum

Chronic valvulitis or insufficiency due to vegetations

What happens in volvulus

Although volvulus may occur anywhere in a bowel segment long enough to twist, the most common site, as the illustration depicts, is the sigmoid colon, causing oedema within the closed loop and obstruction at its proximal and distal ends.

Normal bowel segment

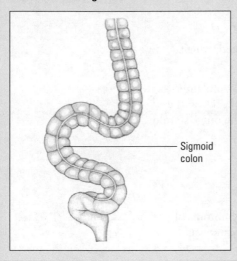

Sigmoid colon

Volvulus

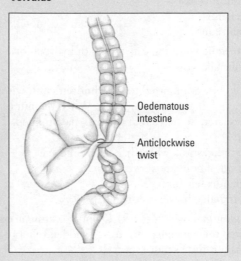

Oedematous intestine

Anticlockwise twist

What to do

The child and parents will need reassurance because the child may be in extreme pain. Because tests may be required on an emergency basis, tell the child what's being done, step-by-step, as each test is being performed.

When the child is relatively comfortable and able to listen or understand, prepare for surgery with age-appropriate explanations about what will happen. In addition, follow these steps:
• Monitor bowel sounds and bowel movements.
• Give pain medications as prescribed.
• Keep NBM until surgery is performed; begin administration of IV fluids to prevent dehydration.
• Insert an NG tube to decompress the stomach.

Post-operative care
• Maintain the administration of IV fluids until the bowel has healed and bowel sounds return.
• Monitor the effects of opioid analgesics that may decrease GI motility.
• Educate the parents about preventing constipation (e.g. increasing the intake of oral fluids, increasing activity, adding high-fibre foods to the diet and the proper use of stool softeners).

Quick quiz

1. A 2-month-old male infant is admitted with a diagnosis of pyloric stenosis. Due to projectile vomiting he's at risk for:
    A. metabolic acidosis.
    B. metabolic alkalosis.
    C. hyperkalemia.
    D. hypernatremia.

Answer: B. Projectile vomiting causes loss of hydrochloric acid, which results in metabolic alkalosis.

2. A 12-year-old boy is admitted to the children's unit with complaints of RLQ abdominal pain and vomiting. When the nurse checks on the child 2 hours later, he states that the pain has stopped. The nurse should suspect that:
    A. he had indigestion, which has been relieved.
    B. he's afraid of going to surgery.
    C. his appendix has ruptured.
    D. he has irritable bowel syndrome.

Answer: C. Abdominal pain in the RLQ and vomiting are symptoms of appendicitis. When the appendix ruptures, a sudden relief of pain occurs, after which the pain resumes more severely.

3. An 18-month-old child is admitted to the children's unit with intussusception. As the nurse is preparing the child for a barium contrast reduction, he passes a soft brown stool. What should the nurse do?
    A. Notify the doctor in order to cancel the procedure.
    B. Prepare the child for emergency surgery.
    C. Take vital signs and monitor for abdominal sounds.
    D. Administer an enema to clear the rectal area for testing.

Answer: A. Passing a normal-looking brown stool indicates that the child no longer has an invaginated section of bowel.

4. The nurse is completing discharge teaching for a child and her parents regarding diet to treat coeliac disease. Which meal selection would be appropriate for this child?
    A. A cheese sandwich on whole wheat bread, a chocolate chip cookie and a glass of milk
    B. A vegetable pizza, an apple and a diet cola
    C. A beefburger, cooked vegetables and a glass of fruit juice
    D. A hot dog on a roll, celery and carrot sticks and a chocolate milk shake

Answer: C. Coeliac disease is intolerance to wheat, barley, rye and oats. Some of these children also have lactose intolerance, especially when they have an acute episode of the disease.

Scoring

☆☆☆ If you answered all four items correctly, congratulations! You've thoroughly digested the material in this chapter.

☆☆ If you answered three items correctly, good job! Your knowledge of GI disorders is unobstructed.

☆ If you answered fewer than three items correctly, don't give yourself an ulcer! Swallow your pride and prepare for the last three quizzes.

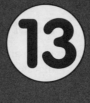

Endocrine and metabolic problems ⑬

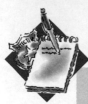

Just the facts

In this chapter, you'll learn:
♦ function of the glands of the endocrine system
♦ tests used to diagnose endocrine and metabolic problems
♦ treatments of children with endocrine and metabolic problems
♦ disorders of the endocrine system and metabolic function.

Anatomy and physiology

The endocrine system is comprised of glands that secrete hormones necessary for normal metabolic function. Along with the nervous system, the endocrine system regulates and integrates the body's metabolic activities. (See *Endocrine system components*, page 447.)

Too little, too much

Altered endocrine function involves a hyposecretion or hypersecretion of hormones, which affects the body's metabolic processes and function. Nursing care involves measures to support hormonal secretion, such as hormone replacement, or curtail secretion, such as radiation therapy. Inborn errors of metabolism involve a biochemical alteration that affects metabolism.

Glands

The major glands of the endocrine system are:
• pituitary gland
• thyroid gland

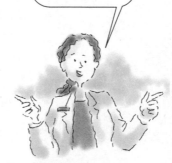

Altered endocrine function involves hyposecretion or hypersecretion of hormones.

Endocrine system components

Endocrine glands secrete hormones directly into the bloodstream to regulate body function. This illustration shows the locations of the major endocrine glands (except the gonads).

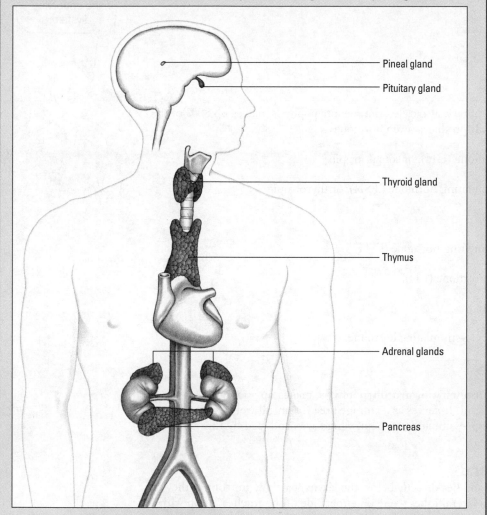

- Pineal gland
- Pituitary gland
- Thyroid gland
- Thymus
- Adrenal glands
- Pancreas

- parathyroid glands
- adrenal glands
- pancreas
- ovaries and testes.

Pituitary gland

The pituitary gland (also called the hypophysis or master gland) rests in the sella turcica, a depression in the sphenoid bone at the base of the brain.

Small but mighty

This pea-sized gland connects with the hypothalamus via the infundibulum, from which it receives chemical and nervous stimulation. The pituitary has two main regions:

👌 anterior pituitary

👌 posterior pituitary.

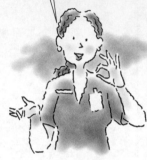

The pituitary may be petite, but it's the master gland of the endocrine system.

Prolific producer

The anterior pituitary, also called the adenohypophysis, makes up 80% of the pituitary gland. It produces seven hormones:

👌 growth hormone (GH), or somatotropin

✌️ thyroid-stimulating hormone (TSH), or thyrotropin

🤟 corticotropin

🖖 follicle-stimulating hormone (FSH)

🖐 luteinising hormone (LH)

🖐👌 prolactin

🖐✌️ melanocyte-stimulating hormone.

Hormones in storage

The posterior pituitary, or neurohypophysis, makes up about 20% of the pituitary gland. It serves as a storage area for antidiuretic hormone (ADH), or vasopressin, and oxytocin, which are produced by the hypothalamus.

Thyroid gland

The thyroid gland lies directly below the larynx, partially in front of the trachea. Its two lateral lobes – one on either side of the trachea – join with a narrow tissue bridge, called the isthmus, to give the gland its butterfly shape.

Thyroid lobe duo

The two lobes of the thyroid gland function as one unit to produce the hormones triiodothyronine (T3), thyroxine (T4) and calcitonin. T3 and T4 are collectively referred to as thyroid hormone (TH), the body's major metabolic hormone. It regulates metabolism by speeding cellular respiration.

The calcitonin–calcium connection

Calcitonin maintains the blood calcium level by inhibiting the release of calcium from bone. Secretion of calcitonin is controlled by the calcium concentration of the fluid surrounding the thyroid cells.

Parathyroid glands
The parathyroid glands are the body's smallest known endocrine glands. These glands are embedded on the posterior surface of the thyroid, one in each corner.

PTH: A parathyroid production

Working together as a single gland, the parathyroid glands produce parathyroid hormone (PTH). The main function of PTH is to help regulate the blood's calcium balance. This hormone adjusts the rate at which calcium and magnesium ions are removed from urine. PTH also increases the movement of phosphate ions from the blood to urine for excretion.

Adrenal glands
There are two adrenal glands in the body; each gland is situated on top of a kidney. These almond-shaped glands contain two distinct structures – the adrenal cortex and the adrenal medulla – that function as separate endocrine glands.

Adrenal cortex
The adrenal cortex is the large outer layer of the adrenal gland and forms the bulk of the gland. It has three zones, or cell layers:

zona glomerulosa, the outermost zone, which produces mineralocorticoids, primarily aldosterone

zona fasciculata, the middle and largest zone, which produces the glucocorticoids cortisol (hydrocortisone), cortisone and corticosterone as well as small amounts of the sex hormones androgen and oestrogen

zona reticularis, the innermost zone, which produces mainly glucocorticoids and some sex hormones.

Adrenal medulla
The adrenal medulla, or inner layer of the adrenal gland, functions as part of the sympathetic nervous system and produces two catecholamines:

adrenaline

noradrenaline.

A leading role

Because catecholamines play an important role in the autonomic nervous system, the adrenal medulla is considered a neuroendocrine structure.

Pancreas

The pancreas, a triangular gland, is nestled in the curve of the duodenum, stretching horizontally behind the stomach and extending to the spleen. The pancreas performs endocrine and exocrine functions. Acinar cells make up most of the gland and regulate pancreatic exocrine function.

Clusters of islets

The endocrine cells of the pancreas are called the islet cells, or islets of Langerhans. These cells exist in clusters and are found scattered among the acinar cells. The islets contain alpha, beta and delta cells that produce important hormones:
* Alpha cells produce glucagon.
* Beta cells produce insulin.
* Delta cells produce somatostatin.

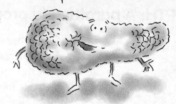

Check out my job description; it includes endocrine functions, exocrine functions, and hormone production. I deserve a raise!

Gonads

The gonads include the ovaries in the female and the testes in the male.

Ovaries

The ovaries are oval-shaped glands in females located on either side of the uterus. They produce ova (eggs) as well as oestrogen and progesterone.

It's a girl thing

Oestrogen and progesterone are responsible for:
* promoting the development and maintenance of female sex characteristics
* regulating the menstrual cycle
* maintaining the uterus for pregnancy
* preparing the mammary glands for lactation.

Testes

The testes in males are located in the scrotum. They produce the male hormone testosterone, which stimulates and maintains male sex characteristics. They also produce spermatozoa.

Hormones

Hormones are complex chemical substances that trigger or regulate the activity of an organ or a group of cells. They include pituitary hormones, THs, adrenal hormones, and androgens and oestrogens. (See *Effects of altered hormonal function*.)

Pituitary hormones

Pituitary hormones include the anterior pituitary hormones (GH, TSH, FSH, LH and prolactin) and the posterior pituitary hormones (ADH and oxytocin). Each of these hormones has a particular function:

Effects of altered hormonal function

This chart shows the effects that may result from excessive or deficient secretion of select hormones.

Hormone	Hypofunction	Hyperfunction
Anterior pituitary hormones		
Growth hormone	• Epiphyseal fusion with cessation of growth • Prepubertal dwarfism • Pituitary cachexia (Simmonds' disease) • Generalised growth retardation • Hypoglycaemia	• Pre-pubertal gigantism • Acromegaly (after full growth is attained) • Diabetes mellitus • Post-pubertal hypoproteinaemia
Thyroid-stimulating hormone	• Hypothyroidism • Marked delay of puberty • Juvenile myxedema	• Hyperthyroidism • Thyrotoxicosis • Graves' disease
Corticotropin	• Acute adrenocortical insufficiency (Addison's disease) • Hypoglycaemia • Increased skin pigmentation	• Cushing's syndrome
Gonadotropins	• Absent or incomplete spontaneous puberty	• Precocious puberty • Early epiphyseal closure
Follicle-stimulating hormone	• Hypogonadism • Sterility • Absence or loss of secondary sex characteristics • Amenorrhoea	• Precocious puberty • Primary gonadal failure • Hirsutism • Polycystic ovary • Early epiphyseal closure
Luteinising hormone	• Hypogonadism • Sterility • Impotence • Absence or loss of secondary sex characteristics • Ovarian failure	• Precocious puberty • Primary gonadal failure • Hirsutism • Polycystic ovary • Early epiphyseal closure
Prolactin	• Inability to lactate • Amenorrhoea	• Galactorrhoea • Functional hypogonadism
Melanocyte-stimulating hormone	• Diminished or absent skin pigmentation.	• Increased skin pigmentation.
Posterior pituitary hormone Antidiuretic hormone or vasopressin	• Diabetes insipidus	• Syndrome of inappropriate antidiuretic hormone secretion • Fluid retention • Hyponatraemia

(continued)

Effects of altered hormonal function (continued)

Hormone	Hypofunction	Hyperfunction
Thyroid hormones Thyroxine and triiodothyronine	• Hypothyroidism • Myxedema • Hashimoto thyroiditis • Greatly reduced general growth (extent depends on age at which deficiency occurs) • Mental retardation (in infants)	• Exophthalmic goiter (Graves' disease) • Accelerated linear growth • Early epiphyseal closure
Parathyroid gland hormone Parathyroid hormone	• Hypocalcaemia (tetany)	• Hypercalcaemia (bone demineralisation) • Hypophosphataemia
Adrenal hormones Aldosterone	• Adrenocortical insufficiency	• Electrolyte imbalance • Hyperaldosteronism
Glucocorticoids (cortisol and corticosterone)	• Addison's disease • Acute adrenocortical insufficiency • Impaired growth and sexual function.	• Cushing's syndrome • Severe impairment of growth with slowing in skeletal maturation

• GH, secreted by the anterior pituitary gland, affects most body tissues. It triggers growth by increasing protein synthesis and fat mobilisation and decreases carbohydrate use.

• TSH is secreted by the anterior pituitary gland and stimulates the thyroid.

• FSH, secreted by the anterior pituitary gland, stimulates the graafian follicles to mature and secrete oestrogen in the female. In males it stimulates development of the seminiferous tubules.

• LH, secreted by the anterior pituitary gland, produces the rupture of the follicle, which results in the discharge of a mature ovum in the female. In the male, it stimulates the production of androgens, particularly testosterone.

• Prolactin is secreted by the anterior pituitary gland and stimulates milk secretion.

• ADH is secreted by the posterior pituitary gland. It controls the concentration of body fluids by altering the permeability of the distal convoluted tubules and collecting ducts of the kidneys to conserve water.

• Oxytocin, secreted by the posterior pituitary gland, stimulates the contraction of the uterus and the letdown reflex in lactating women.

Thyroid hormones

The THs are T3 and T4. These hormones are necessary for normal growth and development, and act on many tissues to increase metabolic activity and protein synthesis.

Adrenal hormones

The adrenal hormones are cortisol, aldosterone, androgens and oestrogen:
• Cortisol is a glucocorticoid that stimulates glucogenesis and increases protein breakdown and free fatty acid mobilisation; it also suppresses the immune response and provides for an appropriate response to stress.
• Aldosterone, a mineralocorticoid, regulates the resorption of sodium and the excretion of potassium by the kidneys; it's affected by corticotropin and is regulated by angiotensin II, which is regulated by renin (together, aldosterone, angiotensin II and renin may be implicated in the pathogenesis of hypertension).
• Androgens are male sex hormones; they promote male traits, especially secondary sex characteristics, such as facial hair and a low-pitched voice.
• Oestrogens are responsible for the development of secondary female sex characteristics.

Pancreatic hormones

The islets of Langerhans are small clusters of endocrine cells in the pancreas. These structures contain cells that produce insulin, glucagon and somatostatin:
• Insulin: a hormone that raises the blood glucose level by triggering the breakdown of glycogen to glucose
• Glucagon: lowers the blood glucose level by stimulating the conversion of glucose to glycogen
• Somatostatin: inhibits the release of GH, corticotropin and certain other hormones.

Hormone release and transport

Although all hormone release results from endocrine gland stimulation, release patterns of hormones vary greatly.
• Secretion of PTH (by the parathyroid gland) and prolactin (by the anterior pituitary) occurs fairly evenly throughout the day.
• Corticotrophin (secreted by the anterior pituitary) and cortisol (secreted by the adrenal cortex) are released in spurts in response to body rhythm cycles; levels of these hormones peak in the morning.
• Secretion of insulin by the pancreas has both steady and sporadic release patterns.

Hormonal action

When a hormone reaches its target site, it binds to a specific receptor on the cell membrane or within the cell. Polypeptides and some amines bind to membrane receptor sites. The smaller, more lipid-soluble steroids and THs diffuse through the cell membrane and bind to intracellular receptors.

Right on target!

After binding occurs, each hormone produces unique physiological changes, depending on its target site and its specific action at that site. A particular hormone may have different effects at different target sites.

Hormonal regulation

To maintain the body's delicate equilibrium, a feedback mechanism regulates hormone production and secretion. The mechanism involves hormones, blood chemicals and metabolites and the nervous system. The feedback mechanism may be simple or complex.

For normal function, each gland must contain enough appropriately programmed secretary cells to release active hormone on demand.

Unsupervised cells

Secretary cells need supervision. A secretary cell can't sense on its own when to release the hormone or how much to release. It gets this information from sensing and signalling systems that integrate many messages. Together, stimulatory and inhibitory signals actively control the rate and duration of hormone release.

It's nice to be recognised

When released, the hormone travels to target cells, where a receptor molecule recognises it and binds to it. The sensitivity of a target cell depends on how many receptors it has for a particular site. The more receptor sites, the more sensitive the target cell.

Diagnostic tests

Diagnostic tests are used to assess endocrine system problems and metabolic function in children:
• Blood glucose tests are used to diagnose type 1 and type 2 diabetes mellitus. Blood glucose tests commonly used for children include the fasting blood glucose test and the oral glucose tolerance test (OGTT).
• GH tests are used to determine pituitary function. The human growth hormone (hGH) test helps detect hypopituitarism, while the GH suppression test is used to diagnose pituitary hyperfunction.
• Neonatal screening consists of tests for a variety of diseases. Typically, neonatal screens are performed for commonly occurring diseases that may cause severe developmental delay or death without early detection and treatment. These tests are all done by blood spot. A very small amount of blood is required and is usually obtained by a heel prick.
• Thyroid function tests are used to determine thyroid function and include T3 and T4 studies.

Glucose, fasting plasma

The fasting plasma glucose test (also known as the fasting blood sugar test) is commonly used to screen for diabetes mellitus. It measures plasma glucose levels after an 8-hour fast.

To fast or not to fast

In the fasting state, plasma glucose levels decrease, stimulating the release of the hormone glucagon. Glucagon then acts to raise plasma glucose by accelerating glycogenolysis, stimulating glyconeogenesis and inhibiting glycogen synthesis. Normally, secretion of insulin checks this rise in glucose levels. In diabetes, however, absence or deficiency of insulin allows persistently high glucose levels.

And the level is …

The normal range for fasting plasma glucose varies according to the laboratory procedure. Normal values after a fast of at least 8 hours differ according to the age of the child:
• Premature neonates – 2.2 to 3.6 mmol/L
• Young children (birth to age 2 years) 3.3 to 6.1 mmol/L
• Children (ages 2 to 18 years) – 3.3 to 5.6 mmol/L.

Glucose tells all

A fasting plasma glucose level of 7 mmol/L or higher obtained on two or more occasions confirms provisional diabetes mellitus. A borderline or transiently elevated level requires a 2-hour post-prandial plasma glucose test or an OGTT to confirm the diagnosis and a positive result is a level above 11 mmol/L.

Nursing considerations
• Explain the procedure to the parents and the child, and encourage the parents to stay with the child.
• Determine how long the child must fast.
• Determine if the timing of the child's medication will interfere with the test results and withhold medication if indicated.

Backup plan

• Apply a topical anaesthetic (when possible) to two spots so an alternate puncture site will be available if the first one isn't successful.
• Specify on the laboratory request the time the child last ate, the sample collection time and the time they received the last pretest dose of insulin.

Glucose tolerance, oral

The OGTT measures carbohydrate metabolism after ingestion of a challenge dose of glucose. A 2-hour OGTT is typically done to diagnose diabetes mellitus in children. (See *Administering oral glucose solutions*.)

Up to the challenge?

The body absorbs the challenge dose rapidly, causing plasma glucose levels to rise and peak within 30 minutes to 1 hour. The pancreas responds by secreting more insulin, causing glucose levels to return to normal after 2 to 3 hours.

Administering oral glucose solutions

The oral glucose load in a glucose tolerance test usually varies from 50 to 100 g. Usually a glucose dose of 40 g/m^2 of body surface area is used, as calculated by a nomogram based on height and weight. Other authorities advocate a glucose load of 1.75 g/kg of body weight, which is especially useful in testing children.

Glucose in disguise

Many children become nauseated after drinking the overly sweet glucose solution. One way to make the solution more palatable is to dissolve it in water, flavour it with lemon juice and chill it.

During this period, plasma and urine glucose levels are monitored to assess insulin secretion and the body's ability to metabolise glucose. Occasionally, glucose levels are monitored for an additional 2 to 3 hours to aid in the diagnosis of hypoglycaemia and malabsorption syndrome.

A little intolerant

In a child with mild or diet-controlled diabetes (type 2), fasting plasma glucose levels may be in the normal range; however, insufficient secretion of insulin after ingestion of carbohydrates causes plasma glucose levels to rise sharply and return to normal slowly. This decreased tolerance for glucose helps confirm mild diabetes.

Nursing considerations

Explain to the child and parents that the test usually requires five blood samples and five urine specimens. Provide the child with coping mechanisms, and help them deal with the multiple blood samples by giving a small reward, such as a sticker, after each blood sample.

In addition, follow these steps:
• Instruct the parents that the child must fast for 8 to 12 hours before the test because the first blood test is a fasting glucose level.
• Send blood and urine samples to the laboratory immediately, or refrigerate them.
• Specify blood and urine collections times, and the time the child last ate.
• As appropriate, record the time that the child received their last pretest dose of insulin or oral antidiabetic drug.

Blood totals

• If the child is an infant or young child, keep an ongoing record of repeated specimen collection and a total of the amount of blood collected.
• As ordered, resume administration of medication withheld before the test.

Growth hormone, human

The hGH test is used to detect hypopituitarism. Also known as growth hormone and somatotropin, hGH is a protein secreted by the anterior pituitary and is the primary regulator of human growth. Children generally have higher hGH levels than adults; these levels can range from undetectable to 16 mcg/L.

The hGH test, a quantitative analysis of plasma hGH levels, is usually performed as part of an anterior pituitary stimulation or suppression test. Such testing is crucial because clinical manifestations of an hGH deficiency can rarely be reversed by therapy.

The lowdown on levels

Increased hGH levels may indicate a pituitary or hypothalamic tumour (commonly an adenoma), which causes gigantism in children and acromegaly in adults and adolescents.

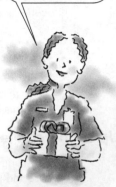

Small rewards, such as stickers, can help make the five needle pricks needed for blood glucose testing a little sweeter.

The highs …

Children with diabetes mellitus sometimes have elevated hGH levels without acromegaly. Suppression testing is necessary to confirm the diagnosis.

… and the lows

Pituitary infarction, metastatic disease, and tumours may reduce hGH levels. Dwarfism may be caused by low hGH levels, but confirmation of the diagnosis requires stimulation testing with arginine or insulin.

Nursing considerations

Prepare the child for the test with an age-appropriate explanation. Tell the child and parents that another sample may have to be taken the following day for comparison. Explain to the parents that the laboratory requires at least 2 days for analysis.

In addition, follow these steps:
- Withhold all medications that affect hGH levels, such as pituitary-based steroids, as prescribed. If these medications must be continued, note this on the laboratory request.
- Make sure the child is relaxed and lying down for 30 minutes before the test because stress and physical activity elevate hGH levels. Explain that the child must fast and limit physical activity for 10 to 12 hours before the test.
- Between 6 a.m. and 8 a.m. on 2 consecutive days, or as ordered, take venous blood samples into a 7-ml clot-activator tube, and send it to the laboratory.

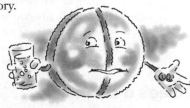

As a pituitary-based steroid, I'm off-limits before a growth hormone test. I do my job so well that I could alter the results.

Growth hormone suppression

The GH suppression test, also known as the glucose loading test, is used to diagnose pituitary hyperfunction. It evaluates excessive baseline levels of hGH from the anterior pituitary by measuring the secretory response to a loading dose of glucose.

Failure to suppress

Normally, hGH raises plasma glucose and fatty acid concentrations; in response, insulin secretion increases to counteract these effects. A glucose load should suppress hGH secretion. In a child with excessive hGH levels, the failure to suppress hGH indicates anterior pituitary dysfunction and confirms a diagnosis of acromegaly or gigantism.

Glucose normally suppresses hGH to levels ranging from undetectable to 3 mcg/L in 30 minutes to 2 hours. In a child with active acromegaly, basal hGH levels are elevated to 75 mcg/L and aren't suppressed to less than 5 mcg/L during the test. In children, rebound stimulation may occur after 2 to 5 hours.

Rest and repeat

When the hGH levels are unchanged or increased in response to glucose loading, hGH hypersecretion is indicated and may confirm suspected acromegaly or gigantism. This response may be verified by repeating the test after a 1-day rest.

Nursing considerations

Explain the test to the child and parents. Tell the child that they may experience nausea after drinking the glucose solution, and prepare them for venepuncture. In addition:
• withhold all steroids; if these or other medications must be continued, note this on the laboratory request
• administer 100 g of glucose solution by mouth; to prevent nausea, tell the child to drink the glucose slowly.

Guthrie screening

The Guthrie screening test, also know as the phenylalanine test, is a screening method used to detect elevated levels of serum phenylalanine, a naturally occurring amino acid essential for growth and nitrogen balance.

Metabolic upset

Elevated levels of phenylalanine may indicate phenylketonuria (PKU), a metabolic disorder inherited as an autosomal-recessive trait. An infant with PKU usually has normal phenylalanine levels at birth, but after feeds commence with breast milk or formula (both of which contain phenylalanine), levels gradually rise because of a deficiency of the liver enzyme that converts phenylalanine to tyrosine. The resulting accumulation of phenylalanine, phenylpyruvic acid and other metabolites hinders normal development of central nervous system cells, causing cognitive and developmental delay.

Three's a charm

The serum phenylalanine screening test detects abnormal phenylalanine levels through the growth rate of *Bacillus subtilis*, an organism that needs phenylalanine to thrive. To ensure accurate results, the test must be performed after at least 3 full days of breast milk or formula feeding but is most usually performed after a week.

Danger ahead

Growth of *B. subtilis* on the filter paper indicates that serum phenylalanine levels are high enough to overcome the antagonist. Such a positive result suggests the possibility of PKU; diagnosis requires exact serum phenylalanine measurement and urine testing. A phenylalanine reading of 240 μmol/L requires further investigation and therefore sampling of phenylalanine and tyrosine should be undertaken using a different analytical method. A positive test may also result from hepatic disease, galactosaemia (an inherited, autosomal-recessive disorder of galactose metabolism) or delayed development of certain enzyme systems. (See *Confirming PKU*.)

Confirming PKU

After the Guthrie screening test detects the possible presence of phenylketonuria (PKU), serum phenylalanine and tyrosine levels are measured to confirm the diagnosis. Phenylalanine hydroxylase is the enzyme that converts phenylalanine to tyrosine. If this enzyme is absent, increasing phenylalanine levels with concomitant decreasing tyrosine levels indicate PKU.

Samples are obtained by venipuncture (femoral or external jugular). Serum phenylalanine levels greater than 4 mg/dl and tyrosine levels less than 0.6 mg/dl – with urinary excretion of phenylpyruvic acid – confirm PKU.

Nursing considerations

Explain the test to the parents. In addition, follow these steps:
• Perform a heel prick and allow the blood to drip onto the filter paper, filling each circle.
• Reassure the parents of a child who may have PKU that early detection and continuous treatment with a low-phenylalanine diet can prevent permanent developmental delay.
• Note the infant's name and birth date and the date of the first breast milk or formula feeding on the laboratory request; send the sample to the laboratory immediately.

Neonatal galactosaemia

Galactosaemia is a genetic disorder. A child with galactosaemia lacks the liver enzyme galactose-1-phosphate uridyltransferase (GALT), which converts galactose into glucose. The child's galactose levels remain abnormally high. Ultimately, galactosaemia may cause hepatomegaly, kidney failure, cataracts or brain damage. If the disorder goes untreated, death may result in 75% of infants with the disorder. In the UK Galactosaemia is not routinely screened for, although it is in the Republic of Ireland.

From sea to shining sea

To detect galactosaemia, two tests may be run on the filter paper blood sample:

First, the level of galactose in the blood is determined.

If this test is abnormally high (usually considered total galactose levels greater than 10 mg/dl), a Beutler assay is performed on the sample to measure GALT enzyme activity.

Where's the GALT?

Galactosaemia is diagnosed if there's no detectable GALT enzyme activity. After the diagnosis is made, treatment must begin immediately.

Nursing considerations

• Screening will provide the best results if it's done after the infant has received a formula-based feed.
• Be sure to indicate the infant's feed and blood transfusion status on the filter paper blood sample.
• Protect the filter paper blood sample from heat, which may damage the GALT enzyme. (See *Galactosaemia interference*.)

Neonatal T4 and TSH blood-spot test

T4 test is performed as part of the neonatal screening with the sample placed as a blood-spot on filter paper. A low T4 level (less than 6 mg/dl) must be

---

Galactosaemia interference

Factors that may alter galactosemia test results include:

• use of aspirin, sulfonamides, nitrofurantoin, vitamin K derivatives, primaquine and fava beans, which decrease galactose-1-phosphate uridyl transferase enzyme activity and precipitate haemolytic episodes
• performing the test after a haemolytic episode or a blood transfusion, which can cause false-negative results
• failure to use a collection tube containing the proper anticoagulant or to adequately mix the sample and anticoagulant
• haemolysis caused by rough handling of the sample.

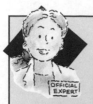

Advice from the experts

Collecting a filter paper sample

To collect a specimen for neonatal thyroid-stimulating hormone testing using the filter paper method, gather the following equipment and follow the easy steps below.

Equipment

- Alcohol swabs
- Sterile lancet
- Specially marked filter paper
- Sterile gauze pads
- Adhesive bandage
- Labels
- Gloves.

Steps

- Assemble the necessary equipment, wash your hands thoroughly and put on gloves.
- Wipe the infant's heel with an alcohol swab; then dry it thoroughly with a gauze pad.
- Perform a prick and squeeze the infant's heel gently, filling the circles on the filter paper with blood, while making sure the blood saturates the paper.
- Gently apply pressure with a gauze pad to ensure haemostasis at the puncture site.
- Allow the filter paper to dry, label it appropriately and send it to the laboratory.

followed by a TSH level, which may be performed on the same blood sample or from a separate sample. (See *Collecting a filter paper sample*.)

The birth surge

Also known as the neonatal thyrotropin test, the neonatal TSH test confirms congenital hypothyroidism. TSH levels normally surge after birth and trigger a rise in TH, which is essential for neurological development. At age 1 to 2 days, TSH levels are normally 25 to 30 μIU/ml (SI, 25 to 30 mU/L). Thereafter, levels are normally less than 25 μIU/ml (SI, 25 mU/L).

Failure to respond

In primary congenital hypothyroidism, the thyroid gland doesn't respond to TSH stimulation, which results in lower TH levels and higher TSH levels. Early detection and treatment of congenital hypothyroidism are critical to prevent developmental delay and cretinism.

Neonatal TSH levels must be interpreted in light of T4 concentrations. Elevated TSH that's accompanied by decreased T4 indicates primary congenital hypothyroidism. Depressed TSH and depressed T4 may be present in secondary congenital hypothyroidism. When TSH is normal and is accompanied by depressed T4, hypothyroidism due to a congenital defect or transient congenital hypothyroidism due to prematurity or prenatal hypoxia may be the cause. A complete thyroid workup must be done to confirm the cause of hypothyroidism before treatment can begin. (See *Neonatal TSH interference*.)

Neonatal TSH interference

Several factors may alter thyroid-stimulating hormone (TSH) levels, or the results of tests used to measure TSH levels in the neonate:

- Corticosteroids, triiodothyronine and thyroxine lower TSH levels.
- Lithium carbonate, potassium iodide, excessive topical resorcinol and TSH injection raise TSH levels.
- Failure to let a filter paper sample dry completely may alter results.
- Rough handling of a serum sample may cause haemolysis, which may alter results.

Nursing considerations

Explain the test to the parents. The T4 test is performed using samples collected from filter paper. This is performed at the same time as the Guthrie test so requires similar explanations.

Thyroxine test (serum)

T4 is an amine secreted by the thyroid gland in response to TSH from the pituitary and, indirectly, to thyrotropin-releasing hormone (TRH) from the hypothalamus.

Cons, pros and suspects

The rate of secretion is normally regulated by a complex system of negative and positive feedback involving the thyroid, the anterior pituitary and the hypothalamus. T4 is the suspected precursor (or prohormone) of T3 and is converted to T3 mainly in the liver and kidneys.

The T4 that binds

Only a fraction of T4 (about 0.3%) circulates freely in the blood; the rest binds strongly to plasma proteins, primarily to thyroxine-binding globulin (TBG). This minute fraction of free circulating T4 is responsible for the clinical effects of TH. TBG binds so tenaciously that T4 survives in the plasma for a relatively long time, with a half-life of about 6 days. This test measures the total circulating T4 level when TBG is normal.

More testing ahead

Serum T4 testing is performed to evaluate thyroid function and to monitor thyroid replacement therapy.

Abnormally elevated levels of T4 are consistent with primary and secondary hyperthyroidism, including excessive T4 (levothyroxine) replacement therapy. Overt signs of hyperthyroidism require further testing and, in doubtful cases of hypothyroidism, the TSH or TRH test may be indicated. (See *Thyroxine levels in children*.)

Thyroxine levels in children

Thyroxine levels change as the child grows:

- cord blood – 95 to 168 nmol/L
- younger than age 1 month – 90 to 292 nmol/L
- ages 1 month to 1 year – 93 to 213 nmol/L
- ages 1 to 5 years – 94 to 194 nmol/L
- ages 5 to 10 years – 83 to 192 nmol/L
- ages 10 to 15 years – 72 to 151 nmol/L.

Nursing considerations

Explain the test to the child and parents. In addition, follow these steps:
• As ordered, withhold medication that may interfere with test results. If medication must be continued, note this on the laboratory request. (If the test is being performed to monitor thyroid therapy, the child should continue to receive daily thyroid supplements.)
• Perform a venepuncture, collect a sample and send this to the laboratory immediately.

Triiodothyronine test (serum)

The T3 test is a highly specific immunoassay that measures total serum content of T3 to investigate clinical indications of thyroid dysfunction. It helps diagnose T3 toxicosis, hypothyroidism or hyperthyroidism and helps monitor the course of thyroid replacement therapy.

T3 is the more potent TH. At least 50% and as much as 90% of T3 is thought to be derived from T4. The remaining 10% or more is secreted directly by the thyroid gland. Like T4 secretion, T3 secretion occurs in response to TSH released by the pituitary and, secondarily, to TRH from the hypothalamus.

A little T3 goes a long way

Although T3 is present in the bloodstream in minute quantities and is metabolically active for only a short time, its impact on body metabolism dominates that of T4. T3 binds less firmly to TBG, so it persists in the bloodstream for a short time; half of it disappears in about 1 day, whereas half of T4 remains for 6 days.

It's all on the level

Normally, serum T3 levels in children are:
• neonate – 1.16 to 4 nmol/L
• children ages 1 to 5 years – 1.54 to 4 nmol/L
• children ages 5 to 10 years – 1.39 to 3.7 nmol/L
• children ages 10 to 15 years – 1.23 to 3.23 nmol/L.

A tandem rise

Serum T3 and T4 levels usually rise and fall in tandem. However, in T3 toxicosis, only T3 levels rise, while total and free T4 levels remain normal. T3 toxicosis occurs in children with Graves' disease, toxic adenoma or toxic nodular goitre. T3 levels also surpass T4 levels in children receiving thyroid replacement containing more T3 than T4. In iodine-deficient areas, the thyroid may produce larger amounts of the more cellularly active T3 than T4 in an effort to maintain the euthyroid state.

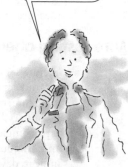

When it comes to potency, T3 has T4 beat. Its effect on body metabolism dominates the effect of T4.

Nursing considerations

Explain the test to the child and parents, Apply local anaesthetic cream for the appropriate time before the test. Encourage a parent to be present during the venepuncture. In addition, follow these steps:

• Withhold medication that may influence thyroid function, such as steroids and propranolol. If such medication must be continued, record this information on the laboratory request.

• Perform a venepuncture, collect the sample and send it to the laboratory immediately.

• If a child must receive thyroid preparations, such as T3 note the time of drug administration on the laboratory request form.

Treatments and procedures

Common treatments and procedures used in the care of a child with an endocrine and metabolic system disorder include radioactive iodine (^{131}I) therapy and thyroidectomy.

^{131}I therapy

A form of radiation therapy, ^{131}I therapy is used to treat hyperthyroidism in children, particularly Graves' disease. It shrinks functioning thyroid tissue, decreasing circulating TH levels.

After oral ingestion, ^{131}I is rapidly absorbed and concentrated in the thyroid as if it were normal iodine, resulting in acute radiation thyroiditis and gradual thyroid atrophy. ^{131}I causes symptoms to subside after about 3 weeks and exerts its full effect only after 3 to 6 months.

Nursing considerations

Explain the procedure and check the child's history for allergies to iodine.

Expecting a glow

The idea of ingesting a radioactive material may be frightening to the child and parents, especially when they hear about the precautions that must be taken. Reassure the child and parents that this treatment will affect only the thyroid, and that all the radioactive material will be excreted from the body.

In addition, follow these steps:

• Unless contraindicated, instruct the parents to stop TH antagonists 4 to 7 days before ^{131}I administration because these drugs reduce the sensitivity of thyroid cells to radiation.

• Tell the parents to ensure the child is fasted overnight as food may delay ^{131}I absorption.

Until my nurse explained my ^{131}I treatment, I thought I was going to be Radioactive Man!

• If the child received an unusually large dose of ^{131}I or if treatment was for cancer, they may stay in the hospital for monitoring. In such cases, observe radiation precautions for 3 days.
• Pregnant nurses should not care for the child.
• Encourage the child to drink plenty of fluids for 48 hours to speed excretion of ^{131}I.

At home with radioactive iodine

If the child will be discharged after treatment, instruct the parents about observing radiation precautions at home:
• Tell the parents that the child must urinate into a lead-lined container for 48 hours.
• Tell the parents that the child must use disposable eating utensils, and avoid close contact with young children and pregnant women for 7 days after therapy.
• Advise the parents to dispose of urine, saliva and vomit properly; urine and saliva will be slightly radioactive for 24 hours and vomitus will be highly radioactive for 6 to 8 hours after therapy.

Thyroidectomy

Thyroidectomy (removal of all or part of the thyroid gland) is performed to treat hyperthyroidism and respiratory obstruction from goitre. Subtotal thyroidectomy, which reduces secretion of TH, is used to correct hyperthyroidism when drug therapy fails or radiation therapy is contraindicated. After surgery, the remaining thyroid tissue usually supplies enough TH for normal function, although hypothyroidism may occur later.

Nursing considerations

Prepare the child for surgery with an age-appropriate explanation, including the post-operative appearance of the site of surgery. Tell the child that their throat may be sore for a few days after surgery, and that medication will be given to make them feel better. Keep in mind that the child may be fearful of having their 'throat cut'; provide clarification and answer all questions.

In addition, follow these steps:
• Iodine preparations are typically administered before surgery; to improve the taste of the preparation, mix it with fruit juice.
• Check for laryngeal nerve damage by asking the child to speak as soon as they awaken from anaesthesia.
• Watch for signs of respiratory distress. Tracheal collapse, mucous accumulation in the trachea, laryngeal oedema and vocal cord paralysis can all cause respiratory obstruction with sudden stridor and restlessness.

Just in case

• Keep a tracheostomy tray at the bedside for the first 24 hours after surgery and be prepared to assist with emergency tracheotomy if necessary.

- Assess for signs of haemorrhage, which may cause shock, tracheal compression and respiratory distress.
- Check the child's dressing and palpate the back of their neck (where drainage tends to flow).

Dribbling drainage patrol

- Expect only scant drainage after 24 hours.
- As prescribed, administer analgesia to relieve a sore neck or throat; reassure the child that this discomfort should resolve within a few days.
- Test for positive Chvostek's (or Weiss') and Trousseau's signs, indicators of neuromuscular irritability from hypocalcaemia; keep calcium gluconate available for emergency IV administration.

Storm's a'brewin'

- Be alert for signs of thyroid storm, a rare but serious complication in children, characterised by sudden and dangerous signs and symptoms, including severe tachycardia (increased heart rate), severe irritability, vomiting, diarrhoea, hyperthermia and hypertension.

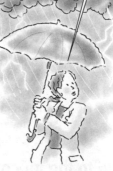

A sudden increase in thyrotoxicosis symptoms is a sign of thyroid storm.

Endocrine and metabolic disorders

Endocrine and metabolic disorders that may affect children include congenital hypothyroidism, Cushing's syndrome, diabetes mellitus, galactosaemia, Graves' disease and PKU.

Congenital hypothyroidism

Congenital hypothyroidism is a deficiency of TH secretion during foetal development or early infancy. If left untreated, it will seriously affect mental development. Congenital hypothyroidism is three times more common in girls than in boys.

The early bird catches the best prognosis

Early diagnosis and treatment produces the best prognosis. Infants treated before age 3 months usually grow and develop normally. Athyroid children (born without a thyroid gland) who remain untreated beyond age 3 months and children with acquired hypothyroidism who remain untreated beyond age 2 years suffer irreversible mental retardation. Skeletal abnormalities are reversible with treatment.

What causes it

Congenital hypothyroidism is caused by defective embryonic development (most common cause), causing congenital absence or underdevelopment of the thyroid gland. It can also occur as an inherited autosomal-recessive defect in the synthesis of T4 (next most common cause).

Mum's meds

Congenital hypothyroidism in infants can result if the mother took antithyroid drugs during pregnancy. Other causes include chronic autoimmune thyroiditis and iodine deficiency during pregnancy.

How it happens
Hypothyroidism in infants and children is related to decreased TH production or secretion, which may result from one of several causes:
• Loss of functional thyroid tissue can be caused by an autoimmune process.
• Defective thyroid synthesis may be related to congenital defects; thyroid dysgenesis (defective development) is the most common defect.
• Hypothyroidism may also be related to decreased TSH secretion or resistance to TSH.
• If left untreated, lack of adequate TH levels seriously affects the nervous system and bone growth.

What to look for
The signs of untreated hypothyroidism usually appear at 6 weeks:
• The infant with hypothyroidism may sleep more than usual; older children may show signs of lethargy.
• They may have noisy respirations due to tongue enlargement. (The tongue may also be dry.)

Cold to the touch

• The extremities may be cold and the overall body temperature may be lower due to decreased metabolism.
• The child's neck will be short and thick.
• The extremities appear short and fat; the legs appear shorter in relation to trunk size.

Constipation consternation

• The abdomen becomes enlarged because of intestinal obstruction from constipation (which results from hypotonia of the intestinal tract).
• Other signs include delayed dentition; dry, scaly skin; easy weight gain and slow pulse.

Whoa, horsey

Infants may have a hoarse cry, persistent jaundice and respiratory difficulties. Older children may exhibit bone and muscle dystrophy, cognitive impairment (which develops as the disorder progresses) and stunted growth or dwarfism (short stature with the persistence of infant proportions).

What tests tell you

Elevated TSH level associated with low T3 and T4 levels points to congenital hypothyroidism. Because early detection and treatment can minimise the effects of congenital hypothyroidism, it is routinely tested for in the UK.

• Thyroid scan and ^{131}I uptake tests show decreased uptake levels and confirm the absence of thyroid tissue in athyroid children.

• Increased gonadotropin levels accompany sexual precocity in older children and may coexist with hypothyroidism.

• An electrocardiogram shows bradycardia and flat or inverted T waves in untreated infants.

• Hip, knee and thigh X-rays reveal the absence of the femoral or tibial epiphyseal line and delayed skeletal development that's markedly inappropriate for the child's chronological age.

Complications

If hypothyroidism isn't treated by 3 months of age, skeletal malformations and irreversible mental retardation can occur; treatment helps to prevent developmental delay. Learning disabilities and accelerated or delayed sexual maturation may also occur.

How it's treated

The treatment of congenital hypothyroidism is lifelong therapy with synthetic TH (levothyroxine, liothyronine). Supplemental vitamin D may also be prescribed to prevent rickets resulting from rapid bone growth. Surgery may be performed for the underlying cause such as a pituitary tumour. The child should have routine monitoring of T4 and TSH levels as well as periodic evaluation of growth to ensure that thyroid replacement is adequate.

What to do

The child and parents will need ongoing support and encouragement. They should be encouraged to express their concerns and feelings, and may need help to develop effective coping mechanisms. Referral to a support group may be extremely helpful. In addition, follow these steps:

• When caring for a neonate, make sure screening has been done to allow for early detection of the disorder.

• Stress to the parents the importance of lifelong treatment, including TH replacement therapy as well as routine blood tests to adjust the medication as the child grows.

• Administer prescribed medication

• Offer support and encouragement to the parents.

Too high, too low

• After initiation of treatment of infantile hypothyroidism, monitor blood pressure and pulse rate, and report hypertension and tachycardia immediately. (Normal infant heart rate is approximately 120 beats/minute.)

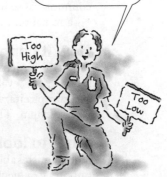

Heed the signs! Parents – and nurses – need to know when the TH replacement dosage is too high or too low.

These signs as well as fever, irritability and sweating indicate that the dose of TH replacement medication is too high.
• Teach the parents to look for signs and symptoms of inadequate treatment (a dose that's too low), including fatigue, lethargy, decreased appetite and constipation.

Plan ahead

• Adolescent girls require ongoing counselling that stresses the importance of adequate TH replacement during pregnancy.
• If the infant's tongue is unusually large, position them on the side and observe frequently to prevent airway obstruction.

Don't delay

If treatment is delayed and signs and symptoms develop:
• help the child and parents develop effective coping skills
• provide meticulous skin and mucous membrane care
• check the child's temperature every 2 to 4 hours; keep the child warm, as needed.

Cushing's syndrome

Cushing's syndrome is a disorder of adrenal hyperfunction. It results from excessive levels of adrenocortical hormones (particularly cortisol) or related corticosteroids and, to a lesser extent, androgens and aldosterone. Cushing's syndrome is most common in females.

Prognosis depends on the underlying cause. The prognosis is poor without treatment and in children with untreatable, ectopic corticotropin-secreting carcinoma or metastatic adrenal carcinoma.

What causes it

Adrenal hyperfunction can be caused by:
• pituitary hypersecretion of corticotropin (Cushing's disease)
• corticotropin-secreting tumour in another organ
• administration of excessive or prolonged synthetic glucocorticoids (most common cause in children)
• adrenal tumour.

How it happens

A loss of normal feedback inhibition by cortisol occurs in Cushing's syndrome. Elevated levels of cortisol don't suppress hypothalamic and anterior pituitary secretion of corticotropin-releasing hormone and corticotropin. The result is excessive levels of circulating cortisol.

What to look for

The unmistakable signs of Cushing's syndrome include adiposity of the face (moon face), neck and trunk, and reddish purple striae on the skin (especially the abdomen). In addition, a child with some or all of the following signs may have Cushing's syndrome:

- weight gain
- muscle weakness
- fatigue
- irritability and emotional instability
- sleep disturbances
- water retention
- amenorrhoea
- thin hair and thin, fragile skin (ruddy complexion)
- thinning extremities with muscle wasting and fat mobilisation
- bruising, petechiae and ecchymoses
- delayed wound healing
- hirsutism
- truncal obesity.

What tests tell you

A low-dose (overnight) dexamethasone suppression test, elevated 24-hour urine free cortisol levels and high night-time cortisol levels (indicating the absence of circadian rhythm) confirm the diagnosis of Cushing's syndrome. The cause can be determined with a plasma corticotropin test and a high-dose dexamethasone suppression test.

Stealth corticotropin

With an adrenal tumour, corticotropin levels aren't detectable and steroid levels aren't suppressed. Ectopic corticotropin syndrome shows elevated corticotropin or unsuppressed steroid levels. Normal to elevated corticotropin with steroid suppressed to less than 50% of baseline indicates Cushing's disease.

Ultrasonography, computed tomography (CT) scanning or angiography localise adrenal tumours. CT scanning or magnetic resonance imaging of the head helps localise pituitary tumours.

Complications

Complications of Cushing's syndrome include:

- osteoporosis and pathological fractures
- peptic ulcer
- impaired glucose tolerance
- frequent infections
- dyslipidemia
- diabetes mellitus
- slow wound healing
- mental health problems ranging from mood swings to psychosis
- suppressed inflammatory response
- hypertension
- ischaemic heart disease, heart failure
- menstrual disturbances.

How it's treated

Radiation, drug therapy or surgery may be necessary to restore hormone balance and reverse the effects of Cushing's syndrome.

Cushing's combo

These management approaches may be used in combination:
• Drug therapy may include antifungal agents, antihypertensives, diuretics, glucocorticoids, potassium supplements, antineoplastic or antihormone agents.
• An adrenal tumour is treated with bilateral adrenalectomy.
• Non-endocrine corticotropin-secreting tumours require excision.
• Hypophysectomy may be needed.

Pre-operative preparation

Before surgery, the child with cushingoid signs and symptoms needs special management to control hypertension, oedema, diabetes and cardiovascular manifestations and prevent infection. Glucocorticoid administration on the morning of surgery can help prevent acute adrenal insufficiency during surgery.

What to do

Children with Cushing's syndrome require painstaking assessment and supportive care:
• Frequently monitor vital signs, especially blood pressure; carefully observe the hypertensive child who also has cardiac disease.
• Check laboratory reports for hypernatraemia, hypokalaemia, hyperglycaemia and glycosuria.

What goes in might not come out!

• Check for oedema and carefully monitor daily weight and intake and output; the cushingoid child is likely to retain sodium and water.
• To minimise weight gain, oedema and hypertension, the dietician will recommend a diet high in protein and potassium but low in calories, carbohydrates and sodium.

Infection prevention

• Use protective measures to prevent infection (a significant problem in Cushing's syndrome).
• Carefully perform passive range-of-motion exercises for children who have osteoporosis and are on bedrest.

Post-operative care

After hypophysectomy using the transsphenoidal approach:
• keep the head of the bed elevated at least 30 degrees
• maintain nasal packing
• provide frequent mouth care

- avoid activities that increase intracranial pressure (ICP)
- monitor for cerebral fluid leaks.
  After bilateral adrenalectomy or hypophysectomy, assess the child for:
- changes in neurological and behavioural status
- severe nausea, vomiting, and diarrhoea
- bowel sounds
- adrenal hypofunction
- increased ICP
- transient diabetes insipidus
- haemorrhage
- shock.

Diabetes mellitus

Diabetes mellitus is a chronic disease of absolute or relative insulin deficiency or resistance.

Absolutely insufficient

Type 1 diabetes mellitus (characterised by absolute insulin insufficiency) is the most common childhood endocrine disorder. Although rare, the incidence of type 2 diabetes mellitus in childhood is rising because of the increase in childhood obesity and sedentary lifestyles. It's characterised by insulin resistance with varying degrees of insulin secretory defects.

Diabetes mellitus can occur at any age but has a peak incidence between 10 and 15 years. Seventy-five per cent of cases diagnosed in children occur before 18 years. Boys seem to have a slightly higher prevalence of the disease than girls.

What causes it

Diabetes mellitus is caused by genetic factors and autoimmune factors (type 1), and may also develop as a result of a viral infection.

Genetic factors

Type 1 isn't inherited but predisposition plays a part in its development.

Blame it on dad

Children born to fathers who have type 1 are about three times more likely to develop diabetes mellitus than children born to mothers with type 1.

Autoimmune factors

About 70% to 85% of newly diagnosed type 1 diabetes mellitus children are found to have pancreatic islet cell antibodies.

Straggler antibodies

These antibodies disappear in most people after diagnosis. It's thought that the presence of these antibodies makes the immune

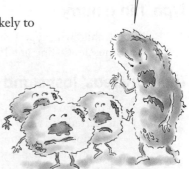

Don't hate me because I'm a virus. Injuring islet cells and triggering type 1 diabetes is my job – it's what I do.

system vulnerable to a trigger event, such as a virus, bacteria or chemical irritant.

Viral infection

Several viruses, including coxsackie B, mumps and congenital rubella, have been associated with the development of type 1 diabetes mellitus.

Vulnerable to viruses

The pancreatic islet cells are susceptible to injury by these viruses and can suffer damage or be changed. This alteration triggers an autoimmune response. The virus becomes a trigger to the development of type 1 diabetes mellitus.

How it happens

Diabetes mellitus is characterised by disturbances in carbohydrate, protein and fat metabolism. Insulin allows glucose transport into the cells for use as energy or storage as glycogen.

Free the fatty acids!

Insulin stimulates protein synthesis and free fatty acid storage in adipose tissues. Deficiency of insulin or insulin resistance and secretory defects compromise the body tissues' access to essential nutrients for fuel and storage.

What to look for

The three cardinal signs of diabetes mellitus are polyuria, polydipsia and polyphagia. Other general signs and symptoms may include:
- weakness and fatigue
- nocturia in a child who has already attained nighttime control
- dehydration (dry mucous membranes and poor skin turgor)
- weight loss and hunger
- vision changes (retinopathy or cataract formation)
- frequent skin and urinary tract infections
- skin changes (cool temperature, and dry, itchy skin, especially on the hands and feet).

Type 1 in a hurry

A child with type 1 diabetes mellitus will have rapidly developing symptoms, muscle wasting and loss of subcutaneous fat.

The pancreas' last stand

A onetime remission of symptoms may occur shortly after insulin treatment is started. It's a last-ditch effort by the pancreas to produce insulin. The child may not need insulin for up to 1 year but may need oral antidiabetic drugs. Symptoms of hyperglycaemia will reappear, and the child will be insulin-dependent for life.

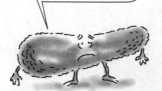

Even in the face of diabetes mellitus, I respond to therapy by making insulin one last time. It's my insulin swan song.

Vaguely type 2

In children with type 2 diabetes mellitus, vague, long-standing symptoms develop gradually. These include and are associated with:
- severe viral infection
- other endocrine diseases
- recent stress or trauma
- use of drugs that increase blood glucose levels
- obesity, particularly in the abdominal area.

What tests tell you

Two fasting plasma glucose tests above 7 mmol/L or, with normal fasting glucose, two blood glucose levels above 11 mmol/L during a 2-hour glucose tolerance test confirm the diagnosis. Other findings include:
- 2-hour post-prandial blood glucose level greater than 11 mmol/L
- increased glycosylated haemoglobin level
- urinalysis that may show acetone or glucose
- diabetic retinopathy, which may be revealed by an ophthalmic examination.

Complications

Diabetic ketoacidosis (DKA) and hypoglycaemia may occur as well as hyperosmolar hyperglycaemic nonketotic syndrome (HHNS). Long-term complications of diabetes mellitus are nephropathy, retinopathy and neuropathy.

If the diabetes isn't well controlled, complications can occur as early as 2 to 3 years after diagnosis. Therefore, good control and regimen compliance are necessary to postpone or prevent complications.

How it's treated

Treating the child with diabetes mellitus requires a multidisciplinary approach and should follow the NICE guidelines on the diagnosis and management of type 1 diabetes in children, young people and adults (2004/2010) as well as the standards from the National Service Framework for Diabetes (2001/02).

Team diabetes

The child, parents and health care professionals (including a paediatrician, dietician and a children's diabetes nurse specialist) should all be involved in the child's care plan. It may also be necessary for a mental health professional to be included as the care plan can have an impact on the child's emotional and psychological health.

Meal planning, exercise and, as needed, insulin or oral antidiabetic agents are prescribed to normalise carbohydrate, fat and protein metabolism and avert long-term complications while preventing hypoglycaemia.

Type 1 diabetes

Childs with type 1 diabetes must take insulin daily because of their absolute insulin deficiency. The insulin needs changes and is affected by emotions,

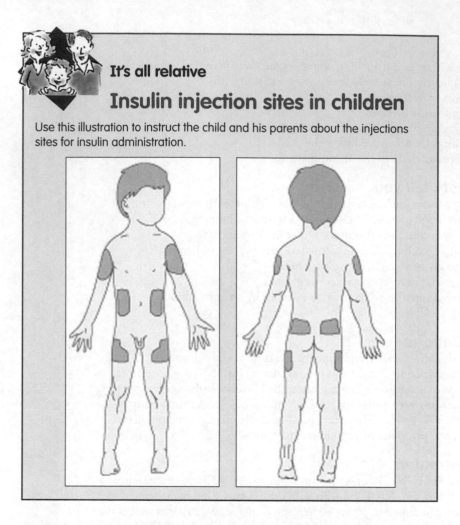

It's all relative

Insulin injection sites in children

Use this illustration to instruct the child and his parents about the injections sites for insulin administration.

nutritional intake, activity, illness and events such as puberty. (See *Insulin injection sites in children*.)

Insulin dosages are based on home blood glucose monitoring. Insulin can be administered as one or two injections per day or by insulin pump (continuous subcutaneous administration).

Type 2 diabetes

Childs with type 2 diabetes may require insulin to control blood glucose levels unresponsive to diet and oral antidiabetic agents, or during periods of acute stress. Children with other types of diabetes commonly require daily insulin therapy to achieve blood glucose control. (See *Insulin therapy*.)

What to do

The child with diabetes may be facing lifelong treatment and restrictions for a chronic disease, with the prospect of setbacks (until control is established)

Insulin therapy

Insulin is administered as prescribed. There are several routes of administration and devices for injection.

Subcutaneous route

Insulin is usually given by subcutaneous (IV) injection with a standard insulin syringe. SC insulin can also be given with a penlike injection device that uses a disposable needle and replaceable insulin cartridges, eliminating the need to draw insulin into a syringe. More recently disposable pen devices have been introduced making it easier for the child and family.

Jet-propelled

Jet-injection devices are expensive and require special cleaning procedures, but they disperse insulin more rapidly and speed absorption. These devices draw up insulin from standard containers, which enables the patient to mix insulins, if necessary, but requires a special procedure for drawing it up. After the insulin is drawn up, it's delivered into the subcutaneous tissue with a pressure jet.

Pump it up!

Multiple-dose regimens may use an insulin pump to deliver insulin continuously into subcutaneous tissue. The infusion rate selector automatically releases about half of the total daily insulin requirement evenly over 24 hours. The patient releases the remainder in bolus amounts before meals and snacks.

Ready, set, rotate!

When administering insulin injections SC, the injection sites should be rotated. Because absorption rates differ at each site, diabetic educators recommend rotating the injection site within a specific area such as the abdomen.

IV and IM routes

Regular insulin or insulin lispro may also be administered IM or IV during severe episodes of hyperglycemia. These are the only types of insulin that should ever be administered by these routes.

Investigational routes

Researchers are working on newer, more efficient ways of administering insulin. Two newer methods of insulin administration are the intranasal delivery method and the programmable implantable medication system (PIMS). Both methods are still experimental.

Up your nose with an aerosol

Intranasal administration uses aerosolised insulin combined with a surfactant; it's administered as a nasal spray. Because nasal solutions are less potent than SC insulin, dosages are higher.

Batteries included

Now undergoing clinical trials, the PIMS has an implantable infusion pump unit that holds and delivers the insulin, and a delivery catheter that feeds insulin directly into the peritoneal cavity.

The pump, encased in a titanium shell, contains a tiny computer to regulate dosages and runs on a battery with a 5-year life span. The patient uses a handheld external radio transmitter to control insulin release. Because the PIMS has no built-in blood glucose sensor, the patient must monitor his glucose levels several times per day.

and serious complications. The child and parents will need a great deal of ongoing support and assistance.

Rebel with restrictions

As the child grows, compliance may become an issue. A child or young person may simply become overwhelmed or tired of taking medication and adhering to dietary restrictions. Equally they may enter a period of rebellion, experimentation and use alcohol. These feelings and behaviours should be recognised as essentially normal and so health care professionals and parents will need to support the young person through this. Referral to a support group may help the child and parents cope with the diagnosis and its implications; however, research has shown that peers are a crucial support mechanism for young people.

In addition, follow these steps:
• Emphasise that adherence to the care plan is essential; it's crucial to bring the child's blood glucose level within an acceptable range and alleviate or prevent DKA or hypoglycaemia.
• For the child with unstable diabetes who isn't experiencing DKA or HHNS, monitor blood glucose levels several times each day as prescribed until they stabilise.

Like a hawk!

• Monitor the child closely for signs and symptoms of DKA or HHNS. Suspect DKA or HHNS if the child exhibits Kussmaul's respirations, develops a fruity odour on their breath and shows signs and symptoms of severe dehydration. Notify medical staff immediately and follow paediatric life support guidelines.
• If the child has DKA or HHNS, treatment may include fluid and electrolyte replacement, increased insulin therapy and therapy to reduce acidosis. Administer doses of IV insulin as prescribed. (Monitor blood glucose levels frequently during insulin infusion.)
• Monitor the child closely for signs and symptoms of hyperglycaemia and hypoglycaemia (caused by an excessively rapid reduction in blood glucose level). Teach these signs and symptoms to the child and parents and provide specific instructions on how to handle each condition. (See *Hypo or hyper?*)
• Make sure the child and parents understand that meal plans should be based on a balanced diet that incorporates the six basic food groups. The dietician will help with this.

Fitting in

• Concentrated sweets are discouraged, so teach the child and parents about alternate snack ideas to help them feel more like their peers. (See *Diabetes mellitus teaching tips*.)

Show and tell

• Demonstrate to the child how to check their blood glucose; it's especially necessary for the child on a tightly controlled regimen. Be aware though for the development of needle phobia.

Galactosaemia

Galactosaemia is an inborn error of carbohydrate metabolism and is a rare disorder affecting approximately 1 in 70,000 children in the UK.

Hypo or hyper?

It's generally difficult to distinguish between hypoglycaemia and hyperglycaemia.

Too little …

Hypoglycaemia symptoms include:

• lethargy
• hunger
• sweating
• pallor
• seizures
• coma.

… too much

Hyperglycaemia symptoms include:

• sweet, fruity breath (acetone)
• dehydration
• decreased sodium, potassium, bicarbonate, chloride and phosphate levels
• vomiting
• abdominal pain
• coma.

It's all relative

Diabetes mellitus teaching tips

Long-term management of diabetes mellitus requires extensive family education:

- Review the ditary plans and teach the child and family how to adjust the child's diet when engaged in extra activity.
- Advise the child and parents about aerobic exercise programs; explain how exercise affects blood glucose levels, and provide safety guidelines.
- Instruct the child on insulin administration, if prescribed, including type, peak times, dosage, using pen device, administration technique, site rotation, sharps disposal and storage.
- Teach the child and parents how to perform blood glucose monitoring.
- Instruct the child on oral antidiabetic therapy, if prescribed, including dosage, frequency and time of administration and potential adverse reactions.
- Tell the child and parents about the Internet as a source of information, and about the Diabeties UK web site. This site offers significant information for the child with diabetes, their family and health care professionals, along with general information about diabetes (advice on exercise, nutrition and daily meal planning) specifically aimed at the UK population.

What causes it

Galactosaemia is inherited as an autosomal-recessive trait.

How it happens

In galactosaemia, the hepatic enzyme GALT is absent. This enzyme is one of three needed to metabolise galactose to glucose. Without GALT, galactose accumulates in the blood, which leads to hepatic dysfunction, cirrhosis and subsequent jaundice. The jaundice is noticeable during the first few weeks of life. Portal hypertension occurs as the spleen becomes involved.

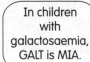

In children with galactosaemia, GALT is MIA.

What to look for

Infants with the disorder appear normal at birth. Soon after ingesting milk, which is high in lactose, they begin to vomit and lose weight. Findings include:

- lethargy
- hypotonia
- diarrhoea
- vomiting
- jaundice
- development of bilateral cataracts.

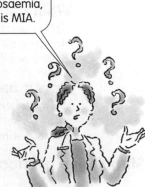

What tests tell you

Genetic screening is positive for the disorder. Galactose levels are increased in the blood and urine (galactosuria), and levels of GALT activity in erythrocytes are decreased or absent.

Complications

Complications of galactosaemia include ovarian dysfunction, cataracts, abnormal speech, cognitive impairment, motor delay and growth retardation.

How it's treated

The disorder is treated by eliminating dietary galactose (generally available as lactose), including breast milk. Lactose-free or soy protein formulas are recommended and, as the child grows, a balanced, galactose-free diet must be maintained. (See *Diet for galactosaemia*).

What to do

Nursing care focuses on education:
• Teach the child and parents about the disorder and provide emotional support and counselling; psychological and emotional problems may result from the difficult dietary restrictions.
• Teach the child and parents about the critical importance of adhering to the diet.
• Teach the parents about normal physical and mental growth and development to help them recognise developmental delay.
• Help the mother deal with feelings of loss, and even guilt, that may result from the inability to breast-feed.

Graves' disease

Graves' disease, also called hyperthyroidism in childhood, is associated with exophthalmos and an enlarged thyroid gland. Most cases occur in children between 6 and 15 years of age. The disease may be present in infants whose mothers were thyrotoxic during pregnancy.

What causes it

Graves' disease is caused by an autoimmune response to TSH receptors. However, no specific etiology has been identified. There also seems to be a familial predisposition for the disease.

How it happens

In Graves' disease, T4 production is increased and the thyroid gland is enlarged (called a goitre). It's characterised by autoantibodies that attach to and then stimulate TSH receptors on the thyroid gland.

Stimulation overload

A goitre may be the result of increased stimulation of the thyroid gland or a response to increased metabolic demand. The latter occurs in

It's all relative

Diet for galactosaemia

A child with galactosaemia must follow a lactose-free diet.

Diet do's

• Fish and animal products (except brains and mussels)
• Fresh fruits and vegetables (except peas and lima beans)
• Breads and rolls made from cracked wheat

Diet don'ts

• Dairy products
• Puddings, cookies, cakes, pies
• Food colouring
• Instant potatoes
• Canned and frozen foods (if lactose is listed as an ingredient)

iodine-deficient areas of the world, where the incidence of goitre increases during puberty (a time of increased metabolic demand). These goitres commonly regress to normal size after puberty in males but not in females.

What to look for

Symptoms of Graves' disease begin gradually and develop on and off during a period of 6 to 12 months. Irritability and excessive motion are the most prominent symptoms. The child may also exhibit:

- hyperactivity
- short attention span
- insomnia
- tremors
- weight loss despite a tremendous appetite
- rapid, pounding pulse (even during sleep)
- skin warm and flushed
- widened pulse pressure
- cardiomegaly
- exophthalmos.

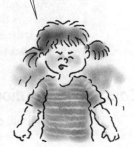

Just because I'm irritable and can't sit still, my parents think I have a behavioural problem! They don't realise these behaviours can be symptoms of Graves' disease.

What tests tell you

- A thyroid scan reveals increased ^{131}I uptake.
- Immunometric assay shows suppressed sensitivity of TSH levels.
- Orbital sonography and CT scans show subclinical ophthalmopathy.
- Radioimmunoassay testing shows elevated T4 levels.

Complications

Complications of Graves' disease include muscle wasting, atrophy and paralysis; vision loss or diplopia and heart failure or cardiac arrhythmias.

How it's treated

Graves' disease is treated with antithyroid medications, such as carbimazole or propylthiouracil to suppress the formation of T4. Hypermetabolic symptoms will subside 4 to 8 weeks after therapy begins, but remission of Grave's disease requires continued therapy for 6 months to 2 years. The child must be monitored closely for signs of leukopenia and thrombocytopenia. If these conditions occur, the medication is discontinued until the counts return to normal levels.

Ablation to the rescue

If the child is unable or unwilling to comply with the medication regimen, or if they have a toxic reaction to the medication, ablation therapy with ^{131}I is used to reduce the size of the thyroid gland.

When in doubt, take it out

Surgical removal of all or most of the thyroid may be necessary. After ablation or surgical removal of the thyroid, the child must remain on lifelong thyroid replacement therapy.

What to do

Explain the disorder to the child and parents and prepare the child for all treatments and procedures:

• Teach the parents of a child being treated with antithyroid drugs or radioisotope therapy to identify and report symptoms of hypothyroidism.

Keep it cool

• Encourage a cool, quiet environment that's conducive to rest until there's a response to drug therapy; restrict physical activity.
• Advise the child with exophthalmos or other ophthalmopathy to wear sunglasses or eye patches to protect the eyes from light; moisten the conjunctiva frequently with isotonic eyedrops.
• To meet the child's increased metabolic demand, provide a balanced diet with six meals per day.

Cough with caution

• Tell the child who has had ^{131}I therapy not to expectorate or cough freely; their saliva is radioactive for 24 hours; stress the need for repeated measurement of serum T4 levels and reassure the child and parents (who may be frightened by the term 'radioactive').
• Instruct the child taking medication (and parents) to have these drugs with meals to minimise GI distress, and to avoid over-the-counter cough preparations because many contain iodine.
• Stress the importance of regular medical follow-up visits after discharge because hypothyroidism may develop 2 to 4 weeks post-operatively and after ^{131}I therapy.

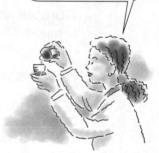

Some over-the-counter products contain iodine. Teach parents to be label-readers and, when in doubt, to ask the pharmacist.

Long-term commitment

• Explain that the child will need lifelong TH replacement. (Encourage them to wear medical identification and to carry medication with them at all times.)

Phenylketonuria

PKU is an inborn error in amino acid (specifically phenylalanine) metabolism. It results in high serum levels of phenylalanine, increased urine concentrations of phenylalanine and its by-products, cerebral damage and mental retardation.

An error by any other name

PKU is also called phenylalaninemia and phenylpyruvic oligophrenia. The disorder occurs in 1 of approximately 12,000 births in the UK. About 1 person in 50 is an asymptomatic carrier.

The case for early detection

Although blood phenylalanine levels approach normal at birth, they begin to increase within a few days. By the time they reach significant levels cerebral damage has begun. Such irreversible damage is probably complete by age 2 or 3 years. Early detection and treatment can minimise cerebral damage.

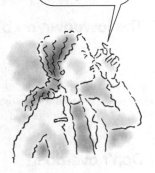

The Guthrie screening test for PKU detection is mandatory in neonates. No studying is required!

What causes it
PKU is transmitted through an autosomal-recessive gene.

How it happens
In PKU, an almost totally deficient activity of phenylalanine hydroxylase, an enzyme that acts as a catalyst in the conversion of phenylalanine to tyrosine, results in phenylalanine accumulation in the blood and urine. This accumulation leads to brain damage and mental retardation.

What to look for
The child may have a family history of PKU. Typically, the history reveals no apparent abnormalities at birth.

Brain on hold

By 4 months, the untreated child begins to show signs of arrested brain development, including cognitive delay and, later, personality disturbances (schizoid and antisocial personality patterns and uncontrollable temper). About one-third of children have a history of seizures, which usually begin between 6 and 12 months of age. Many children also show a precipitous decrease in IQ in their first year.

Got the blues?

On inspection, the child typically has a lighter complexion than unaffected siblings and may have blue eyes. They may also exhibit macrocephaly, eczematous skin lesions, or dry, rough skin.

Hyper, irritable and repetitive

The child is usually hyperactive and irritable exhibiting purposeless, repetitive motions and has an awkward gait. A musty odour from the skin and urinary excretion of phenylacetic acid may also be noted.

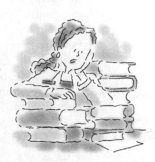

What tests tell you
Testing for PKU is part of the national neonatal screening programme. See Guthrie test discussed earlier in the chapter.

Complications
Phenylalanine accumulation causes mental retardation.

How it's treated

To prevent or minimise brain damage, phenylalanine blood levels are kept between:
- 0 to 5 years: 120 to 360 μmol/L
- 5 to 10 years: 120 to 480 μmol/L
- Above 10 years: 120 to 480 μmol/L.

With increasing age, compliance with diet can be a challenge and the young person may have higher values up to 700 μmol/L.

The lowdown on phenylalanine

During the first month of life, a special, low-phenylalanine amino acid mixture is substituted for most of the protein in the diet, supplemented with a small amount of natural foods. An enzymatic hydrolysate of casein, such as Lofenalac powder or Pregestimil powder, is substituted for milk in the diets of affected infants. Dietary restrictions are required throughout life.

Don't overdo it!

Such a diet calls for close monitoring. The body doesn't make phenylalanine, so overzealous dietary restriction can induce phenylalanine deficiency, causing lethargy, anorexia, anaemia, skin rashes and diarrhoea.

What to do

Teach the parents about PKU, and provide emotional support and counselling. Psychological and emotional problems may result from the difficult dietary restrictions. In addition, follow these steps:
- If the child is experiencing seizures or has some mental dysfunction, implement safety measures to prevent injury; refer the parents and child to appropriate community resources.

Just say 'no' to chicken and cheese

- Teach the child and parents about the critical importance of adhering to the diet; the child must avoid breads, cheese, eggs, flour, meat, poultry, fish, nuts, milk, legumes, and aspartame (NutraSweet). Also, the child will need frequent tests for urine phenylpyruvic acid and blood phenylalanine levels to evaluate the effectiveness of the diet.
- Refer the family to a paediatric dietician.
- Teach the parents about normal physical and mental growth and development to help them recognise developmental delay from excessive phenylalanine intake.

Rebel with a cause

As the child grows older and is supervised less closely, parents have less control over what they eat. As a result, deviation from the restricted diet

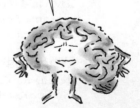

Dietary phenylalanine restriction is the best way to protect me in a child with PKU.

becomes more likely, which increases the risk of further brain damage. Encourage the parents to allow the child some choices in the kinds of low-protein foods eaten to help make them feel trusted and more responsible, which will encourage compliance.

Quick quiz

1. The purpose of the endocrine system is to:
    A. deliver nutrients to the body's cells.
    B. regulate and integrate the body's metabolic activities.
    C. eliminate waste products from the body.
    D. stimulate secondary sex characteristics.

Answer: B. Along with the nervous system, the endocrine system regulates and integrates the body's metabolic activities.

2. The midwife or nurse takes blood from the heel of an infant for a Guthrie screening test. This test is used to diagnose which inborn error of metabolism?
    A. Absence of GALT
    B. PKU
    C. Galactosaemia
    D. Hypothyroidism

Answer: B. The Guthrie screening test is a bacterial inhibition assay used to diagnose PKU. *Bacillus subtilis*, present in the culture medium, grows if the blood contains an excessive amount of phenylalanine.

3. The gland that produces glucagon is the:
    A. pancreas.
    B. thymus.
    C. adrenal.
    D. pituitary.

Answer: A. The alpha cells of the pancreas produce glucagon, a hormone that raises the blood glucose level by triggering the breakdown of glycogen to glucose.

4. An infant with congenital hypothyroidism shows which sign or symptom?
    A. Shrill cry
    B. Diaphoresis
    C. Hypothermia
    D. Diarrhoea

Answer: C. Hypothermia is one common finding in congenital hypothyroidism. Other common findings include lethargy, poor feeding, prolonged jaundice, vomiting, constipation, mottling, coarse facial features, hoarse cry, large fontanelles and hypotonia.

5. Which food shouldn't be eaten by a child with galactosaemia?
   A. Instant potatoes
   B. Chicken
   C. Whole wheat bread
   D. Apples

Answer: A. The child with galactosaemia must follow a lactose-free diet. Appropriate foods for his diet include fish and chicken, fresh fruits and vegetables and bread made from whole wheat. The child should avoid dairy products and other lactose-containing foods such as instant potatoes.

Scoring

☆☆☆ If you answered all five items correctly, astonishing! Your brain cells must be on steroids!

☆☆ If you answered three or four items correctly, wow! You've just won a trip to the islets of Langerhans! Bon voyage!

☆ If you answered fewer than three items correctly, don't moan over these hormones! Two more quick quizzes are ahead.

14 Haematological and immunological problems

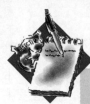

Just the facts

In this chapter, you'll learn:

♦ anatomy and physiology of the haematological and immune systems

♦ normal function of blood cells and the role of genetics in the haematological and immune systems

♦ tests used to diagnose haematological and immunological problems

♦ treatments and procedures for children with haematological and immunological problems

♦ haematological and immunological disorders that affect children.

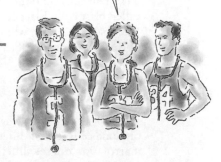

The haematological and immune systems work as a team to reach the same goal!

Anatomy and physiology

The haematological and immune systems are separate but interrelated. They help the body fight infection or invaders through different mechanisms, but usually work together for the same goal. Both systems essentially arise from an organ known as bone marrow which, although housed within the bones, has little relationship with the skeletal system.

Haematological system

Bone marrow contains the essential element in the haematological system: the stem cell. The stem cell is sometimes referred to as the pluripotential stem cell, meaning it has the ability to transform into more than one type of blood cell. Every blood cell in the body arises from a stem cell.

Did you say tissue?

Although it's a fluid, blood is one of the body's major tissues. It continually circulates through the heart and blood vessels, carrying vital elements to every part of the body.

Blood formation

Early in utero, the process of blood formation, called haematopoiesis, occurs in the liver and spleen. These organs retain some haematopoietic ability throughout life. After birth, the red bone marrow becomes the main site of haematopoiesis.

Yellow with age

In infants and young children, all bones contain red bone marrow (red from the production of red blood cells [RBCs]) and are, therefore, capable of haematopoiesis. However, as the child approaches adolescence and bone growth ceases, the bone marrow in many bones can't form blood cells because the marrow has transformed to yellow bone marrow (yellow from fat deposits), although it can usually revert to red bone marrow during times of increased blood cell demand. Only the ribs, sternum, vertebrae and pelvis continue to contain red bone marrow and produce blood cells.

Have a blast

The stem cells contained in the red bone marrow create primitive blood cells called blast cells. Blast cells are the least mature form of blood cell and are the precursors to RBCs, white blood cells (WBCs) and platelets. These cells are normal and shouldn't be confused with the blast cells seen in leukaemia and other cancers.

Like a fine wine ...

These blast cells then stay in the bone marrow to mature. The maturation of blood cells, called differentiation, occurs in stages; thus, in normal bone marrow you can see different forms of all the blood cell lines. (See *Human blood cell development*.) Mature blood cells travel by blood throughout the body to perform specific functions.

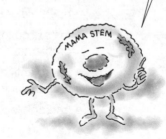

A mother's work is never done! It's from me that new cells are created for all three main blood cell types.

MAMA STEM

Human blood cell development

All blood cell types originate from the same stem cell. The chart below shows how this stem cell becomes differentiated, developing into each blood cell type.

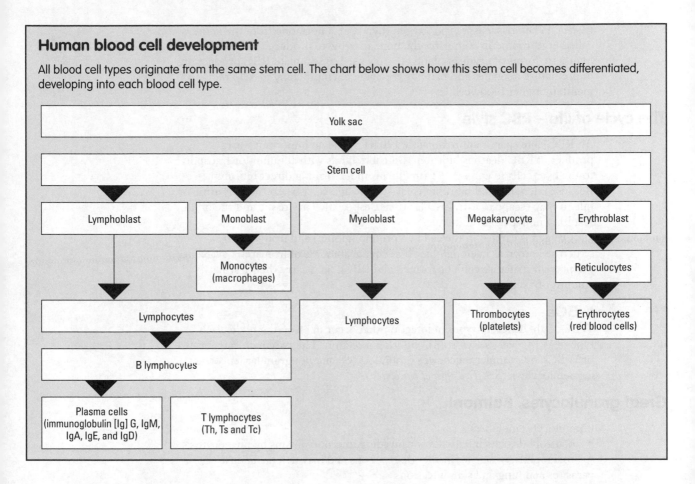

Blood components

Blood is composed of plasma and cells. Plasma is the fluid portion of the blood. It's 90% water and 10% solutes, such as proteins, electrolytes, albumin, clotting factors, anticoagulants, antibodies and dissolved nutrients. The three main cell types in the blood originate from blast cells and include:

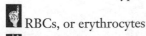 RBCs, or erythrocytes

WBCs, or leucocytes

platelets, or thrombocytes.

RBCs

In addition to the bone marrow, some RBCs are stored in the liver or spleen. RBCs carry oxygen to the tissues and carry carbon dioxide away from tissues. When tissue is low on oxygen (hypoxia), a hormone from the kidneys called erythropoietin stimulates the bone marrow to produce more RBCs. Synthetic forms of erythropoietin are now used to stimulate RBC production in premature neonates and patients receiving chemotherapy to help them maintain higher blood cell levels.

The cycle of life – RBC style

An RBC's life span is approximately 120 days, and an important waste product of RBC death is bilirubin. Bilirubin binds with albumin for transport to the liver cells to conjugate with glucuronide, forming direct bilirubin. Because unconjugated bilirubin is fat-soluble and can't be excreted in urine or bile, it may escape to extravascular tissue, especially fatty tissue and the brain, resulting in hyperbilirubinemia.

Oxygen is carried in the cell in a protein (globin) and iron (haem) structure known as haemoglobin. If adequate amounts of iron aren't available, the protein structure can't be formed and RBCs can't carry their normal amount of oxygen.

WBCs

WBCs fight different types of infection that occur in or on the body; each type of WBC has its own role in fighting infection. The two main categories of WBCs are granular leucocytes (granulocytes) and nongranular leucocytes (agranulocytes). (See *Two types of leucocytes*.)

Great granulocytes, Batman!

Granulocytes include:
• neutrophils, which help devour invading microorganisms by phagocytosis
• eosinophils, which act in allergic reactions and may defend against parasites and lung and skin infections
• basophils, which release heparin and histamine, are involved in inflammatory and infectious reactions, and are known as mast cells when they exist in body tissues.

Not a granule to be found

Agranulocytes include:
• lymphocytes, which are the main cells that fight infections and include B cells and T cells
• monocytes, which, along with neutrophils, help devour invading microorganisms by phagocytosis, and also form macrophages in the body tissues.

Platelets

Platelets adhere to one another and plug holes in vessels or tissues where there's bleeding. This action is part of a larger coagulation (clotting) process. Platelets also release serotonin at injury sites. Serotonin, a vasoconstrictor, decreases blood flow to the injured area.

Two types of leucocytes

Leucocytes vary in size, shape and number. The two types of leukocytes are granular and nongranular.

Granular

Granular leucocytes (granulocytes) are the most numerous. They include:

- *basophils*, which contain cytoplasmic granules that stain readily with alkaline dyes
- *neutrophils*, which are finely granular and recognisable by their multinucleated appearance
- *eosinophils*, which stain with acidic dyes.

Nongranular

Nongranular leucocytes have few, if any, granulated particles in the cytoplasm. They include:

- lymphocytes
- monocytes.

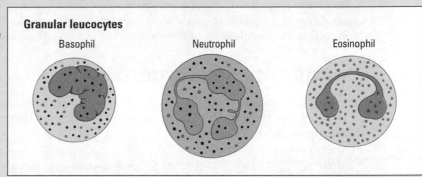

Granular leucocytes

Basophil Neutrophil Eosinophil

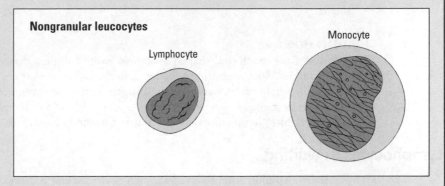

Nongranular leucocytes

Lymphocyte Monocyte

Haemostasis

Haemostasis is a complex process by which the body controls bleeding. When a blood vessel ruptures, local vasoconstriction and platelet clumping (aggregation) at the injury site initially help prevent haemorrhaging.

Like a waterfall

Activation of the coagulation system, called the extrinsic cascade, involves the release of thromboplastin from the damaged tissue cells. However, formation of a more stable clot requires initiation of the complex clotting mechanism known as the intrinsic cascade system.

When endothelial vessel injury or a foreign body in the bloodstream activates the intrinsic cascade, activating factor XII triggers clotting. Finally, prothrombin is converted to thrombin and fibrinogen to fibrin, which is necessary for creation of a fibrin clot.

Immune system

The body protects itself from foreign invaders, such as bacteria, viruses, parasites and fungi, through the organs and cells of the immune system. The components of the immune system work together to recognise 'self' from 'non-self' and to rid the body of those substances recognised as 'non-self'.

Immune system organs

Immune system organs and tissues are described as lymphoid because they're all involved with the growth, development and dissemination of lymphocytes. These organs and tissues include:
- lymph nodes
- thymus
- spleen
- tonsils.

Lymph nodes
Lymph nodes are small, oval-shaped structures located along a network of lymph channels. Most abundant in the head, neck, axillae, abdomen, pelvis, and groin, they help remove and destroy antigens (substances capable of triggering an immune response) that circulate in the blood and lymph. Lymph nodes filter lymphatic fluid and return it to the bloodstream.

Lymphocytes in waiting

These nodes also filter foreign invaders, such as viruses and bacteria, and can serve as waiting stations for lymphocytes that might be needed in that area to fight infection.

Nodes of concern

In children, the lymphatic system grows rapidly between ages 3 and 6 years. At this age, swollen lymph nodes in the neck and groin areas are common. Lymph nodes that should cause concern are:
- enlarged (greater than 2 cm in diameter), firm, painless and fixed to the skin (malignancy)
- painful, soft and producing heat (local inflammation or infection).

Thymus
The thymus is located in the mediastinal area of the chest and may look quite large on the chest X-ray of a neonate. After birth, the thymus slowly shrinks and may not be visible on chest X-rays by 6 months.

The thymus uses hormones to enable maturation of lymphocytes, produced by the bone marrow, into T lymphocytes (T cells). The mature T cells can then function normally.

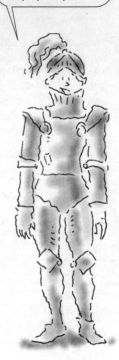

Never fear – the immune system is here! It protects the body from invaders with its army of lymphocytes.

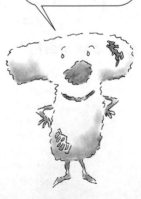

Once I mature in the thymus, I'm ready and willing to function normally.

Spleen

The spleen functions as a reservoir for blood and blood cells. It also acts like a screen to filter out unwanted invaders and help break up old RBCs that lose their elasticity with age and can't squeeze through the fine mesh of the spleen. The spleen is particularly good at filtering out one specific bacteria called *Streptococcus pneumoniae*. Children without a spleen or with a non-functioning spleen (such as those with sickle cell anaemia) should be put on prophylactic penicillin and will need immediate antibiotics if they have a fever.

Tonsils

The tonsils consist of lymphoid tissue that serves as a storage site for lymphocytes and can also produce some. In children, the tonsils may normally be slightly enlarged between 3 and 6 years old (while the immune system is at its peak of development).

Sounds of silence?

Parents of a 3- to 6-year-old child will commonly report that they snore. Snoring at this age is usually due to the enlarged tonsils partially obstructing the airway during sleep.

Immune system cells

All immune system cells are produced in bone marrow. The main cells of the immune system are B cells (B lymphocytes), phagocytes and T cells (T lymphocytes).

B cells

B cells, which are involved in humoral immunity, produce antibodies. Each B cell is programmed to make a specific antibody. In humoral immunity, a B cell will divide and differentiate into plasma cells when it encounters its triggering antigen. The plasma cells will secrete antibodies to the antigen.

To find and bind

These antibodies then travel in the blood and lymph, which circulate throughout the body. When the antibodies find the antigen, they bind to it to tag it so other immune system cells can destroy it.

Gobs of globulins

Some antibodies are proteins that perform special functions and are called immunoglobulins. There are five types of immunoglobulins (Igs) produced by B cells:

IgA defends external body surfaces and is present in colostrum, saliva, tears and nasal fluids as well as respiratory, GI and genitourinary secretions

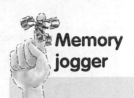

Memory jogger

If humoral immunity is all Greek to you, you're right! To remember what humoral immunity is, think Greek. B-cell antibodies travel in the blood and lymph, which the ancient Greeks called the *humors* of the body.

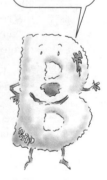

I'm the great antigen hunter. I release the hounds (antibodies) on invading forces!

(neonates have small amounts of this immunoglobulin and are more susceptible to an overgrowth of organisms in mucous membranes).

IgD is found on the surface of B cells and functions in controlling lymphocyte activation or suppression.

IgE is the antibody responsible for hypersensitivity reactions; it has an immediate response to an antigen and stimulates the release of heparin and histamine from mast cells.

IgG makes up the majority of plasma antibodies and is the main antibacterial and antiviral antibody; transfusions of IgG specific for viral diseases, such as varicella (chickenpox), are useful in treating children who are exposed but have decreased immune function (such as those on chemotherapy).

IgM is the first immunoglobulin produced during an immune response; because it's very large, IgM is usually seen only in the blood and can't pass into tissues to fight infections.

Phagocytes

Phagocytes are immune cells that engulf, kill and digest particulate matter and foreign invaders. Phagocytes include neutrophils, monocytes and macrophages. Macrophages are a type of monocyte; they're versatile scavenger cells found in tissues throughout the body. In addition to their phagocytic action, macrophages:

activate T cells

secrete various blood products, including clotting factors, enzymes and regulatory molecules.

T cells

T cells are responsible for cell-mediated immunity. Lymphocytes derived from bone marrow migrate to the thymus, where they mature into T cells. In cell-mediated immunity, T cells directly attack antigens, including bacteria, viruses and other pathogens. They have the ability to identify an antigen (target cell) and produce lymphokines that attack the target directly. Cell-mediated immunity is also responsible for tissue and transplant incompatibility rejections and delayed hypersensitivity reactions (such as a positive tuberculin test response).

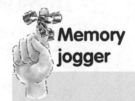

Memory jogger

To remember where B cells and T cells mature, mind your Bs and Ts:
B cells = Bone marrow
T cells = Thymus

There's definitely a T in team

Different types of T cells work together to create the best immune response possible. Helper T cells (CD4+ cells) stimulate B cells to mature into plasma cells that produce immunoglobulins to fight antigens and to also remember them if they occur again in the future.

Search and destroy

The helper T cells also help the killer T cells (CD8+ cells) to more readily recognise the antigen and attack directly. Killer T cells bind to the surface of the invading antigen and disrupt the cell membrane, causing the antigen's destruction.

> Immunoglobulins are like me – they never forget! Once they fight an antigen, they remember it as the enemy if it ever has the nerve to show up again.

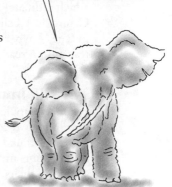

Complement system

The complement system is composed of several proteins that are important in the inflammatory process. It's activated by the antigen–antibody complexes (classic pathway) or toxins released by antigens (alternate pathway). The complement system is one of the body's primary defences; it immediately assists in mast cell degradation, which enhances vascular permeability and assists in attracting neutrophils to the site.

Hypersensitivity

Hypersensitivity reactions are one of the body's immune responses to an antigen and may be immediate (occurring within minutes) or delayed (may take several hours). There are four types of hypersensitivity reactions, each serving a specific function.

Type I: Atopy or anaphylaxis

In some people, certain antigens (allergens) induce B-cell production of IgE, which binds to receptors on mast cell surfaces. The mast cells degranulate and release various mediators, including heparin, histamine and prostaglandins. These mediators cause vasodilation, bronchospasm, oedema and mucus secretion, leading to such symptoms as wheezing, hives and rhinorrhoea.

Second time around

IgE is produced in sufficient quantities only with repeated exposure and, therefore, may have little effect with occasional allergic reactions. Because severe reactions may not occur with the first exposure to a drug or allergen, the body may only produce antibodies, which will react with the second exposure. In severe reactions, anaphylaxis may occur, resulting in respiratory and cardiac arrest.

Type II: Cytotoxic response

IgG and IgM are involved in tissue-specific hypersensitivity reactions (type II). The type II hypersensitivity response generally involves the destruction of a target cell by an antibody directed against cell-surface antigens.

Deadly complement

Binding of an antigen and an antibody activates the complement system, which ultimately disrupts the cellular membranes, causing cell death. Cytotoxic T cells and natural killer cells also contribute to tissue death in type II hypersensitivity. Examples of type II hypersensitivity include transfusion reactions and haemolytic disease in the neonate.

Type III: Immune complex

Immune complex-mediated (type III) reactions are similar to type II in that the complex recognises the same type of antigen. However, in type II the antigen is found on the cell or organ surface, while in type III the antigen is free-floating and is attacked regardless of where it's located. If the antigens are left in the circulatory system, they may cause inflammatory reactions that can result in vessel wall damage and changes in permeability.

Attack first, ask questions later

Autoimmune disorders are caused by type III reactions in which the immune complexes have difficulty distinguishing between normal and abnormal tissue and may attack both. These disorders include systemic lupus erythematosus (SLE), juvenile rheumatoid arthritis and glomerulonephritis.

Type IV: Cell-mediated hypersensitivity

In type IV hypersensitivity, antigen is processed by macrophages and presented to T cells.

Release the lymphokines!

T cells function by releasing lymphokines, which recruit and activate other lymphocytes, monocytes, macrophages and polymorphonuclear leucocytes. The coagulation (kinin) and complement pathways also contribute to tissue damage in this type of reaction. The most serious reactions occur with transplantation when the transplanted tissue is perceived as foreign and attacked. Type IV reactions also occur with exposure to plants or substances that trigger a response resulting in contact dermatitis.

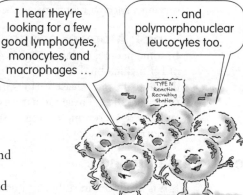

Diagnostic tests

Tests used to diagnose haematological and immunological problems in children include allergy skin testing, bone marrow aspiration and biopsy and full blood count (FBC) with differential.

Allergy skin testing

Children commonly have short-term allergic problems that may disappear as the child grows older. A child older than 2 years with a history of chronic allergic symptoms, such as coughing, runny nose, watery eyes and upper respiratory congestion, may need to be evaluated for allergies. Symptom management with medication (such as antihistamines) is recommended until the child reaches 4 years or older. If symptoms persist beyond this age, testing may be warranted.

RAST to the rescue

Allergy skin testing examines specific allergic antigens. The radioallergosorbent test (RAST) identifies antigens in the blood that are causing an immunological reaction mediated by IgE. The quantity of circulating IgE correlates well with the clinical severity of the allergic symptoms.

The family tree of allergy

When testing is started, a paediatric dermatologist obtains a detailed history from the family and child in an attempt to identify the specific antigen. Allergy skin testing entails injecting small amounts of common allergic antigens under the skin (intradermal) to assess for localised reaction. RAST is recommended when there's a strong suspicion that a specific substance is responsible for the allergy problem.

Nursing considerations
Allergy skin testing runs the risk of causing an anaphylactic reaction, and the nurse should be prepared to provide life support. The child should be closely monitored for at least fifteen minutes after the injections for any signs of an anaphylactic reaction.

A song and a wiggle

The child should be prepared for injections (for testing and treatment) and given a 'job' to do such as keeping very still. Distraction techniques (such as telling the child to wiggle their toes or sing a song) may help reduce the child's anxiety and enhance cooperation.

Bone marrow aspiration and biopsy

Bone marrow aspiration and bone marrow biopsy are slightly different tests that are usually done for the same reason. Both tests are done to view the integrity of function of the bone marrow as an organ.

Bone bank withdrawal

In bone marrow aspiration, a specially designed needle with a stylet is inserted into the centre of the bone to withdraw bone marrow. The front and back crests of the iliac bone are most commonly sampled in children. In a bone marrow biopsy, a section of bone is taken, revealing all levels of bone and bone marrow.

To aspirate or biopsy – that is the question

Ideally, the marrow should show a wide variety of cell types in various stages of maturation. Primary, malignant, blast leukaemic cells with few normal cells are seen in leukaemia. When a solid tumour, such as neuroblastoma or rhabdomyosarcoma, has metastasised to the bone marrow, a biopsy may be more helpful in showing the clumps of tumour cells among some normal cells. Both tests show whether the bone marrow is functioning normally.

Nursing considerations

Bone marrow aspiration or biopsy can be performed under light general anaesthesia or with a local injection to numb the area. An oral or IV sedative may be given before the procedure. Prepare the child for the test with an age-appropriate explanation, and monitor for sedation or adverse effects of anaesthesia. Tell the child that a parent may stay during the test.

In addition, follow these steps:
- Apply a pressure dressing after the procedure, which should be sufficient to stop blood loss.
- Be aware of the proper handling and labelling of the specimens to prevent the need to repeat the aspiration; multiple tests may be performed on the specimens obtained.
- Provide a mild analgesic as ordered; post-procedural pain is short-term after aspiration and consists of a dull ache for a few days after the biopsy.

FBC with differential

One of the most important tests for general screening for haematological and immune problems is the full blood count. An additional test that may be ordered is the differential, which is used to determine the percentage of WBCs that are present.

Decrease = disorder

In general, the FBC reveals the numbers of the three main blood cells (WBCs, RBCs and platelets). Decreased values in any cell line may be an

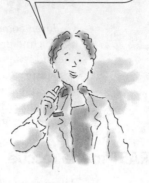

Bone marrow *aspiration* is used to withdraw a small amount of bone marrow. In bone marrow *biopsy*, a small section of bone is removed.

indication of a disorder related to the bone marrow or the immune system, or may be the result of infection.

What's up with the whites?

WBC counts vary with age.
- A healthy neonate typically has higher counts of 15,000 to 20,000/mm³.
- The typical adult WBC count of 5,000 to 10,000/mm³ is generally present in children older than 2 years.
- Counts over 15,000/mm³ in children older than 6 months should be considered high and abnormal (although this doesn't necessarily indicate serious illness).

Seeing red

While the RBC count is included in the FBC, the haemoglobin level and haematocrit are usually used as a gauge of the number of RBCs present:
- Haemoglobin is a molecule responsible for carrying oxygen to the tissue, and is somewhat affected by age. Higher levels of 15 to 20 g/dl are present in the neonate but, within 2 months, the normal range will be 12 to 15 g/dl.
- Haematocrit is approximately three times the level of haemoglobin, and normal ranges are 35% to 45%. This level is affected by hydration level and may be elevated with dehydration and decreased if the child has fluid overload.

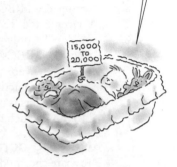

Don't be alarmed! A WBC count of 15000 to 20000/mm³ is normal in a healthy neonate like me.

Paediatric and parental platelets

Platelet counts should be between 150,000 and 500,000/mm³, regardless of age.

Nursing considerations

Prepare the child for venepuncture using a topical anaesthetic such as Ametop or EMLA and allow the parent to be present to comfort the child. After the venepuncture, monitor the site for signs of continued bleeding.

Treatments and procedures

Treatments and procedures used for children with haematological and immunological problems include blood transfusion and bone marrow transplantation.

Blood transfusion

Blood transfusion is necessary if levels of blood cells become too low or if the child is experiencing symptoms caused by a decrease in the number of available cells.

Pump up the vascular volume

Generally, transfusions are aimed at increasing volume within the vascular system, increasing RBCs to improve oxygenation, or increasing the number of platelets to reduce or correct bleeding problems:

• Whole blood is transfused if trauma with bleeding occurs and the risk of shock is present because of decreased intravascular volume. Blood loss from surgery may also require whole blood to replace cells and plasma.

• In children who have decreased levels of RBCs only, transfusion with packed RBCs is indicated. Because plasma is removed from these concentrated RBCs, transfusion increases intravascular volume only minimally (only small amounts of WBCs and platelets are contained in the transfused RBCs).

• Platelets are transfused when counts are below 60,000/mm^3 with symptoms of active bleeding. If the count is below 20,000/mm^3, transfusion with platelets is recommended due to the risk of spontaneous intracranial bleeding, which can lead to death.

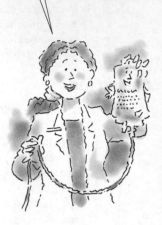

Blood product screening has come a long way, baby! Reassure the child and parents that the blood used for transfusion is safe.

Nursing considerations

Prepare the child and his parents for the procedure. Reassure the parents (and the child, if old enough) about the measures that are taken to ensure the safety of transfused blood products.

In addition, follow these steps:

• Following local policy double-check the child's name, identification number, name bracelet, ABO group and Rh status with another nurse to help prevent haemolytic transfusion reactions. If there's a discrepancy, don't administer the blood product and notify the blood bank immediately.

• Start the blood transfusion within 30 minutes after it arrives from the blood bank. If you can't start the transfusion in this timeframe, return the blood product to the blood bank.

• Take baseline vital signs just before the start of the transfusion, and every 15 minutes during the transfusion.

• Monitor for suspected reactions to the transfusion, including fever, chills, rash, respiratory distress or a change in the child's behaviour. If any occur, stop the transfusion immediately, take the child's vital signs and notify medical staff.

Bone marrow transplantation

Bone marrow transplantation is used to treat such diseases as acute leukaemia, aplastic anaemia and severe combined immunodeficiency disease. The haematopoietic stem cells may be malignant themselves or may have been destroyed by aggressive therapy for malignant disease.

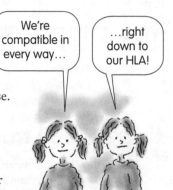

We're compatible in every way…

…right down to our HLA!

Share and share alike

With transplantation, marrow or stem cells are transplanted from a twin or another human leukocyte antigen (HLA)-identical donor (usually a sibling) in the hope that the new stem cells will produce normal, healthy cells. Autologous bone marrow transplantation is another option for some patients. In this procedure, the patient's own marrow or stem cells are harvested from healthy tissues or harvested and then treated to remove malignant cells. The cells are then returned to the patient.

A harvest of plenty

During bone marrow harvest, marrow is extracted from a matched donor with multiple bone marrow aspirations; 200 to 500 ml of marrow are collected, processed and purified.

Getting ready to receive

The recipient is given high-dose chemotherapy to destroy the malignant marrow and WBCs that might cause a reaction. Prior to the transplantation, the recipient may be given total-body radiation to further destroy components of the malignant bone marrow, and to destroy WBCs throughout the body that may identify the transfused cells as foreign and destroy them.

From harvest to seed

The collected donor marrow, which looks like a blood product, is then transfused through an IV line. If the transfusion is successful, the transplanted stem cells will reseed the bone marrow and start producing normal blood cells.

Graft battles host

A great risk after bone marrow transplantation is that the new bone marrow may produce B cells that interpret the normal body tissue as being foreign and attack it. This is commonly seen in the skin, eyes, liver and other organs, and is known as graft-versus-host disease (GVHD). The donated cells must be HLA-matched to prevent GVHD. Typically, this complication will start after the stem cells have engrafted (about 2 weeks after the transplant).

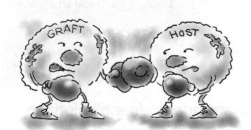

While some GVHD may be beneficial and act against recurrence of the malignancy, if the stem cells continue to produce cells that attack tissue, the effect can be dramatic, with sloughing of skin, organ malfunction or failure and eventual death.

Nursing considerations

The donor and the recipient should be prepared for the procedure with age-appropriate explanations. In addition, follow these steps:
• Administer immunosuppressants, such as steroids and cyclosporine, as prescribed to control GVHD.

- Monitor the child for signs of GVHD, such as changes in skin colour or appearance, haematuria, diarrhoea, jaundice and a change in mental status (even after they leave the hospital).
- Because the child is at high risk for infection immediately after the transplantation, monitor closely for signs of infection. Usually the child will be nursed in a single room with positive pressure until their blood counts recover
- Prevent skin breakdown by using pressure-relieving or pressure-reducing beds or mattresses; turn the child frequently.
- Support the child and his family throughout this stressful time because the child will be critically ill with the potential for life-threatening complications.

Haematological and immunological disorders

Haematological and immunological disorders that may affect children include acquired immunodeficiency syndrome (AIDS), aplastic anaemia, haemophilia, Hodgkin's disease, iron deficiency anaemia, leukaemia, sickle cell anaemia, SLE and thalassaemia. Other immunological disorders include allergic rhinitis discussed here and atopic dermatitis, which is in the next chapter.

AIDS

The identification of the human immunodeficiency virus (HIV) in the 1980s foreshadowed a worldwide epidemic that crosses all ethnic, cultural and age barriers. While the initial cases were primarily among homosexual men, the virus then expanded into all groups, including infants and children. In the 1990s, women and children were the fastest growing population with HIV.

What causes it

HIV, a retrovirus, has the ability to enter a cell and incorporate itself into the cell's ribonucleic acid, essentially changing the genetic structure and causing the cell to slowly die.

A stranger in friend's clothing

Because HIV becomes part of the cell, the body's normal defence mechanisms (from the immune system) don't recognise it as foreign, and the virus goes unchallenged.

Out of control

From the first single cell, the virus replicates and then enters other cells, eventually infecting several cells and rendering them non-functional. When a large number of cells become infected, the normal ability to control common organisms is compromised, and the person develops AIDS.

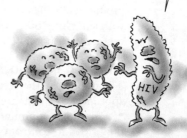

After I enter a single cell, I replicate – and the rest fall like dominoes!

How it happens

Transmission of HIV occurs by contact with infected blood or body fluids, and is associated with identifiable, high-risk behaviours, including sexual intercourse with multiple partners, IV drug use and pregnancies in HIV-infected women.

It's different for kids

The mode of transmission in children has always been different from that in adults. Although transmission in adolescents may occur from sexual contact or IV drug use, these issues aren't common factors in transmission to the younger child. Common sources of infection in children include:
• being born to an infected mother
• breast-feeding from an untreated, infected mother
• blood transfusions with HIV-tainted blood products (haemophiliacs with contaminated factor VIII or other factor products that were pooled from multiple donors before blood donations were routinely screened).

Destructive domino effect

The HIV virus has a particular affinity for the CD4+ helper T cell as well as monocytes and macrophages. The virus invades these cells and renders them non-functional, resulting in suppressed cell-mediated and humoral immunity. The degree of immunosuppression will progress and, eventually, result in opportunistic infection and even death.

What to look for

In adults, the diagnosis of AIDS was historically based on CD4+ counts and the presence of indicator diseases, which are opportunistic infections associated with HIV disease. (See *Indicator diseases and HIV*, page 502.)

In children, these diseases are less common until the infection is more severe. However, infants and children are particularly susceptible to fungal diseases. Children who are HIV positive tend to have repeated bacterial infections, such as otitis media, that don't respond to antibiotics.

The incubation period for children averages only 17 months, and the signs and symptoms of HIV resemble those in adults. Initially, the child may have flu-like symptoms, and then may remain asymptomatic for years. As the disease progresses, neurological signs from HIV encephalopathy and symptoms of an opportunistic infection may manifest. (See *HIV classification in children*, page 503.)

What tests tell you

Testing for the presence of HIV can be performed by assessing for the presence of the antibodies to the virus. Commonly testing for HIV occurs 1 month after a possible exposure. Antibody tests in neonates may be unreliable because transferred maternal antibodies persist for up to 18 months, causing a false-positive result. Therefore, in infants, testing may include viral culture, polymerase chain reaction testing or p24 antigen detection.

Indicator diseases and HIV

This chart describes some common infections associated with human immunodeficiency virus (HIV) disease in children, along with their characteristic signs and symptoms and their treatments.

Infection	Signs and symptoms	Treatment
Bacterial		
Mycobacterium avium complex A primary infection acquired by oral ingestion or inhalation; can infect the bone marrow, liver, spleen, GI tract, lymph nodes, lungs, skin, brain, adrenal glands and kidneys; is chronic and may be localised and disseminated in its course of infection	Multiple, non-specific symptoms consistent with systemic illness (fever, fatigue, weight loss, anorexia, night sweats, abdominal pain and chronic diarrhoea); *physical examination findings:* emaciation, generalised lymphadenopathy, diffuse tenderness, jaundice and hepatosplenomegaly; *laboratory findings:* anaemia, leukopenia and thrombocytopenia	Treatment regimens vary and can include two to six drugs. The Centers for Disease Control and Prevention currently recommend that every patient take either azithromycin or clarithromycin. Many experts prefer ethambutol as a second drug. Additional drugs include rifabutin, rifampin, ciprofloxacin and, sometimes, amikacin.
Fungal		
Candidiasis A disease caused by the fungus *Candida albicans* that exists on teeth, gingivae and skin and in the oropharynx, vagina and large intestine; majority of infections are endogenous and related to interruption of normal defence mechanisms; possible human-to-human transmission, including congenital transmission in neonates (who develop thrush after vaginal delivery)	*Thrush* (the most prevalent form in HIV-infected individuals): creamy, curd-like, white patches surrounded by an erythematous base, found on any oral mucosal surface; *nail infection:* inflammation and tenderness of tissue surrounding the nails or the nail itself; *vaginitis:* intense pruritus of the vulva and curd-like vaginal discharge	Nystatin suspension and clotrimazole troches are administered for thrush; nystatin suspension or pastilles, clotrimazole troches, fluconazole or itraconazole for oesophagitis; topical clotrimazole, miconazole or ketoconazole for cutaneous candidiasis; oral fluconazole or ketoconazole for candidiasis of nails and topical clotrimazole, miconazole or oral fluconazole for vaginitis.
Protozoan		
Pneumocystis carinii pneumonia Pneumonia caused by *P. carinii*; also has properties of fungal infection; exists in human lungs and is transmitted by airborne exposure; the most common life-threatening opportunistic infection in individuals with acquired immunodeficiency syndrome (AIDS)	Fever, fatigue and weight loss for several weeks to months before respiratory symptoms develop; *respiratory symptoms:* dyspnea (usually noted initially on exertion and later at rest) and cough (usually starting out dry and non-productive and later becoming productive)	Co-trimoxazole may be given orally or IV, although about 20% of patients with AIDS are hypersensitive to sulfa drugs. IV pentamidine may be given but can cause many adverse effects, including permanent diabetes mellitus. Dapsone (DDS) with trimethoprim, clindamycin, primaquine, atovaquone or corticosteroids are also used. Prophylaxis for disease-prevention and following treatment includes co-trimoxazole, atovaquone or dapsone.
Cryptosporidiosis An intestinal infection caused by the protozoan *Cryptosporidium;* transmitted by person-to-person contact, water, food contaminants and airborne exposure; small intestine is the most common site	Abdominal cramping, flatulence, weight loss, anorexia, malaise, fever, nausea, vomiting, myalgia and profuse, watery diarrhoea	No treatment currently exists that can eradicate the infecting organism. Treatment consists mainly of supportive measures to control symptoms. These measures may include fluid replacement, total parenteral nutrition (occasionally), correction of electrolyte imbalances and administration of analgesic, antidiarrhoeal and antiperistaltic agents. Paromomycin and octreotide are used.

(continued)

Indicator diseases and HIV (continued)

Infection	Signs and symptoms	Treatment
Viral		
Herpes simplex virus Chronic infection caused by a herpes virus; usually a reactivation of an earlier herpes infection	Red, blister-like lesions occurring in oral, anal and genital areas; also found on the oesophageal and tracheobronchial mucosa; pain, bleeding and discharge	Acyclovir, famciclovir or valacyclovir are given IV or orally. Low-maintenance dosages may be given to prevent recurrence of symptoms.
Cytomegalovirus (CMV) A viral infection of the herpes virus that may result in serious, widespread infection; most common sites are the lungs, adrenal glands, eyes, central nervous system, GI tract, male genitourinary tract and blood	Unexplained fever; malaise; GI ulcers; diarrhoea; weight loss; swollen lymph glands; hepatomegaly; splenomegaly; blurred vision; floaters; dyspnea (especially on exertion); dry, non-productive cough and vision changes leading to blindness in patients with ocular infection	Ganciclovir or foscarnet is used to treat CMV. Ganciclovir has shown some anti-HIV properties. Foscarnet or intraocular ganciclovir implants may be used to treat CMV retinitis.

HIV classification in children

The Centers for Disease Control and Prevention's revised classification system for human immunodeficiency virus (HIV)-infected children is based on three categories.

Category	Symptoms and criteria
Category A	A child is *mildly symptomatic* when he has two or more symptoms, such as enlarged lymph nodes, liver or spleen or recurrent or persistent upper respiratory infections, sinusitis or otitis media.
Category B	A child is *moderately symptomatic* if he has developed more serious illnesses, such as oropharyngeal candidiasis, bacterial meningitis, pneumonia, sepsis, cardiomyopathy, cytomegalovirus infection, hepatitis, herpes simplex virus, bronchitis, pneumonitis or esophagitis, herpes zoster (shingles), lymphoid interstitial pneumonia, pulmonary lymphoid hyperplasia complex or toxoplasmosis.
Category C	A child is *severely symptomatic* if he has developed serious bacterial infections, such as septicemia, pneumonia, meningitis, bone or joint infections or abscess of an internal organ or body cavity or infections, such as candidiasis (esophageal or pulmonary), encephalopathy, herpes simplex lasting longer than 1 month, histoplasmosis, lymphoma, mycobacterium (tuberculosis) or *Pneumocystis carinii* pneumonia. Unlike adults, children rarely develop Kaposi's sarcoma.

Screen with ELIZA, confirm with the blot

The recommended protocol is initial screening with an enzyme-linked immunosorbent assay (ELIZA). After checking and re-checking the results, findings are confirmed by the Western blot test or an immunofluorescence assay.

Back-up blood tests

Other blood tests support the diagnosis and are used to evaluate the severity of immunosuppression:
• The CD4+ and CD8+ cell subset counts determine the risk of HIV being converted to AIDS. As the CD4+ level lowers, the risk of AIDS conversion increases, with levels below 200 cells/l considered diagnostic of AIDS (with or without the presence of another disease or condition).
• CD8+ killer T cell counts are monitored, as is the ratio of CD4+ to CD8+, which may give an indication of decreased percentage of CD4+ cells, and AIDS conversion.
• A FBC may provide an overall view of the health of the child. (See *Cell counts and disease progression*.)

Complications

Complications of HIV infection may include opportunistic infections, failure to thrive and nutritional deficits, malignancies and HIV encephalopathy. In addition to treatment of HIV itself, the child may be on various drugs to treat or control opportunistic infections, including antibiotics for bacterial infection, steroids for control of symptoms and chemotherapy if malignancies are present. These drugs can cause an array of severe adverse reactions, including peripheral neuropathy, seizures, nausea, vomiting, neutropenia and thrombocytopenia.

How it's treated

There's no cure for HIV infection; however, several types of drugs are used to treat the disease and prolong life. Many treatment protocols combine

Cell counts and disease progression

The chart below lists CD4+ cell counts and how they relate to progression of human immunodeficiency virus in children.

Immunologic category	Up to 12 months	1 to 5 years	6 to 12 years
No evidence of suppression	>1,500 cells/μl	>1,000 cells/μl	>500 cells/μl
Evidence of moderate suppression	750 to 1,499 cells/μl	500 to 999 cells/μl	200 to 499 cells/μl
Severe suppression	<750 cells/μl	<500 cells/μl	<200 cells/μl

Centers for Disease Control. USPHS/IDSA guidelines for prevention of opportunistic infections in persons infected with HIV. *Morbidity and Mortality Weekly Report* 46(12):1, 1997.

three or more drugs to produce the maximum benefit with the fewest adverse reactions. Combination therapy also helps to inhibit the production of mutant HIV strains resistant to particular drugs.

Do-good drugs

Drugs known to be effective against HIV include:
• nucleoside reverse transcriptase inhibitors, such as zidovudine, lamivudine, stavudine and didanosine
• non-nucleotide reverse transcriptase inhibitors, such as efavirenz and delavirdine
• protease inhibitors, such as indinavir, ritonavir and lopinavir
• anti-infective drugs, such as dapsone and rifabutin
• antineoplastic drugs, such as methotrexate to combat opportunistic infections and associated cancers.

What to do

Many parents and children equate this diagnosis with a death sentence. Despite the increasing numbers of people who are living with AIDS (because of new treatments), the diagnosis is likely to be terrifying and devastating to the entire family.

A listening ear

The diagnosis is also profoundly distressing because of the disease's social impact and the discouraging prognosis. Listen to the child and his parents because they may feel alone and isolated, and may need a safe person with whom they can talk.

In addition, follow these steps:
• Use standard precautions to reduce the risk of HIV transmission.
• Monitor the child for changes in vital signs, especially low-grade fevers (above 38°C).

Infection detection

• Observe for evidence of infection or lesions, including signs of skin breakdown, cough, sore throat and diarrhoea.
• Maintain strict confidentiality as a stigma remains with this disease and the family may not want the diagnosis to be common knowledge.
• Refer the family, if they wish, to counsellors and support groups that can help them cope with the diagnosis and living with the condition.

Haemophilia

A hereditary bleeding disorder, haemophilia results from a deficiency of specific clotting factors. Haemophilia A (classic hemophilia) results from deficiency of factor VIII; haemophilia B (Christmas disease) results from deficiency of factor IX. There are two less common types of haemophilia.

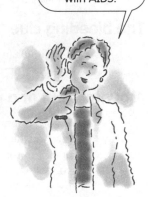

Sometimes, having someone just listen is the best medicine for a family dealing with AIDS.

Haemophilia C is a deficiency of factor XI. Von Willebrand's disease includes a factor VIII defect and poor platelet aggregation.

What causes it

The inheritance pattern is X-linked recessive in about 80% of all haemophilia cases. Haemophilia C is transmitted by an autosomal-recessive trait in both sexes. Von Willebrand's disease is transmitted as an autosomal-dominant disorder.

How it happens

Haemophilia produces mild-to-severe abnormal bleeding. After a platelet plug develops at a bleeding site, the lack of clotting factor prevents a stable fibrin clot from forming. Although haemorrhaging usually doesn't occur immediately, delayed bleeding is common.

A matter of degrees

Haemophilia may be severe, moderate or mild, depending on the degree of normal clotting (factor VIII) activity:
- In severe disease, there's less than 1% normal clotting activity.
- In moderate disease, there's 1% to 5% normal clotting activity.
- In mild disease, there's 5% to 50% normal clotting activity.
Most children with haemophilia (60% to 70%) demonstrate the severe form.

What to look for

There's usually a family history of haemophilia or bleeding problems in men.

The bleeding clue

Bleeding can occur spontaneously, and the neonate may have prolonged bleeding times with routine blood collection for neonate tests.

Mountain out of a molehill

Later, spontaneous or disproportionately severe bleeding after minor trauma may produce large subcutaneous and deep intramuscular hematomas. Signs and symptoms of decreased tissue perfusion include restlessness, anxiety, confusion, pallor, cool and clammy skin, chest pain, decreased urine output, hypotension and tachycardia.

What tests tell you

- A coagulation screen shows a normal prothrombin time (PT) with a prolonged partial thromboplastin time (PTT).
- Factor VIII coagulant activity is decreased in haemophilia A and is normal in haemophilia B.
- Factor IX is decreased in haemophilia B and normal in haemophilia A.
- Platelet aggregation and platelet count is normal in both haemophilia A and B.

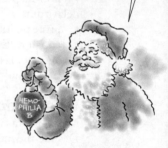

Ho, ho, haemophilia B is known as *Christmas disease*. (Don't expect any factor IX under the tree.)

Complications

Any type of haemophilia puts the child at risk for bleeding – even with normal activities – making it extremely important to take safety precautions during activities that could place the child at risk.

Head's up!

The greatest risk is with a head injury with intracranial bleeding or bleeding into joints. Joint mobility may be affected with repeated joint injury and may cause decreased range of motion. Any injury may cause bleeding into tissue that may require clotting factor transfusion and hospitalisation for monitoring.

The incredible expanding spleen

Injury of the spleen with resulting bleeding may be life-threatening as the spleen expands with blood, causing hypovolemic shock. Historically, haemophiliacs were infected in large numbers with HIV and hepatitis C before screening for these viruses in blood products was started.

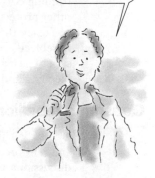

Parents of a child with haemophilia must become safety experts!

How it's treated

Haemophilia isn't curable, but treatment can prevent crippling deformities and prolong life. Increasing plasma levels of deficient clotting factors helps prevent disabling deformities caused by repeated bleeding into muscles, joints and organs.

Everyone in the pool!

Haemophilia A or B can be treated with pooled factor obtained from blood products. Historically, these products ran a risk of transmitting viral illness, but current recombinant factor VIII and IX are safe and free from viral infection. Desmopressin acetate (DDAVP) is a synthetic vasopressin analog. It has a minimal antidiuretic effect but does increase the factor VIII level up to fourfold. It has no effect on factor IX. Haemophilia C and von Willebrand's disease are treated with DDAVP, and factor VIII replenishment may also help in von Willebrand's disease.

What to do

The nurse's role involves educating the parents about safety issues while monitoring the child for acute problems. The child must become accustomed to restrictions in activities and precautions that may make them feel different from their peers. Counselling may be needed to help the child deal with these issues and to help ensure compliance. In addition, follow these steps:

• Observe for evidence of bruising, bleeding or change in mental status.
• If transfusions are ordered, monitor for blood product reactions, such as fever, chills or irritability.

Do try this at home

- Because home infusions are commonly done (minimising the need for hospitalisation), educate the parents about the process. They will be referred to a community children's nursing service for support.
- Teach the family about age-appropriate safety measures, including padding cots and other hard surfaces and, later, wearing a bicycle helmet and other protective gear during sports activities.
- Teach the parents to recognise signs of bleeding by monitoring for nosebleeds and colour of stool. Fresh blood in stool or black, tarry stool is sign of gastric bleeding; excessive swallowing during sleep may be a sign of bleeding and swallowing the blood.

Quash the rebellion

- As the child grows older, assess their participation in new activities and reinforce the need for safety measures. Including the child in these discussions and allowing them as much choice as possible will help keep the growing child's normal tendency to rebel against restrictions in check.
- Make families aware of such support groups as the UK Haemophilia Society, and inform them about any local support sources.

Iron deficiency anaemia

Iron deficiency anaemia is a disorder of oxygen transport in which the production of haemoglobin is inadequate. Without sufficient iron, the body can't produce the haemoglobin molecule because the haem component is primarily iron.

Some heavy competition

Excesses of other heavy metals (such as lead) may compete for iron-binding sites and cause a lack of haemoglobin that may mimic iron deficiency. Iron deficiency anaemia is most common in the youngest and oldest children in the paediatric age range (infants and toddlers, and adolescents).

What causes it

Iron deficiency anaemia can be caused by inadequate intake of iron in the diet, malabsorption of iron through the GI tract or chronic blood loss.

A gift from mum

In the last trimester of pregnancy, the foetus draws what iron it needs from the mother. In the last month, it draws enough iron stores for approximately 6 to 12 months. If the mother is deficient in iron or the neonate is more than 4 weeks premature, the infant may not have sufficient iron stores and,

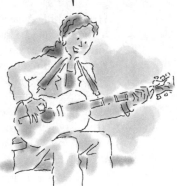

Heavy metals compete for iron-binding sites and lack of haemoglobin can mimic iron deficiency. I think I'll stick with folk music!

eventually, becomes anaemic. This condition is usually evident in the second year of life but can occur earlier if the child is more premature, especially less than 32 weeks' gestation.

How it happens

Despite the concern about adequate intake of iron in the diet, about 80% of the iron used in building haemoglobin is actually reabsorbed in the GI tract from dead RBCs that have broken up. Therefore, problems with GI absorption cause iron deficiency.

> Who knew? Most of the iron used to build haemoglobin comes from the GI tract, where it's resorbed from dead RBCs.

Got milk?

Cow's milk allergy due to heat-labile protein in cow's milk causes inflammation of the GI tract with chronic blood loss and decreased absorption. This allergy is a common source of iron deficiency anaemia. In adolescents, iron deficiency anaemia is commonly related to fad dieting and overconsumption of snack foods containing little or no iron.

You are what you eat

Girls in the adolescent period are at risk for iron deficiency anaemia during their growth spurt and at the beginning of menses, especially if periods are irregular. Boys are at a lower risk, although boys and girls may have poor dietary habits or eat faddy diet foods. Vegetarians aren't at increased risk if they plan their diets with adequate sources of iron.

What to look for

Clinical symptoms may be mild until anaemia is severe, causing a pale appearance and decreased activity. Toddlers may have a history of prematurity and poor weight gain. Other symptoms include:
- fatigue
- inability to concentrate
- palpitations
- dyspnoea on exertion
- craving for non-nutritive substances such as ice
- tachycardia
- dry, brittle nails
- concave, or 'spoon-shaped', fingernails.

What tests tell you

A FBC and haemoglobin level is needed to establish the presence of anaemia.

Bleached out bull's eye

Iron deficiency anaemia is a microcytic, hypochromic anaemia, meaning the RBCs are small and pale. RBCs with decreased iron appear bleached out, resembling a bull's eye target. Because the cells are small, the mean corpuscular volume, the mean corpuscular haemoglobin and the mean corpuscular haemoglobin concentration are low. Serum iron levels are decreased.

Complications

Untreated iron deficiency anaemia can cause stress on all body tissue, with decreased oxygenation. Severe anaemia poses the greatest risk to the respiratory and cardiovascular systems. Increasing evidence suggests that children with even mild iron deficiency have less ability to concentrate and greater difficulty in school. Overtreatment with replacement iron can occur when toxic levels of iron build up, which may cause excessive iron deposits, affecting the liver, heart, pituitary glands and joints. Pica may lead to eating lead-based paint and can result in lead poisoning, although this is very rare.

How it's treated

The main treatment is correction of the underlying problem. If chronic blood loss or GI bleeding is suspected, appropriate intervention is needed.

In with the iron

If the problem is nutritional, the child's diet should be adjusted to increase iron intake. Cultural considerations may be important here if there are any required restrictions. Good sources of dietary iron include red meat, legumes (such as kidney beans), green leafy vegetables, raisins and dried apricots as well as iron-fortified cereals and formula. Milk has little iron and may actually cause the anaemia by preventing the intake of other iron-rich foods (if the child fills up on milk).

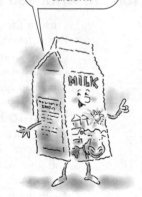

Contrary to popular belief, I'm not a good source of iron. Check back with me when you need some calcium.

It's supplementary, my dear Watson!

In addition to dietary changes, the child may be placed on oral iron supplementation, although iron supplements aren't absorbed as well as iron from dietary sources. Commonly children with haematocrit below 34% (haemoglobin level less than 11.3 g/dl) are prescribed supplemental iron.

Ascorbic acid may be added to the supplement because it helps with iron absorption, or encourage the child to take it with orange juice. Breast milk has low levels of iron, but is extremely well absorbed and is adequate for most infants. Formula should be iron-fortified.

What to do

Nursing care focuses on educating the parents about diet and treatment regimens:
• Monitor the child's compliance with the prescribed iron supplement therapy.
• Teach the parents of infants the importance of using iron-fortified infant cereals and breast milk or iron-fortified formula.
• Teach the parent or young person about good iron sources in the normal diet; if the child is a vegetarian, explain the importance of incorporating iron-rich vegetable sources into the diet.

- Caution the child and parents that taking iron supplements may result in dark green or black stool; supplements can also cause constipation.
- Make sure the parents understand the dosage and administration of oral iron supplements; stress the importance of storing the supplements safely because they're a major source of poisoning in children.

Hodgkin's disease

Hodgkin's disease is a malignancy of lymph nodes. In the paediatric age-group, it affects primarily adolescents, although children as young as 3 years have been diagnosed with the disease. This type of cancer causes painless, progressive enlargement of the lymph nodes, spleen and other lymphoid tissue.

And the good news is ...

Although the disease is fatal if untreated, recent advances have made Hodgkin's disease potentially curable, even in advanced stages. With appropriate treatment, about 90% of children live at least 5 years. Children with early stage I and II diseases have a long-term survival rate of more than 90%.

What causes it

Like most malignancies, the exact cause is unknown. It's found worldwide and can occur at any age but is most common after the second decade of life. Many with Hodgkin's disease have had infectious mononucleosis, so an indirect relationship may exist between this form of cancer and the Epstein–Barr virus.

How it happens

Lymph nodes, most typically in the chest and neck area, take a malignant turn and don't grow into normal lymphatic tissue. The malignant nodes become hard and enlarged, leading to firm-to-hard masses in the neck and chest.

Bigger isn't better

Enlargement of the lymph nodes, spleen and other lymphoid tissues results from proliferation of lymphocytes, histiocytes and, rarely, eosinophils. Patients also have distinct chromosome abnormalities in their lymph node cells.

What to look for

Hard, swollen lymph nodes of the supraclavicular or axillary areas that aren't erythematous or tender are classic characteristics of Hodgkin's disease.

Spreading swelling

The painless swelling of the lymph nodes then progresses to the axillary, inguinal, mediastinal and mesenteric regions. (See *Staging Hodgkin's disease*, page 512.)

Staging Hodgkin's disease

Treatment of Hodgkin's disease depends on its stage (the number, location and degree of involved lymph nodes). The Ann Arbor classification system, adopted in 1971, divides Hodgkin's disease into four stages. Each stage is subdivided into categories. Category A includes those without defined signs and symptoms, and category B includes those who experience such defined signs as recent, unexplained weight loss, fever and night sweats.

Stage I

Hodgkin's disease appears in a single lymph node region or a single extralymphatic organ.

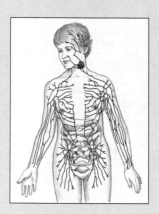

Stage II

Hodgkin's disease appears in two or more nodes on the same side of the diaphragm and in an extralymphatic organ.

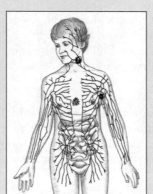

Stage III

Hodgkin's disease spreads to both sides of the diaphragm and, perhaps, to an extralymphatic organ, the spleen, or both.

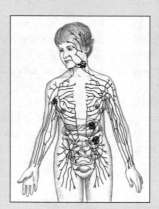

Stage IV

Hodgkin's disease disseminates, involving one or more extralymphatic organ or tissues, with or without associated lymph node involvement.

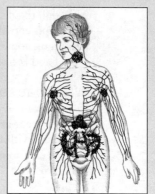

In addition to the symptoms of the primary disease, secondary symptoms associated with Hodgkin's disease (any of which warrants bone marrow biopsy to assess for more extensive disease) may include:
• unexplained fever above 38°C
• night sweats without fever
• unexplained weight loss of more than 10% of total body weight in the previous 6 months
• severe pruritus causing skin excoriation.

What tests tell you

FBC is usually normal unless the child has anaemia from malnutrition or bone marrow involvement. The erythrocyte sedimentation rate (ESR) may be elevated but this test is non-specific and ESR may be elevated with any infection. Bone marrow biopsy may rule out or confirm metastatic disease.

Verify, then confirm

A chest X-ray that verifies the presence of a mediastinal mass remains the easiest way to confirm the diagnosis, but further evaluation with enhanced computed tomography (CT) scanning or magnetic resonance imaging (MRI) will confirm the presence of other enlarged nodes throughout the body. Bone, liver and spleen scans may help determine whether metastatic disease is present.

It's a hoot!

A lymphangiogram has historically been used to identify enlarged nodes but is less valuable now that improved radiological studies are available. The diagnosis must be confirmed by lymph node biopsy showing the presence of Reed–Sternberg cell (a double nucleus cell that looks like an owl) or malignant lymphatic tissue consistent with a histological type of Hodgkin's disease.

> Chest X-ray makes diagnosis of a mediastinal mass a snap. CT scanning and MRI can confirm enlarged nodes in other areas.

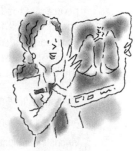

Complications

Hodgkin's disease will cause enlarging nodes that may restrict lung movement and create respiratory distress. The nodes may also press against the heart, causing cardiac arrhythmias if the mass is large and untreated. Metastatic disease may cause anaemia and decreased blood counts if bone marrow disease is extensive. It may invade and compromise bone, the liver or the spleen.

When treatment gets complicated

Today, most complications are related more to therapy, with short- and long-term consequences:
• Short-term radiation may cause severe, localised skin reactions, although usually less severe than those seen in adult malignancies as doses are lower in children.
• Immunosuppression with decreased ability to fight all types of infection is common with decreased blood counts from chemotherapy.
• Anaemia is common, although transfusion may not be required.
• Lowered platelet counts are seen but usually aren't severe and rarely cause major bleeding problems. If the platelet count is below 60,000/mm^3 or haemoglobin is below 8 g/dl, transfusion with the relevant blood product may be considered.

Long-term legacy

One of the most severe, long-term problems of Hodgkin's disease is secondary malignancies, which develop in up to 5% of long-term survivors; acute myeloid leukaemia is the most common. Sterility is another severe long-term complication and is caused by alkylating chemotherapeutic agents (e.g. cyclophosphamide) It is usual to provide sperm banking where a boy is an appropriate age. Some centres also offer egg banking for girls. Radiation may cause decreased bone and tissue growth, which can be a major cause of scoliosis and kyphosis in childhood survivors.

How it's treated

Hodgkin's disease was one of the first malignancies to demonstrate the superiority of treatment with multiple chemotherapeutic agents (versus a single agent).

Mopping the floor with Hodgkin's

The mechlorethamine, Oncovin (vincristine), procarbazine and prednisone (MOPP) research protocol of the mid 1960s immediately changed the prognosis for Hodgkin's disease to a survival rate of more than 50% in adults and children. The drugs from the MOPP protocol remain staples of therapy, although the less toxic cyclophosphamide may be used in place of mechlorethamine. Drug treatment is based on the stage of the disease and individual needs but common regimes include:

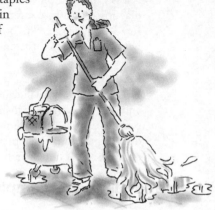

Combination therapy with the MOPP protocol is the mainstay of chemotherapy for Hodgkin's disease.

Chlorambucil, Vinblastine, Procarbazine, Prednisolone	ChIVPP
Adriamycin, Bleomycin, Vinblastine, Dacarbazine	ABVD
Vincristine, Etoposide, Epirubicin, Prednisolone	VEEP

What to do

Care of children with malignancies is coordinated through one of several paediatric oncology centres. Nursing care is based on the treatment protocol and understanding the adverse effects of the drugs and therapies used:
• Watch for and promptly report adverse effects of radiation and chemotherapy (particularly anorexia, nausea, vomiting, diarrhoea, fever and bleeding).
• Minimise adverse effects of radiation therapy by maintaining good nutrition, encouraging fluid intake, pacing activities to counteract therapy-induced fatigue and keeping the skin dry in irradiated areas.
• Prepare the child (and parents) for all tests and treatments, including adverse effects of therapy. Encourage the child to express their feelings, which may include fear and anger.
• Provide emotional support and offer appropriate reassurance. Make sure the family know that a variety of charities are available for information, financial assistance and supportive counselling.

Leukaemia

Leukaemia is an abnormal, uncontrolled overproduction of WBCs by the stem cells in bone marrow. The non-functional, leukaemic cells infiltrate the tissues of the body and replace normal cells. Children are most commonly diagnosed with acute lymphocytic leukaemia (ALL), which involves the lymphocytic WBC cell line or acute myeloid leukaemia (AML), which involves the granulocytic–myelocytic WBC cell line.

What causes it

The exact cause of leukaemia is unknown, although specific genes have been identified that can cause leukaemia. In addition, individuals with certain chromosomal disorders are at higher risk. There's an increased incidence of ALL in children with Down's syndrome (trisomy 13). Other risk factors include exposure to large doses of ionising radiation or drugs that suppress bone marrow. Certain viruses, such as human T-cell lymphotrophic virus type I, are also associated with an increased risk for leukaemia.

How it happens

The rapid production of WBCs results in the accumulation of immature, non-functional cells called blast cells. The blast cells multiply continuously, regardless of the body's needs. However, the proliferating blast cells don't attack and destroy normal cells. Rather, they crowd out other healthy, functional cells, robbing them of nutrition essential for metabolism, leading to pancytopenia (reduction in the number of blood cells being produced by all cell lines).

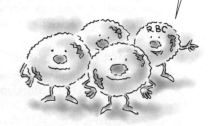

In leukemia, the malignant cells crowd out my buddies – the WBCs and platelets – and me until we become the minority.

Needed: Crowd control

Eventually, the bone marrow becomes packed with the malignant cells, and they spill out into the peripheral blood where they can be seen on microscopic slides.

What to look for

Signs and symptoms of ALL and AML are similar and are related to suppression of elements of the bone marrow:
• RBC and platelet levels are reduced as the stem cells are no longer producing them, which leads to anaemia with decreased haemoglobin.
• A low platelet count leads to bruising, bleeding and multiple nosebleeds; minor trauma, such as bumping into furniture, may cause large bruises.
• Because the WBCs are immature and non-functioning, the ability to fight infection is diminished, and the child may experience high fevers and show signs of sepsis.

What tests tell you

• Blood counts show thrombocytopenia and neutropenia. The WBC count in a FBC will be very high and the differential determines cell type.
• Lumbar puncture is performed to detect meningeal involvement; cerebrospinal fluid analysis reveals abnormal WBC invasion of the central nervous system (CNS).
• Bone marrow aspiration and biopsy confirm the disease, showing mostly malignant blast cells present in large numbers. (These tests are also used to determine whether the leukaemia is lymphocytic or myeloid, which will help determine treatment and prognosis.)

Complications

Because leukaemia and its treatment affect all blood cell lines and the immune system, complications vary and can be severe. Infections are of particular concern.

Fungus alert

Children on long-term immunosuppressive therapy may have overgrowth of fungal infections, such as candida, or little resistance to severe fungal infections such as aspergillus. Disruptions in the child's and the family's routine may cause major problems with school or socialisation as well as stress and anxiety.

How it's treated

Both forms of acute leukaemia are treated with combinations of IV chemotherapy drugs aimed at killing the malignant stem cells plus leukaemia cells that may have migrated to other areas of the body. AML is more resistant; therefore, the treatment regimens are more severe, usually requiring more hospitalisations. Because IV chemotherapy can't penetrate the CNS and spinal fluid, treatment of the CNS involves intrathecal chemotherapy and/or low-dose radiation of the spine and head.

   Treatment may also include:
- antibiotic, antifungal and antiviral drugs
- colony-stimulating factors, such as filgrastim, to spur the growth of granulocytes, RBCs and platelets
- transfusions of platelets to prevent bleeding and RBCs to prevent anaemia.

Transplant to the rescue

Bone marrow transplantation has become a standard treatment of AML when the child is in remission because a transplant improves long-term survival. In ALL, bone marrow transplantation is used after relapse if a second remission can be achieved because a relapse signifies more resistant disease.

What to do

Leukaemia is a devastating diagnosis for the child and his family. The child must deal not only with the disease but also with the adverse effects of treatment. The child should be prepared for all tests and treatments, and emotional support should be offered to his family. Referral to additional support services may be needed.

   In addition, follow these steps:
- Educate the child and family about the disease and treatments (including treatment-related problems).
- Assess for bleeding, bruising, fatigue or signs and symptoms of an impending infection.

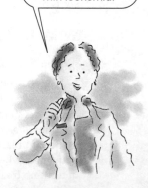

Bone marrow transplantation improves long-term survival. Its use during remission is the standard of care for children with leukemia.

- Coordinate care so the child doesn't come in contact with staff members who also care for patients with infections or infectious diseases.
- Provide guidelines for reducing such adverse effects of chemotherapy as nausea, vomiting and diarrhoea. Make sure the parents understand how to administer medications to treat these adverse effects.
- Make the parents aware that any fever is serious and may be life-threatening; medical staff should immediately evaluate the child with a fever.
- Shared care between the specialist paediatric oncology unit and local health services provides the family with care closer to their home.

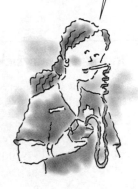

Any fever is cause for concern in a child with leukaemia.

Sickle cell anaemia

Sickle cell anaemia is an inherited, autosomal-recessive genetic disease that affects the RBCs, which become acutely sickle-shaped. They occlude small vessels, causing pain and decreased function. The two common variants of sickle cell anaemia are haemoglobin SS (Hgb SS) and haemoglobin SC (Hgb SC) disease. Symptoms are usually severe with Hgb SS, and moderate or undetectable in Hgb SC.

What causes it

The child must receive the autosomal-recessive gene from both parents to have the condition. The defective haemoglobin (haemoglobin S) takes on the classic sickle shape with decreased oxygen carrying capacity and inability to flow through capillaries. Carriers of sickle cell trait have few symptoms, and only on rare occasions.

How it happens

Sickle cell anaemia occurs as a result of a mutation in the gene that encodes the beta chain of haemoglobin. This mutation causes a structural change in haemoglobin. A single amino acid change from glutamic acid to valine occurs in the sixth position of the beta-haemoglobin chain.

Haemoglobin S is for sickle

When hypoxia (oxygen deficiency) occurs, the haemoglobin S in the RBCs becomes insoluble. As a result, the blood cells become rigid and rough, forming an elongated crescent, or sickle, shape. Sickling can cause haemolysis (cell destruction).

Capillary traffic jam

Sickle cells accumulate in capillaries and smaller blood vessels, causing occlusions and increasing blood viscosity. This increased viscosity impairs normal circulation, causing pain, tissue infarctions (tissue death), swelling and anoxic changes that lead to further sickling and obstruction.

Low on O$_2$

Sickle cell crisis occurs when a patient with sickle cell anaemia experiences cellular oxygen deprivation from, for example, an infection, exposure to cold or high altitude, or overexertion. A chain of events then ensues. (See *Understanding sickle cell crisis*.)

Understanding sickle cell crisis

Sickle cell crisis is triggered by infection, cold exposure, high altitudes, overexertion and other conditions that cause cellular oxygen deprivation. Here's what happens:

- Deoxygenated, sickle-shaped erythrocytes adhere to the capillary wall and to one another, blocking blood flow and causing cellular hypoxia.

- The crisis worsens as tissue hypoxia and acidic waste products cause more sickling and cell damage.
- With each new crisis, organs and tissues are destroyed and areas of tissue die slowly (especially in the spleen and kidneys).

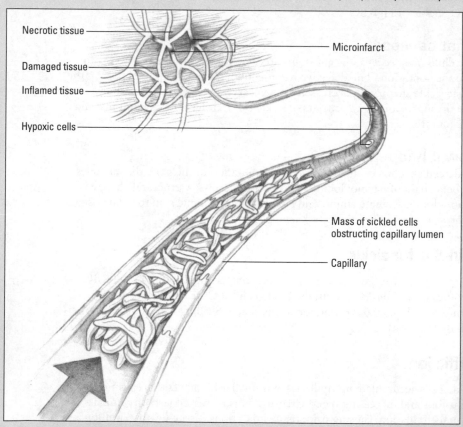

Necrotic tissue —
Damaged tissue —
Inflamed tissue —
Hypoxic cells —
Microinfarct
Mass of sickled cells obstructing capillary lumen
Capillary

What to look for

Signs and symptoms of sickle cell anaemia usually don't develop until after 6 months of age because large amounts of foetal haemoglobin protect infants until then. Foetal haemoglobin has a higher oxygen concentration and inhibits sickling.

A telling history

The history includes chronic fatigue, unexplained dyspnoea or dyspnoea on exertion, joint swelling, aching bones, severe localised and generalised pain, leg ulcers (rare in children) and frequent infections. Inspection may reveal jaundice or pallor. A young child may appear small for their age. The spleen will usually be enlarged and palpable.

Sickle cell crisis

In sickle cell crisis, symptoms include severe pain, haematuria, lethargy, irritability, and pale lips, tongue, palms and nail beds.

Isn't one enough?

Four different types of crisis can occur:

In painful crisis, there is severe abdominal, thoracic, muscle or bone pain and, possibly, increased jaundice, dark urine or a low-grade fever.

Aplastic crisis results from bone marrow depression and is characterised by pallor, lethargy, sleepiness, dyspnoea, possible coma, markedly decreased bone marrow activity and RBC haemolysis.

Acute sequestration crisis, occurring in infants, may cause sudden, massive entrapment of RBCs in the spleen and liver; if untreated, lethargy and pallor progress to hypovolemic shock and death.

Haemolytic crisis results from complications of the disease rather than the disease itself; degenerative changes cause liver congestion and enlargement, and chronic jaundice worsens.

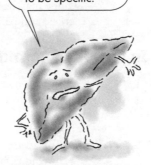

Being trapped inside me definitely qualifies as a crisis – an acute sequestration crisis, to be specific.

What tests tell you

• Haemoglobin levels will be low, and sickle cells will be seen on microscopic slide.
• Additional blood tests show low RBC counts, elevated WBC and platelet counts, a decreased ESR, increased serum iron levels, decreased RBC survival and reticulocytosis.
• Genetic tests will help identify the status of the parents and can be used to assess sibling status. Because of the importance of early diagnosis, it has become standard for all neonates to be tested at birth for both carrier and disease state.

Complications

Clinical manifestations of sickle cell anaemia vary, resulting in a wide range of complications related to occlusion of the blood vessels. These complications can include anaemia, aplastic crisis, sequestration crisis, dactylitis (hand and foot swelling), osteonecrosis from bone infarcts and greater risk for infection. Priapism, the state of constant penile erection, is a complication that can be embarrassing in adolescents as well as very painful.

How it's treated

Treatment of a child in sickle cell crisis consists of following life support guidelines and involves symptom management including:
- oxygen treatment-required if the blood oxygen saturation is low
- immediate pain relief usually with opiate analgesia
- intravenous fluids
- antibiotics.

The primary focus of treatment of SCD is prevention. Education is a key component for both the child and his family. Transfusion may be used in crisis to provide more functional RBCs.

Hydroxyurea a chemotherapeutic drug used in cancer treatment has been shown to decrease the number and severity of crises. Other medications, such as analgesics, may help to relieve the pain of a vasoocclusive crisis. Iron supplements may be given if folic acid levels are low.

What to do

A child who experiences the pain of a crisis will likely be fearful of future crises, as will parents. This may have a significant impact on the child's life. They may be afraid to participate in normal activities for fear of bringing on a crisis, and parents may become naturally overprotective.

In pursuit of normal

Prevention and education are the keys to leading a normal life, and participation in a support group may be extremely helpful in this regard. To prevent sickle crisis, the goal is to maintain as high a state of oxygenation as possible:
- Be aware that excessive exercise or activity may precipitate crisis.
- Avoid tight or restricting clothes such as elastic at the end of sleeves.
- Promote relaxation and stress-reducing activities because mental stress may play a role in crisis.
- Encourage the child to attend school and social functions while being aware that they may be more susceptible to infection.
- Explain the need to avoid flying in unpressurised aircrafts.
- Stress the importance of immediate evaluation of fever; children with sickle cell anaemia are functionally asplenic and are at risk for pneumococcal sepsis.

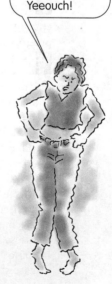

No one has to convince me that tight clothing has an adverse effect on oxygenation. Yeeouch!

Systemic lupus erythematosus

SLE is an autoimmune disease. For unknown reasons, the body turns on itself and attacks healthy cells and tissues leading to inflammation and damage.

It generally affects adolescent girls and women between 15 and 45, but it can be seen at other ages. In children, it typically strikes girls between 9 and 15 years. Neonatal lupus is seen in infants of women with SLE. It rarely affects males.

What causes it

The exact cause of SLE is unknown, although there are likely genetic, environmental and, possibly, hormonal influences. Exposure to ultraviolet light, infections, stress and pregnancy are known precipitating factors. Although no specific gene has been identified, current research is pointing to a genetic basis. Several genes may play a role in the development of this disease.

How it happens

The formation of autoantibodies in lupus occurs for unknown reasons. These autoantibodies join together with antigens to form soluble immune complexes and are deposited in multiple body tissues, including the skin, joints, lungs, heart, kidneys, brain and blood vessels.

A complex reaction

Symptoms appear due to inflammatory reactions and tissue damage that occur after the deposition of these immune complexes. Defects in the body's production of complement and cellular and humoral responses cause increased B-lymphocyte production and autoantibody reactions against T-lymphocytes, rendering them ineffective.

What to look for

SLE is a multisystem inflammatory disease of the joints, serous linings, kidneys, skin and CNS; therefore, symptoms may be widespread. Symptoms vary depending on the severity of the organ involvement. Common findings include:
- painful and swollen joints
- muscle pain
- unexplained fever
- extreme fatigue
- weight loss
- alopecia
- skin rashes, including the characteristic 'butterfly' (malar) rash over both cheeks and the nasal bridge, which are extremely sensitive to sun
- peripheral vasospasm (Raynaud's phenomenon).

Getting involved

As the disease progresses, systemic involvement increases. Hepatosplenomegaly and lymphadenopathy may occur. Inflammation of the lung and heart linings may cause chest pain and dyspnea. CNS involvement can produce seizures, coma, hemiplegia and behavioural disturbances, including psychosis. Renal SLE can progress rapidly and is the leading cause of death in people affected with this disease.

What tests tell you

Antinuclear antibody test is positive in patients who have active untreated disease; however, a negative test doesn't completely exclude SLE.
• ESR is usually elevated; anaemia, leukopenia and thrombocytopenia are commonly seen.
• Proteinuria may be one of the initial signs of renal involvement.
• A CT scan or MRI may identify pathological conditions of the brain due to SLE.

Complications

Complications from SLE are commonly related to treatment. Toxicity from the medications can cause growth failure, adrenal suppression, Cushing's syndrome, osteoporosis and aseptic necrosis. Liver damage and bone marrow suppression can occur with immunosuppressant use. Retinal damage may occur with the use of hydroxychloroquine. Amenorrhoea may result from either the disease itself or the medications used to treat it.

How it's treated

Although SLE can't be cured, young people with the disease can achieve remission and lead a high-quality life. Treatment may include drugs and other approaches:
• Corticosteroids are a mainstay of SLE treatment; they've been shown to significantly reduce mortality and should be used in all patients with renal, cardiac and CNS involvement.
• Immunosuppressants may be added if disease control is inadequate with steroids.
• Anti-inflammatory medications, such as nonsteroidal anti-inflammatory drugs and COX-2 inhibitors, may be used to help decrease the inflammation seen with SLE.
• Hydroxychloroquine is an antimalarial drug used to treat the inflammation associated with this disease.
• Holistic treatment approaches include fostering healthy behaviours, such as diet, rest and exercise.

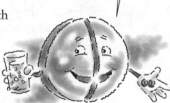

As a corticosteroid, I'm the go-to guy for treatment of SLE.

What to do

Nursing care aims to promote the best possible outcome for the child with a chronic illness. Interventions are directed towards preventing flare-ups, maintaining growth and development, preventing infection and preserving skin integrity:
• Teach the child to avoid such precipitating factors as sun exposure and stress; if necessary, a mental health referral should be made.

• Promote self-esteem, especially in young people; the use of hypoallergenic make-up, wigs and other aids will help cover up the disfiguring effects of this disease.
• Instruct the child to layer clothing and use mittens and sock liners to help decrease the discomfort associated with Raynaud's phenomenon.
• If needed, refer the child and family to support groups that may help them cope with the diagnosis and living with the condition.

Thalassaemia

Thalassaemia is characterised by the defective synthesis of haemoglobin.

Beta-thalassaemia

Beta-thalassaemia is the most common form of this disorder, resulting from defective beta-polypeptide chain synthesis. It occurs in three clinical forms: major, intermedia and minor, and the prognosis depends on which form of beta-thalassaemia the child has:
• Children with thalassaemia major seldom survive to adulthood.
• Children with thalassaemia intermedia develop normally into adulthood, although puberty is usually delayed.
• People with thalassaemia minor can expect a normal life span. (See *Ethnicity and thalassaemia*.)

What causes it

Thalassaemia major and thalassaemia intermedia result from homozygous inheritance of the partially dominant autosomal gene responsible for this trait. Thalassaemia minor results from heterozygous inheritance of the same gene.

How it happens

In each disorder, total or partial deficiency of beta-polypeptide chain production impairs haemoglobin synthesis and results in continual production of foetal haemoglobin, lasting even past the neonatal period.

What to look for

In thalassaemia major, the infant is well at birth but develops severe anaemia, bone abnormalities, faltering growth and life-threatening complications. In many cases, the first signs are pallor and yellow skin and sclera in infants 3 to 6 months of age.

Large but not in charge

Later clinical features include splenomegaly or hepatomegaly with abdominal enlargement, frequent infections, bleeding tendencies and anorexia. These signs and symptoms are also found:
• Children usually have small bodies and large heads.

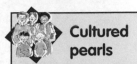

Cultured pearls

Ethnicity and thalassaemia

Thalassaemia is most common in people of Mediterranean ancestry (especially Italians and Greeks) but also occurs in people from southern China, India and Southeast Asia.

- If untreated, older children may have an enlarged maxilla, depressed bridge of the nose and protruding lips.
- Children become susceptible to pathological bone fractures as well as cardiac arrhythmias, heart failure and other complications that result from iron deposits in the heart and other tissues due to repeated blood transfusions.
- Patients with thalassaemia intermedia show some degree of anaemia, jaundice and splenomegaly; thalassaemia minor may cause mild anaemia but usually produces no symptoms and is commonly overlooked.

What tests tell you

Haemoglobin levels and RBC counts are low, and reticulocyte and bilirubin levels are elevated. X-rays of the skull and long bones show thinning and widening of the marrow space because of overactive bone marrow. (See *Skull changes in thalassaemia major*.) Quantitative haemoglobin studies show a significant rise in haemoglobin F. With prolonged disease, there may be increased levels of serum ferritin from RBC lysis and chronic transfusion.

Complications

Complications from the primary disease include heart failure from chronic low oxygenation as well as faltering growth, iron overload from repeated transfusions, osteopenia with fractures and suboptimal quality of life due to fatigue and chronic illness.

How it's treated

Thalassaemia intermedia and thalassaemia minor generally don't require treatment. Treatment of thalassaemia major generally involves repeated packed RBC transfusions to maintain higher haemoglobin levels. Transfusions may be needed as frequently as every 3 weeks.

Don't overdo it!

These transfusions must be administered judiciously to minimise iron overload. Desferrioxamine and deferiprone are chelating agents given to eliminate excess iron from the body. Increased demand for folic acid requires supplements to help maintain normal levels. Splenectomy and bone marrow transplantation have been performed, but their effectiveness hasn't been confirmed.

What to do

Provide emotional support to the parents; encourage them to express their feelings and concerns and make sure that their questions are answered. Explain all tests and procedures. In addition, follow these steps:
- Monitor for adverse reactions during packed RBC transfusions, such as fever, chills and irritability.
- Make the parents aware of the inherited nature of the disorder so they can seek genetic counselling.

Skull changes in thalassaemia major

This illustration of an X-ray shows a characteristic skull abnormality in thalassaemia major: diploetic fibres extending from internal lamina, resembling hair standing on end.

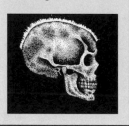

- Educate the parents on the nature of the disease and the symptoms of low haemoglobin, such as fatigue and paleness, and the risk of failure to thrive.
- Encourage a normal lifestyle to the extent possible.
- Provide education about adequate diets, which can reduce the risk of further complications, including anaemia and growth problems.

Allergic rhinitis

Inhaled airborne antigens, such as dust and pollen, may cause an immune response that results in watery eyes (allergic conjunctivitis) or an inflammation of the nasal mucosa (rhinitis). Depending on the allergen, allergic rhinitis may occur seasonally (hay fever) or year-round (perennial allergic rhinitis).

What causes it

Allergic rhinitis is a type I hypersensitivity reaction mediated by IgE. Hay fever occurs in the spring, summer and fall, and is usually induced by airborne pollens from trees, grass and weeds. In the summer and fall, mould spores may also cause it.

It may be difficult to identify the exact source of allergic rhinitis. Major perennial allergens and irritants include:
- house dust, dust mites and their excreta
- feathers
- moulds and fungi
- animal dander
- processed materials or industrial chemicals
- tobacco smoke, directly or from clothes worn while smoking (a major offender in children).

Hope for the future

Children who have allergic symptoms beginning before 2 years may outgrow them or may have reduced symptoms with time.

How it happens

Once the antigen is recognised by the immune system, a type I hypersensitivity reaction occurs. IgE is created by the conversion of B cells to plasma cells. Histamine release results in the swelling of the mucous membranes. Secondary sinus infections and middle ear infections may be triggered, and nasal polyps caused by oedema and infection may increase nasal obstruction.

What to look for

Allergic rhinitis may produce symptoms that vary by age, and may be difficult to distinguish from viral upper respiratory infections:

- The patient complains of sneezing attacks, rhinorrhoea (profuse, watery nasal discharge), nasal obstruction or congestion, itching nose and eyes and headache or sinus pain.
- Allergic rhinitis doesn't normally cause fever unless a secondary infection is present; fever with viral illnesses, such as an upper respiratory infection, isn't uncommon.
- A family history of allergies, asthma and atopic dermatitis (eczema) may indicate that symptoms are IgE mediated.
- Symptoms lasting longer than 2 weeks may indicate a more allergic than infective cause, especially if the child hasn't had a fever. (See *Allergic shiners*.)

What tests tell you

Most laboratory tests aren't helpful in determining if a short-term illness is an allergy. A large number of eosinophils are seen in specimens of sputum and nasal secretions. The activity of the eosinophils isn't completely understood, but they're known to destroy parasitic organisms and play a role in allergic reactions.

Sneezing in your sleep

FBC will be normal with either short- or long-term allergic problems, but may be helpful in ruling out a more serious illness if fever is present. Skin testing for allergies, or RAST, is helpful after the symptoms are present for several weeks and begin to affect the quality of life, especially by causing sleep disturbances. Short-term or less severe allergic rhinitis remains primarily a clinical diagnosis in children.

Complications

Complications of allergic rhinitis are rarely serious but affect the quality of life of the child and his family. The child may have sleep disturbances from a runny nose, frequent sneezing or coughing caused by postnasal drip.

The nose knows

Nosebleeds (epistaxis) may occur as a result of the allergic rhinitis itself or from overuse of medications, which dries mucous membranes. Children with allergic rhinitis are more susceptible to otitis media, sinusitis, bacterial conjunctivitis and other infections of the upper respiratory tract.

How it's treated

Treatment of allergic rhinitis is aimed at controlling the symptoms and preventing infection. Treatment may include removing the environmental allergen and administering drug therapy. Antihistamines block histamine release and decrease the overall reaction and swelling of the tissue. This action reduces the inflammation of the mucous membranes and decreases nasal drainage.

Timing is everything

One adverse effect of antihistamines in children is sedation. Use of antihistamines should be avoided before going to school and is usually more

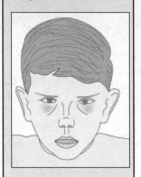

Allergic shiners

In allergic shiners, blood circulation around the eye backs up around the orbit, resulting in dark circles under the eyes or *Dennie's sign* (a peculiar horizontal line).

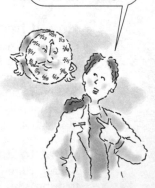

Antihistamines at bedtime help a child be bright-eyed, bushy-tailed and ready (if not willing) for school in the morning.

appropriate at bedtime or naptime. Newer antihistamines, such as loratadine and cetirizine, have been approved for use in older children and are non-sedating.

Up your nose with a nasal spray!

Other therapies may include cromolyn nasal spray to prevent responses to antigen, and topical nasal corticosteroids flunisolide or triamcinolone to control exacerbations. Long-term management may include immunotherapy or desensitisation with injections of allergen extracts administered pre-seasonally, seasonally or annually.

What to do
Stress the importance of taking daily antihistamines, and teach the parents and child about their potential adverse effects, and ways to reduce the child's exposure to the identified environmental allergen:
• Monitor a child who has received an allergy injection for at least 30 minutes to detect adverse reactions.
• Determine if family history is consistent with allergic problems and be aware that asthma is more common with familial history of allergies.

Quick quiz

1. The main function of platelets is to:
    A. provide oxygen to tissue.
    B. fight viral infections and provide immunity.
    C. fight bacterial infections.
    D. form a blood clot.

Answer: D. Platelets adhere to one another and plug holes in vessels or tissues where there's bleeding.

2. Which type of cell induces cell-mediated immunity?
    A. T lymphocytes
    B. Monocytes
    C. Reticulocytes
    D. B lymphocytes

Answer: A. T lymphocytes and macrophages are the chief participants in cell-mediated immunity.

3. What causes ALL?
    A. RBCs are defective and can't fight infection.
    B. Bone marrow stem cells are defective and produce ineffective blast cells.
    C. WBCs mature into only one cell line and fight only one type of infection.
    D. Platelets can't form clots, leading to severe haemorrhaging.

Answer: B. Stem cells start to produce non-functional blast cells for no apparent reason. The blast cells compete with and deprive normal cells of their essential nutrients, and gradually replace them.

4. An example of a type I hypersensitivity reaction is:
   A. anaphylaxis.
   B. transfusion reaction.
   C. autoimmune disorder.
   D. GVHD.

Answer: A. Examples of type I hypersensitivity reactions are anaphylaxis, hay fever (allergic rhinitis) and, in some cases, asthma.

Scoring

☆☆☆ If you answered all four items correctly, bravo! You're obviously immune to incorrect answers.

☆☆ If you answered three items correctly, great work! Your knowledge of haematological and immunological systems is coursing through your blood.

☆ If you answered fewer than three items correctly, don't have an adverse reaction. There's only one more quiz to go!

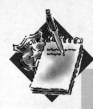

⑮ Dermatological problems

Just the facts

In this chapter, you'll learn:

♦ anatomy and physiology of the integumentary system

♦ tests used to diagnose dermatological problems in children

♦ treatments and procedures for children with skin problems

♦ dermatological disorders that may affect infants, children and adolescents.

Anatomy and physiology

The integumentary system, which consists of the skin and its components, is the largest organ system in the body. At birth, the skin is only 1 mm thick; the dermal layer of the skin doubles in thickness at maturity.

The great protector

The skin protects most of the other organ systems by acting as a mechanical barrier. Other functions include sensory perception, temperature regulation, vitamin synthesis and excretion of wastes through sweating.

Structures of the skin

The skin is composed of layers of tissue. Appendages of the skin include the hair and glands.

> This one's for you, Mr. Skin – our protector and barrier to the outside world. Without you, we'd be out there for the whole world to see!

Skin layers

The skin consists of two layers and a sub-layer, subcutaneous tissue:
• The epidermis, or outermost covering, provides a protective barrier to external trauma and limits the loss of body contents to the environment; dermatological problems are characteristically evident on the epidermis.
• The dermis consists of connective tissue that gives the skin strength and elasticity; it contains blood vessels, lymphatics and nerves.
• The subcutaneous layer lies below the dermis and is composed of loose connective tissue, or adipose tissue. It contains larger blood vessels, lymph channels and nerve trunks. This layer attaches the skin to the underlying bones, acts as a cushion and temperature insulator and determines the skin's contours. (See *Structure of the skin*.)

Structure of the skin

Major components of the skin include the epidermis, dermis and epidermal appendages (hair and glands).

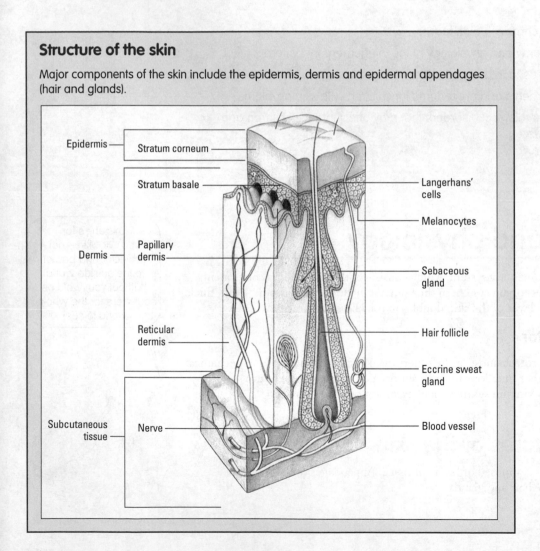

Thin-skinned

Skin layers act to prevent water loss, which varies with environmental temperature and humidity as well as the proportion of body surface exposed. Thus, fluid loss in the preterm neonate is greater than in an adult because the neonate's skin is thinner.

Hair
Hair changes markedly during the stages of development.

Foetal comb-over

Fine body hair, or lanugo, is found in utero over most of the foetus but decreases as the foetus approaches full-term. The neonate's scalp hair varies greatly in amount and is usually lost before growth of permanent hair, which gradually thickens.

Growth spurt

Puberty causes additional growth of hair in the axilla and pubic regions of both genders; boys experience facial hair growth.

Glands
The main glands of the skin are:
•   sebaceous glands, or sebum-producing glands, which contain the hair follicles and keep the skin supple by minimising water loss. They're more prevalent on the scalp, forehead, nose, chin and genitalia.
•   sweat glands, which may be eccrine (function as the body's heat-regulating mechanism by producing sweat) or apocrine (mature at puberty and cause the unpleasant body odour associated with sweating).

Diagnostic tests

Various tests are used to help diagnose skin problems and related systemic diseases and to identify the causes of the disorder.

Potassium hydroxide preparation

Potassium hydroxide (KOH) preparation is an alkalinising agent that's used to prepare clinical specimens for microscopic examination needed to help diagnose fungal disorders.

Fungus finder

A drop of 20% KOH is added to skin scrapings to dissolve debris before the scrapings are placed on a slide. When the slide is heated, the skin cells dissolve, leaving fungal elements visible on microscopic examination.

Nursing considerations

Explain the procedure to the parents and the child. Tell the child what to expect, including discomfort they may experience, and suggest coping strategies such as distraction techniques.

Skin biopsy

Skin biopsy is the removal of a section or an entire lesion for microscopic analysis to determine its cell structure and make a diagnosis. (See *Recognising skin lesions*.) A skin biopsy specimen can be obtained by:
*   shave biopsy
*   punch biopsy
*   excisional biopsy.
    Whichever method is utilised, the child should be given appropriate analgesia, local anaesthetic or sedation. In some cases, this may mean the administration of a GA.

The closest shave

In a shave biopsy, the protruding portion of the growth is excised at skin level and the specimen is sent for microscopic examination.

Pulled and punched

In a punch biopsy, the skin surrounding the lesion is pulled taut, and the punch is introduced firmly into the lesion. The punch is then rotated to obtain a tissue specimen, or plug. The plug is lifted with forceps or a needle and the surgeon severs as deeply as possible into the fat layer. The wound is then sutured closed.

Out, out, darn lesion

In an excisional biopsy, a scalpel is used to excise the lesion completely.

Nursing considerations

Explain the procedure to the parents and child dependent on the biopsy method and the analgesia, sedation or anaesthetic to be used. Tell the child what to expect, including discomfort they may experience, and suggest coping strategies such as distraction techniques.

Post punch, shave and excise

After the procedure:
*   apply a pressure dressing to the site
*   observe the site for bleeding
*   administer analgesics for pain as ordered.

Tzanck test

Tzanck test is a microscopic examination of cells taken from skin lesions to aid in the diagnosis of vesicular diseases. Cells are scraped from the

There's no closer shave than a shave biopsy! The part of the growth that protrudes is shaved off at skin level.

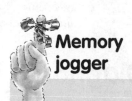
Memory jogger

Need help remembering what to assess when evaluating a skin lesion? Just think about your ABCDs.

Asymmetry
Border
Colour and configuration
Diameter and drainage.

Recognising skin lesions

These illustrations depict the most common primary and secondary skin lesions.

Macule

Flat, pigmented, circumscribed area less than 1 cm in diameter (freckle, rubella)

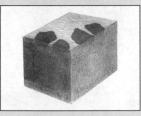

Papule

Firm, inflammatory, raised lesion up to 0.5 cm in diameter, may be same colour as skin or pigmented (acne papule, lichen planus)

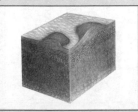

Plaque

Circumscribed, solid, elevated lesion more than 1 cm in diameter; elevation above skin surface occupies larger surface area compared with height (psoriasis)

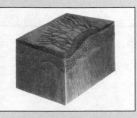

Patch

Flat, pigmented, circumscribed area more than 1 cm in diameter (herald patch [pityriasis rosea])

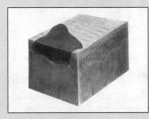

Nodule

Firm, raised lesion; deeper than a papule, extending into the dermal layer; 0.5 to 2 cm in diameter (intradermal nevus)

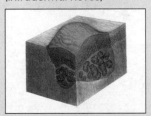

Tumour

Elevated, solid lesion more than 2 cm in diameter, extending into dermal and subcutaneous layers (dermatofibroma)

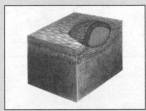

Wheal

Raised, firm lesion with intense localised skin edema, varying in size and shape; colour ranging from pale pink to red, disappears in hours (hive [urticaria], insect bite)

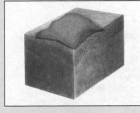

Comedo

Plugged pilosebaceous duct, exfoliative, formed from sebum and keratin (blackhead [open comedo], whitehead [closed comedo])

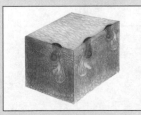

Cyst

Semisolid or fluid-filled encapsulated mass extending deep into the dermis (sebaceous cyst, cystic acne)

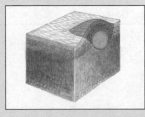

Vesicle

Raised, circumscribed, fluid-filled lesion less than 0.5 cm in diameter (chickenpox, herpes simplex)

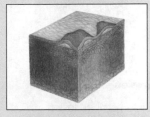

Pustule

Raised, circumscribed lesion usually less than 1 cm in diameter; containing purulent material that makes it a yellow-white colour (acne pustule, impetigo, furuncle)

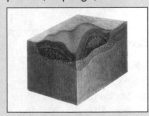

Bulla

Fluid-filled lesion more than 2 cm in diameter; also called a *blister* (severe poison oak or ivy dermatitis, bullous pemphigoid, second-degree burn)

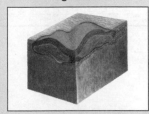

(continued)

Recognising skin lesions (continued)

Atrophy

Thinning of skin surface at site of disorder (striae, aging skin)

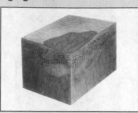

Scale

Thin, dry flakes of shedding skin (psoriasis, dry skin, newborn desquamation)

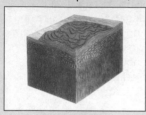

Excoriation

Linear scratched or abraded area, usually self-induced (abraded acne, eczema)

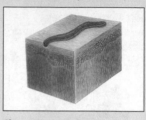

Lichenification

Thickened, prominent skin markings from constant rubbing (chronic atopic dermatitis)

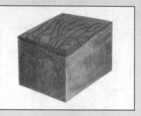

Erosion

Circumscribed lesion involving loss of superficial epidermis (rug burn, abrasion)

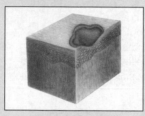

Crust

Dried sebum, serous, sanguineous or purulent exudate overlying an erosion or weeping vesicle, bulla or pustule (impetigo)

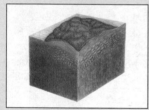

Fissure

Linear cracking of the skin extending into the dermal layer (hand dermatitis [chapped skin])

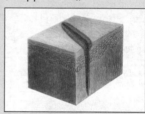

Scar

Fibrous tissue caused by trauma, deep inflammation or surgical incision; red and raised (recent), pink and flat (6 weeks) and depressed (old) (on a healed surgical incision)

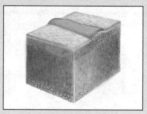

Ulcer

Epidermal and dermal destruction may extend into subcutaneous tissue; usually heals with scarring (pressure ulcer)

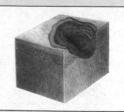

base of a vesicle to obtain moist, cloudy debris or exudate. The cells are then placed on a slide, air-dried and stained with Wright's or Giemsa stain. Multinucleated giant cells are indicative of either herpesvirus or varicella.

Nursing considerations

Explain the procedure to the parents and the child. Tell the child what to expect, including discomfort they may experience, and suggest coping strategies such as distraction techniques.

Treatments and procedures

Management of skin disorders may include a variety of therapeutic procedures, including laser surgery and skin grafting.

Laser surgery

Laser is the common term for light amplification by simulated emission of radiation. Lasers are used in surgery to divide adhesions or to treat lesions of the skin. The most common types of lasers used are the pulsed dye laser, the argon laser and the carbon-dioxide laser, each of which emits light at a different wavelength.

Complications

Complications associated with laser surgery include secondary infections, keloid or pyrogenic granuloma formation, localised dermatitis and hyperpigmentation or hypopigmentation.

Nursing considerations

The procedure may be undertaken under GA or with the use of a local anaesthetic. Explain the procedure to the parents and the child and prepare the child for discomfort they may experience. Make sure to prepare the child (and the parents) for the appearance of the treated area after laser surgery because it will probably look much worse than it does before treatment (some laser treatments leave skin raw and oozing). Reassure the child that this is normal and the area will heal quickly.

After the laser

After laser surgery:
• apply dressings as ordered
• instruct the parents in care of the treated area
• stress to the child and parents the importance of avoiding trauma to the lesion or picking at the scab.
• educate the parents and child on the use and importance of sunblocks.

Skin grafting

During skin grafting, a section of skin is separated from its blood supply and implanted over an area where skin has been lost due to burns, injury or surgical debridement of diseased tissue.

Tis better to give than receive

The area from which the skin is removed is referred to as the donor site. For donor areas in which appearance or joint movement is important, the graft is transplanted intact. In flat areas where appearance is less critical, the graft may be meshed (fenestrated) to cover up to three times its original size. It's then placed on what's known as the recipient site.

A healthy loan

Skin from the patient's own healthy skin (autograft) may be used. If an autograft isn't available, a homograft (cadaver skin) or xenograft (pigskin) may be surgically attached.

Keys to success

The skin graft may be a split-thickness graft (involving the epidermis and superficial dermis) or a full-thickness graft (involving the epidermis and all layers of dermis). To be successful, grafts must have a sufficient blood supply, have contact with the recipient area, be free from infection and mechanical trauma and have minimal bleeding or fluid accumulation.

Nursing considerations

Explain the procedure to the parents and the child. Prepare the child for the post-grafting appearance of the donor site and the recipient site. Reassure the child that the sites will heal, but tell them that this may take some time.

After graft

After grafting, follow these steps:
• Observe the donor and graft sites dressings for fluid drainage and odour; if these occur, notify medical staff.
• Observe the child for pain at the graft sites because this may indicate infection.
• Monitor the child's temperature every 4 hours because a rise in temperature may also indicate the present of infection. Changes should be reported to medical staff.
• Instruct the parents on the care of the donor and recipient sites and include them in the child's care as much as possible (including dressing changes).
• Teach parents to recognise the signs of infection (such as pain, a rise in temperature, fluid drainage and odour) and instruct them to report these signs immediately.

- Stress to the parents (and the child) the importance of protecting the donor and recipient sites from trauma.
- Encourage the parent to hold and comfort the child despite the presence of the bulky dressings; reassure them that the dressings allow them to hold their child without hurting them.

Dermatological disorders

Dermatological disorders that may affect children and young people include scabies, atopic dermatitis (eczema), contact dermatitis and burns.

Scabies

Scabies, a highly transmissible parasitic skin infestation, is characterised by burrows, pruritus and excoriations with secondary infections. It characteristically spreads to family members, intimate contacts and among school children. Prolonged contact is needed to become infected.

What causes it

Scabies is a contagious disease caused by the scabies mite, *Sarcoptes scabiei*, which burrows into the stratum corneum of the epidermis and deposits eggs and faeces. (See *Scabies: Cause and effect*.)

How it happens

The female scabies mite burrows under the skin and forms a small tunnel that's evident as a fine, wavy, dark line with a black dot at the end. The mite

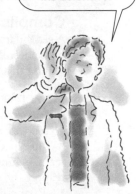

After skin grafting, the parents may need to be reassured that holding and cuddling their child won't hurt him.

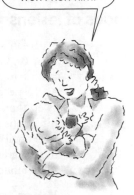

It's human nature. Parents are more likely to listen (and learn) when they aren't put on the defensive.

Scabies: Cause and effect

Infestation with *Sarcoptes scabiei* – the itch mite – causes scabies. The top illustration shows the mite (enlarged); it has a hard shell and measures a microscopic 0.1 mm. The bottom illustration depicts the erythematous nodules with excoriation that appear in patients with scabies.

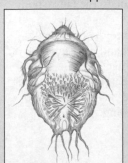
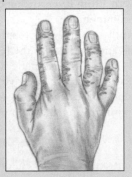

extends the burrow, laying up to three eggs per day as she travels. The eggs hatch in about 2 weeks, thus continuing the process.

What to look for
• The lesions initially produce no symptoms but sensitisation to the mites occurs in about 3 weeks. At that time, intense itching occurs, becoming more severe at night.

Loads of lesions
• Infants have dozens of lesions, while older children commonly have fewer than 10. Children younger than 2 years usually have lesions on the feet and ankles; in older children, most lesions are found on the hands and wrists.
• Inspection reveals characteristic grey-brown burrows, which may appear as erythematous nodules when excoriated; secondary excoriation and bacterial infections commonly obscure the burrows and papules.
• Papules of various sizes may exist simultaneously and are typically distributed in such areas as the finger webs, flexor surfaces of the wrist, elbows and axillary folds, along the belt line and on the lower buttocks.

What tests tell you
• Microscopic examination reveals the characteristic eight-legged scabies mite, eggs or faeces. (Scrapings from an unscratched burrow should be placed in saline or mineral oil. The scrapings shouldn't be placed in KOH because it can dissolve the mites, eggs or faeces.)
• The burrow ink test reveals the presence of burrows. This test involves applying a drop of ink or a blue or black felt-tipped pen to a suspected burrow, wiping off the excess ink with an alcohol pad and examining the area with a magnifying glass for an ink-stained burrow.

Complications
A secondary bacterial infection from scratching is one possible complication of scabies. Post-scabetic syndrome may occur, characterised by lesions and itching that commonly persist for days to weeks following treatment.

How it's treated
Pharmacological treatment with a thin layer of scabicide to the entire body (except the eyes) is usually recommended:
• Be especially careful to gently massage the cream into the fingernails, scalp, behind the ears, all folds and creases and the feet and hands; in 7 days, reapply the cream to the child and all symptomatic contacts.
• Permethrin 5% cream is safer and more effective than malathion, and is safe for infants as young as 2 months; the cream should be left on for 8 to 14 hours, and then removed with bathing and shampooing.

Fighting the mighty mite
• Malathion 1% cream is contraindicated for children younger than 6 months and for those with seizure disorders because it has potential central

nervous system effects. If used, the cream is applied from the neck down, and is left on for 8 to 12 hours before bathing. Treatment is then repeated in 1 week.

What to do

All family members, friends, and school and nursery contacts should undergo treatment, even if they're asymptomatic. Parents should be educated about the course of the disease and told that the rash and itching commonly persist for up to 3 weeks. Children are no longer infectious 24 hours after treatment has started, and may return to school or nursery.

Instruct the parents to:
• wash all bed linens and clothing with hot water, and then dry for 20 minutes in a hot dryer.

Whole-house vacuum

• vacuum the entire house
• store non-washable items in sealed bags for 1 week
• use meticulous hand washing and good hygiene to avoid secondary infections
• trim the child's fingernails short to avoid excoriation from scratching
• use soothing lotions to control itching.

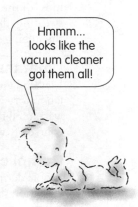

Hmmm... looks like the vacuum cleaner got them all!

Atopic dermatitis

Atopic dermatitis, also called eczema, is a chronic condition of the skin characterised by superficial skin inflammation and intense itching. The skin doesn't hold moisture or oil and becomes dry, scaly and itchy. Although this disorder may appear at any age, it typically begins during infancy or early childhood.

What causes it

The exact cause is unknown but an allergic component is strongly suspected. A family history commonly reveals adults with childhood histories of atopic dermatitis, other forms of allergies or asthma. About 20% of children will also develop asthma at some point. Another theory suggests defective T-cell function.

To make matters worse...

Exacerbating factors include irritants, infections (commonly caused by *Staphylococcus aureus*) and some allergens. Exposure to food allergens may coincide with flare-ups of atopic dermatitis.

How it happens

Scratching the skin causes vasoconstriction and intensifies itching, resulting in reddened, weeping lesions. Eventually, the lesions become scaly and lichenified. Usually, they're located in areas of

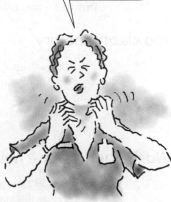

Atopic dermatitis sets up a vicious cycle. Itching leads to scratching, which causes vasoconstriction and makes itching even worse!

flexion and extension, such as the neck, antecubital fossa, popliteal folds and behind the ears. In infants, the lesions are also common on the cheeks and may look like a windburn.

What to look for

Atopic dermatitis begins with skin drying and then cracking, eventually leading to open sores with bleeding. These open sores are susceptible to secondary infections. Children commonly scratch in their sleep and can do most of the skin damage at that time if the itching isn't controlled. Heat, sweating, dry skin and clothing with wool or coarse materials tend to worsen the itching sensation. (See *Infant with atopic dermatitis*.)

What tests tell you

Elevated levels of IgE and eosinophils are seen in this disorder, but routine laboratory values, such as FBC, aren't affected. Allergy testing may be warranted in the older child but avoiding the allergen may not affect the course of atopic dermatitis.

Complications

Atopic dermatitis may disrupt the family in general because it's a chronic condition that requires daily care. The child may have sleep difficulties from constant pruritus.

From scratching to scarring

Skin damage from scratching leaves the child susceptible to secondary infection that may require either topical treatment with antibiotic ointment or systemic antibiotics. Because the upper layers of the skin are most involved, it's rare for scarring to occur, even with excoriation from scratching.

How it's treated

Measures to ease this chronic disorder include meticulous skin care, environmental control of offending allergens and drug therapy. The overall treatment plan is aimed at controlling the symptoms – particularly the pruritus – and restoring moisture to the skin to prevent further drying.

Too clean, too dry

Excessive bathing leads to further reduction in skin oils and worsens the dryness. Once-daily bathing in warm water with cream-based soaps can relieve symptoms. Frequent application of non-irritating topical lubricants, for example, aqueous cream is important, especially after bathing or showering.

Wash, then wear – hold the bleach

Minimising exposure to irritants, such as wool and harsh detergents, also helps control symptoms. New clothes should be washed before wearing to

Infant with atopic dermatitis

Children with atopic dermatitis have papular and vesicular skin eruptions with surrounding erythema. The vesicles rupture and exude yellow, sticky exudate. The secretions form crusts on the skin as they dry.

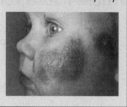

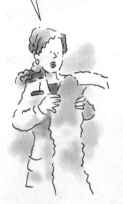

To manage atopic dermatitis, there's a 'laundry' list of do's and don'ts.

avoid exposure to irritating dyes or chemicals. Clothes washed with bleach should be double-rinsed to ensure that all bleach is removed (because it dries and irritates the skin). Hypoallergenic soaps should be used for all laundry, and starch should be avoided. Some children's condition is worsened by the use of biological soap powders. The use of wash balls which do not use any cleaning chemicals may be useful.

Down with itch and inflammation!

Drug therapy involves the use of topical corticosteroids and antipruritics. A mild 1% steroid cream, such as hydrocortisone, can relieve the inflammation and associated itching, and may be massaged into the affected area three or four times per day and after bathing.

Diphenhydramine or hydroxyzine are effective antipruritics but may cause sedation. These medications are especially useful at bedtime to reduce night-time scratching and resulting skin damage.

What to do

The children's nurse plays an important role in the management of atopic dermatitis and is commonly the key source of help for minimising the impact of this condition on the child and their family:

• Instruct all caretakers about the management of the skin lesions.
• Make the family aware that atopic dermatitis is a chronic condition that isn't usually related to an identifiable allergen. Reassure them that the child with a mild case is likely to outgrow it.
• Although avoiding such foods as nuts and eggs is normally recommended for all children younger than 3 years, it may not have an affect on atopic dermatitis.
• Make sure the parents are aware of such serious complications as infection and emphasise the need for evaluation of any open, draining areas.

Contact dermatitis

Contact dermatitis occurs as an acute or chronic inflammatory response due to a hypersensitivity reaction to a natural or synthetic chemical substance. The irritating substance can be a primary irritant or a sensitising agent or allergen.

What causes it

Irritant dermatitis is caused by the toxic effect of the substance directly on the skin. The extent of the rash and itching depends on the length of exposure and the concentration of the irritant. Common irritants include:

• detergents, harsh soaps, bubble bath and baby wipes
• bathing too frequently
• saliva, urine and faeces. (Nappy dermatitis, the most common form of irritant dermatitis, is a reaction to urine and by-products of faeces.)

Allergic annoyances

Allergic dermatitis occurs with exposure to substances that cause an immunological response triggered by an allergen to which the child has become sensitised. Sensitising reactions occur with repeated or prolonged exposure to such substances as:
- plant oils (poison ivy)
- nickel-containing jewellery
- clothing with woollen or rough textures
- topical medications, such as neomycin and lanolin
- perfumed soaps or cosmetics.

How it happens

In primary irritant dermatitis, the toxic substance causes damage to the stratum corneum and the skin's lipid film, impairing the protective barrier mechanism of the skin. The toxic substance is then absorbed into the skin, resulting in vasodilatation, oedema of the upper dermis, inflammatory infiltrates and breakdown of epidermal cells. Vesicles or bullae may develop as a result of the fluid accumulating between the epidermal cells that act as a sponge.

Not immune to an immune response

Allergic dermatitis is due to an immune response caused by the sensitising chemical entering the dermis and combining with epidermal proteins to form a new molecule that acts as an antigen. This antigen enters the local cutaneous lymphoid tissue, causing an inflammatory reaction.

What to look for

A thorough history should elicit information about:
- exposure to new or unusual substances
- repeated exposure to a substance
- history of diarrhoea or infrequent diaper changes
- location of the rash related to specific areas of the body
- treatments or forms of at-home management.

Oozing, scaling and itching – Oh, my!

Mild irritants and allergens produce erythema and small vesicles that ooze, scale and itch. Strong irritants may also cause blisters and ulcerations.

It's a classic

A classic allergic response produces clearly defined lesions with straight lines following the points of contact. A severe allergic reaction also produces marked oedema of the affected area.

What tests tell you

Tests should be reserved for a time when the child isn't experiencing acute, active dermatitis. There are two methods used to determine allergy:

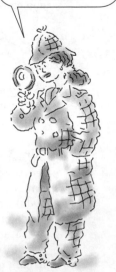

Following the clues from a thorough history will lead you to the prime suspect – the offending substance in contact dermatitis.

• The patch test identifies specific allergens. The suspected substance is applied to a patch left in place on the child's skin for a specified period. If the area under the patch is red and swollen when the patch is removed, the test is positive and the child is considered allergic to the offending substance.
• In skin testing, the suspected allergen is introduced intradermally on the child's back or upper arm.

Complications

Complications of contact dermatitis include secondary infections and trauma from scratching. The child may have serious concerns about his appearance and body image.

How it's treated

The keys to successful treatment are identification and removal or elimination of the causative agent, and appropriate skin care and management. Resolution of contact dermatitis typically takes 2 to 3 weeks.

How offensive!

When the offending substance has been identified and eliminated from the child's environment, management consists primarily of treating and preventing worsening of symptoms:
• For nappy dermatitis, change nappies frequently, use air-drying if possible.
• Hydrocortisone cream 1% should be used sparingly for no more than 5 days.
• Antifungal agents may be necessary if secondary infection develops.

A soak in the bath

• Cool baths and compresses may soothe itching and vesicular rashes.
• Petroleum-based or lanolin and petroleum-based emollients may be applied to dry and chaffed skin, but must be avoided if the skin is inflamed.

Ditch the itch!

• Topical corticosteroids may be administered two to three times per day; oral antihistamines are commonly prescribed for itching.
• Referral to a dermatologist for patch testing may be necessary.

What to do

Management requires problem solving to determine the cause of the skin reaction and to find a mutually agreeable solution:
• Educate the child and family about hygiene practices to prevent infections.
• Teach the parents about antipruritic agents and their proper use to relieve discomfort and itching.

Replace; don't recycle

- Discuss proper use and regular replacement of skin care products.
- Educate the parents and the child about ways to prevent future exposures.

Don't judge

- Establish a professional rapport with the child and parents and provide education in a non-judgemental manner; parents may become defencive and are less likely to listen when they feel they're being judged or their parenting skills are being questioned.
- Encourage the child to express concerns about their appearance and body image.

Burns

Burns are caused by excessive heat, but are also related to exposure to cold, chemicals, electricity or radiation. When the skin is burned, it loses its ability to perform its normal physiological functions.

Educational efforts aimed at burn prevention have significantly decreased the number of burn injuries and deaths among children. However, fire and burn injuries remain the third leading cause of unintentional, injury-related death in children younger than 14 years.

What causes it

Burn injuries result from various causes and represent a severe trauma to the body. Exposure to thermal, chemical and electrical sources can cause burn injuries.

Thermal burns

Thermal burns, the most common type, are usually the result of residential fires, car accidents, children playing with matches, improperly stored petrol, space heater or electrical malfunctions or arson. Other causes include improper handling of fireworks, scalding accidents, kitchen accidents (such as a child climbing on top of a cooker) and access to dangerous items (such as a hot iron).

Chemical burns

Chemical burns result from contact, ingestion, inhalation, or injection of acids, alkalis, vesicants or noxious agents used in cleaning products.

Electrical burns

Electrical burns usually occur after contact with faulty electrical wiring or from inserting conductive objects into electrical outlets. Children can also sustain electrical burns by chewing on electric cords.

Other burns

Burns also may occur from:

- skin being rubbed harshly against a coarse surface (called friction or abrasion burns)
- sun exposure (minor burns)
- child abuse (intentionally inflicted injuries from such actions as immersion in hot water and contact with hot objects such as cigarettes).

How it happens

Children, especially those younger than 5 years, are at greater risk for burn injuries. Developmentally, children have a limited ability to act promptly and properly in a dangerous situation, such as a fire and an explosion, or when they're exposed to dangerous items (such as cookers and hot irons).

Thermal and chemical burns disrupt the normal protective function of the skin, leading to various sequelae. In an electrical injury, the heat generated by the electricity passes through the body, causing injury to the tissues.

Two levels of response to the burn injury occur:

 local

systemic.

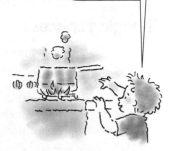

Hey, I'm just a kid! I can't be trusted to make adult decisions about dangerous situations.

Local response

Local response represents local tissue damage to the skin:
- Oedema results from increased capillary permeability and increased hydrostatic pressure forcing water, protein and electrolytes into the interstitial spaces.
- Fluid loss from the burn-injured skin is a result of the inflammatory response.
- Significant circulatory alterations cause capillary stasis in the burned area.
- Thrombi develop, leading to tissue ischemia and necrosis, causing pain and oedema.

Systemic response

Systemic response to burns may involve various body systems:
- Cardiovascular changes occur, such as burn shock caused by dramatic alterations in circulation; tachycardia and tachypnoea occur to compensate for decreasing vascular volume and increased oxygen needs.

A tight squeeze

- Compartment syndrome, requiring surgical correction, may occur when severe oedema causes a tourniquet-like effect that compromises circulation and entraps nerves.
- The respiratory system may be compromised by smoke inhalation; injuries can range from tissue oedema of upper respiratory airways to impaired gas exchange in the alveoli.

Constricted and depressed

- Renal changes occur, such as renal vasoconstriction, reduced renal plasma flow, and depressed glomerular filtration.
- GI ischemia may occur as perfusion to the GI tract and liver is decreased.
- Gastric ileus may occur, with digestion almost ceasing.
- Metabolism is greatly increased, which can lead to prolonged starvation and extensive energy needs.

Changing spaces

- Fluid shifts to the extravascular spaces and altered concentrations of potassium, sodium, chloride and bicarbonate occur.
- Elevated body temperature occurs as a result of increased metabolism, even in the absence of infection.
- The neuroendocrine system attempts to restore equilibrium by secreting trophic hormones to stimulate various organs.

Fragile: Handle with care

- Increased cell fragility and loss of circulatory red blood cells lead to anaemia and the production of lactic acid.
- Growth and development are retarded with severe burn injuries due to growth hormone suppression.
- The child is prone to infections, such as nosocomial infections, due to loss of skin and tissue integrity and an immature immune system.

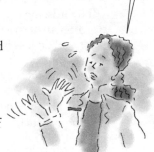

Burns can make you hot all over! When burns occur, metabolism increases and body temperature rises.

What to look for

Assessment of the child with a burn injury should begin basic life support and immediate assessment of the thermal injury and life-threatening sequela. A thorough history should be obtained. A description of events surrounding the burn injury should include the cause and the duration the agent was in contact with the skin. The history also consists of how and when the injury occurred, treatment of the burn and history of previous burns. Assessment of parental interactions with the child as well as the description of events must be undertaken so that any concerns about abuse are considered.

A matter of degree

Burns are assessed according to degree (depth of damage) and extent (percentage of body surface area). One goal of assessment is to determine the depth of skin and tissue damage:

In first-degree burns, damage is limited to the epidermis, causing erythema and pain.

In second-degree burns (partial thickness), the epidermis and part of the dermis are damaged, producing blisters and mild-to-moderate oedema and pain.

Gauging burn depth

One method of assessing burns is determining their depth. As shown in this illustration, a partial-thickness burn damages the epidermis and part of the dermis, whereas a full-thickness burn damages the epidermis, dermis, subcutaneous tissue, and muscle.

In third-degree burns (full thickness), the epidermis and the dermis are damaged; no blisters appear, but white, brown or black leathery tissue and thrombosed vessels are visible.

Fourth-degree burns are rare, and damage extends through deeply charred subcutaneous tissue to muscle and bone. (See *Gauging burn depth*.)

TBSA or not TBSA

Another assessment goal is to estimate the size of a burn, which is usually expressed as a percentage of the total body surface area (TBSA). The TBSA, together with the body part affected, determines morbidity, mortality and management strategies.

10% of TBSA = a hospital stay

For children, burns that make up 10% or more of TBSA are considered critical and require hospitalisation. In addition, significant burns of the hands, feet, face, ears and genitalia also require immediate hospitalisation. Children's larger body surface areas put them at high risk for fluid volume and heat loss leading to dehydration. (See *Estimating the extent of a burn*, page 548)

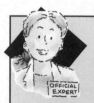

Advice from the experts

Estimating the extent of a burn

To estimate the extent of a burn in a child, use the Lund and Browder chart. To use the chart:

- mentally transfer your patient's burns to the body chart shown here
- then add up the corresponding percentages for each burned body section.

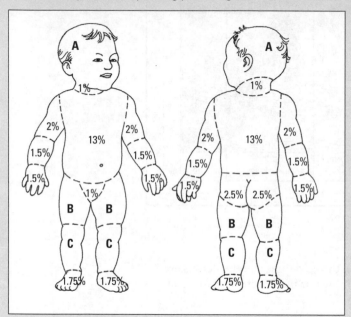

Relative percentages of areas affected by growth

	At birth	0 to 1 yr	2 to 4 yrs	5 to 9 yrs	10 to 15 yrs
A: Half of head	9½%	8½%	6½%	5½%	4½%
B: Half of thigh	2¾%	3¼%	4%	4¼%	4½%
C: Half of leg	2½%	2½%	2¾%	3%	3¼%

Inspect to detect

Inspection reveals other characteristics of the burn as well, including location, pattern and extent. Assess for sensation and degree of pain, and check for blanching and capillary refill of the nail beds.
- Lung auscultation may reveal respiratory compromise, tachypnoea or stridor.
- Assessment of the cardiovascular system may reveal tachycardia, narrow pulse pressure and hypotension.
- The child may have decreased urine output.

Complications

Nursing care of a child with burns is challenging because many organ systems are affected by the burn injury. Potential complications depend on the depth and severity of the burn as well as its specific cause. The most common

complications and leading causes of death are respiratory complications and sepsis. Other possible complications include:
• burn shock
• fluid and electrolyte deficits
• hypothermia
• hypermetabolism
• hypovolemic shock
• infections
• scarring and disfigurement
• contractures
• multisystem organ failure.

How it's treated
Superficial first-degree burn injuries and partial-thickness burns heal spontaneously with reasonable care.

Minor burns
Management of minor burns includes removing burned clothing, cleaning with tepid water and leaving blisters intact. In addition:
• nothing should be applied to the burn except a clean cloth that is (sometimes) treated with antimicrobial ointment or cream
• tetanus prophylaxis is necessary if no history of immunisation is available or if more than 5 years has passed since the last immunisation
• a mild analgesic may be administered.

Moderate or severe burns
If the burn involves a large area of the body surface (above 10%) or critical body parts, it represents severe trauma and usually requires treatment at a specialised burn centre. Emergency management of major burns involves stopping the burning process and placing the child in a horizontal position. In addition:
• establish and maintain a patent airway, initiating advanced life support if necessary
• remove burned clothing, jewellery and any other items while keeping the child warm
• cover the burn to prevent contamination
• until transported to the specialist burn centre, don't allow the child to eat or drink anything; IV fluids should be started and oxygen therapy provided at 100%.

In the unit

Initial management of the major burn in the burn unit includes maintenance of an adequate airway. IV fluid replacement should be started as soon as possible. Intubation and mechanical ventilation may be necessary. In addition:
• a urinary catheter is inserted to adequately measure urine output

- a nasogastric tube may be necessary to decompress the stomach; later, it may be used to administer a high protein, high-calorie diet or total parenteral nutrition (which may be necessary if the GI tract is dysfunctional)
- baseline FBC and blood chemistry
- IV pain medication is administered
- topical wound cleaning is begun to prevent infections
- tetanus prophylaxis is administered if required.

In general

General wound management includes wound debridement, hydrotherapy for dressing removal and debridement, topical antimicrobial therapy, nutritional therapy, physiotherapy focusing on range of motion and contracture prevention and skin grafting.

What to do

Burns are one of the most painful injuries a child can sustain. Severe burns are life-threatening. The child and his parents will need a great deal of emotional support and reassurance.

Every effort should be made to make the child as comfortable as possible during such painful procedures as debridement. Depending on the child's age, it may be difficult to understand why doctors and nurses are inflicting pain during such procedures. The reasons for these treatments should be explained repeatedly and the child should be encouraged to express their feelings, which may include fear and anger.

Referral to a physiotherapist, occupational therapist and a support group may be needed to help the child and parents deal with the traumatic injury because such traumas can have long-lasting psychological effects. Similar referrals are needed if severe scarring or disfigurement is anticipated.

In the heat of the moment

During the acute phase – the first 24 to 48 hours after the burn occurs – nursing care includes:

- treating burn shock
- monitoring respiratory status
- maintaining a patent airway
- monitoring vital signs and fluid status every hour
- maintaining adequate fluid and electrolyte balance
- caring for the burn wound
- managing pain.

When the fire dies down

Ongoing management and rehabilitation should include preventing wound infections and complications (such as heat loss and contractures), promoting wound healing, managing the child's pain and promoting comfort, promoting adequate nutrition and providing psychosocial support for the child and his family. The child and his family should be educated about long-term needs and follow-up care. Education about safety issues, including prevention of future burns, should be conducted in a non-judgemental manner because the parents will likely already have strong feelings of guilt.

Concerns?

Burns are often perpetrated through acts of abuse and so the health care team will utilise all the assessment information to consider whether the child, the history and presenting condition is consistent with the history and explanations. If there are concerns, then local safeguarding children procedures must be followed.

Quick quiz

1. Which statement about the integumentary system and its components is true?

    A. It's the largest organ in the body and serves primarily as an insulator.

    B. It can only protect the body from trauma that's mechanical in nature.

    C. It consists of just the dermis and epidermis.

    D. Its main function is to act as an organ of excretion.

Answer: A. The integumentary system, which consists of the skin and its components, is the largest organ system in the body. It functions to shelter most of the other organ systems, protecting them while acting as a mechanical barrier.

2. The glands that are primarily responsible for the odour associated with sweating are known as the:

    A. endocrine sweat glands.

    B. eccrine sweat glands.

    C. cutaneous sweat glands.

    D. apocrine sweat glands.

Answer: D. The sweat glands consist of the eccrine sweat glands, which function as the body's heat-regulating mechanism by producing sweat, and the apocrine sweat glands, which mature at puberty and cause the body odour associated with sweating.

3. The proportion of a child's body that's burned is typically estimated according to:

    A. Rule of Nines.

    B. TBSA.

    C. depth of injury.

    D. three-dimensional analysis.

Answer: B. One goal in assessing burns is to estimate its size, which is usually expressed as a percentage of TBSA. The TBSA and body part affected determines morbidity, mortality and management strategies.

4. When assessing a child with a rash consistent with irritant dermatitis, which question should the nurse ask?
 A. 'Has your child been playing with children who may have chickenpox?'
 B. 'Has your child been ill lately?'
 C. 'Has your child been exposed to a new or unusual substance?'
 D. 'Has your child eaten anything different?'

Answer: C. Irritant dermatitis is caused by the toxic effect of the substance directly on the skin. Common irritants include detergents, harsh soaps, bubble bath, baby wipes, saliva, urine or faeces or over-bathing.

5. Pruritus caused by contact dermatitis can usually be treated at home with:
 A. cool baths and compresses.
 B. soothing scented bath oils.
 C. ice and heat alternately.
 D. patch skin applications.

Answer: A. Cool baths and compresses may soothe itching and vesicular rashes.

6. Which of the following is true about scabies?
 A. Tzanck testing is done immediately to confirm the scabies mite.
 B. Infants usually have very few lesions on their bodies.
 C. Characteristic lesions are raised greyish brown linear burrows.
 D. Itching is worse during the daytime hours when the child is awake.

Answer: C. Inspection of scabies reveals characteristic greyish brown burrows, which may appear as erythematous nodules when excoriated.

Scoring

★★★ If you answered all six items correctly, hooray! Your knowledge of dermatological problems is more than skin deep.

★★   If you answered four or five items correctly, congratulations! The material in this chapter has gotten under your skin.

★   If you answered fewer than four items correctly, take an oatmeal bath, relax and then re-read the chapter! This is the last quick quiz to irritate you.

Glossary

accessory muscles: thoracic and abdominal muscles used during respiratory distress to help expand and contract the chest so the child can inhale and exhale

allergic salute: pushing up and out on the base of the nose to relieve stuffiness

allergic shiners: dark circles under the eyes from oedema and congestion related to histamine

allergy: hypersensitivity to normal environmental antigens

alveoli: small, saclike structures in the lungs where the exchange of oxygen for carbon dioxide takes place

anaemia: decrease in the number or quality of circulating red blood cells from haemorrhage, haemolysis or lack of production

anorexia: lack or loss of appetite for food

anorexia nervosa: voluntary control of hunger characterised by a refusal to eat and maintain a minimum healthy body weight for age and height, leading to body weight of 85% less than expected or normal

antigen: a substance that stimulates the body to produce antibodies

anuria: absence of urine formation, manifested by no urine output

arteries: large, thick-walled blood vessels that distribute oxygenated blood to the capillaries

astrocytoma: slow-growing tumour in the cerebellum

atelectasis: failure of a portion of the lung to expand, preventing respiratory exchange in that area

atresia: termination or absence of a normal anatomic passageway

autism: psychiatric disorder characterised by a lack of interest in reality, especially in relating to others

azotaemia: excess nitrogenous waste products, such as urea, in the blood

bulimia: multiple episodes of compulsive overeating followed by forced emesis; also called the binge-purge cycle

cancer: multiple and varying alterations in cell function resulting from overproduction of immature and non-functional cells or tissue enlargement for no physiological reason

cardiac output: amount of blood ejected by the heart in one minute

cephalocaudal: head-to-toe direction

chemotherapy: medical treatment with highly toxic doses of medications aimed at interfering with the mitotic division of cancerous cells

chordae tendineae: thin, fibrous bands that attach the leaflets of the tricuspid and mitral valves of the heart to the papillary muscles in the ventricles

chorea: purposeless, rapid, involuntary movements seen as a consequence of rheumatic fever and lasting for months

colic: daily period of crying for 3 hours or more during which the infant is virtually inconsolable; occurs in 10% to 20% of infants

debridement: removal of eschar (dead skin) to allow granulation

dehydration: deficiency in body fluid from decreased intake, output greater than intake, or loss of fluids by vomiting, diarrhoea or diaphoresis

development: acquisition of skills and abilities occurring throughout life

developmental assessment: measurement of physical (motor), cognitive, psychosocial and psychosexual parameters compared to norms for one's chronologic age

diaphoresis: excessive sweating

diffusion: passage of molecules from an area of higher concentration to an area of lower concentration

ductus arteriosus: foetal cardiac structure that connects the pulmonary artery to the aorta, allowing blood to bypass the foetal lungs; when this structure remains patent after birth, it creates an abnormal heart condition known as patent ductus arteriosus

ductus venosus: foetal structure that carries oxygenated blood from the umbilical vein to the inferior vena cava, bypassing the liver

echolalia: verbal pattern of one who repeats whatever is said

electrocardiography: graphic representation of the heart's electrical activity

enuresis: involuntary urination after the age at which control should have been attained

ependymoma: ventricular tumour that results in a non-communicating hydrocephalus; usually benign, but pressure can damage vital organs

epiglottis: a flap-like structure that overhangs the entrance to the trachea

553

erythropoiesis: red blood cell formation

ethnicity: subjective beliefs in common customs, descent, languages and characteristics

Every Child Matters: governmental policy to ensure children and young people meet five outcomes crucial to their well-being and development

faltering growth: failure of an infant to maintain weight, and sometimes length, above the 5th percentile on age- and gender-appropriate growth charts. Previously referred to as failure to thrive

family: structure or relationship of individuals to one another to provide financial and emotional support and for social functioning

family-centred care: incorporating parental and family input and involvement in a child's care

fine motor skills: skills requiring the use of small muscles (primarily those in the hand), such as using the hands and fingers to grasp or manipulate an object

fontanelle: space covered by membranous tissue at the juncture of cranial sutures

foramen ovale: septal opening between the atria of the foetal heart

glioma: slow-growing tumour that's usually inoperable because of its location in the brain stem

glomerular filtration: process of filtering blood as it flows through the kidneys

gross motor skills: skills requiring the use of large muscle groups, such as head control, sitting, standing and walking

growth: increase in size, such as in height or weight

head circumference: measurement of the largest diameter of the head; taken by placing a measuring tape around the head at the level of the frontal bone of the forehead to the occipital prominence at the back of the head

haemarthrosis: bleeding into a joint

haematuria: blood in the urine

human leukocyte antigen: genetically transferred antigenic marker on the cell surface of all nucleated cells that allows the body to recognise self and non-self

hypertrophy: increase in the size of a body organ or structure, sometimes because of an increase in cell size

hypoxia: deficiency of oxygen to the tissue

immunotherapy: using specially treated white blood cell immunopotentiators to replace immunocompetent lymphoid tissue, such as bone marrow and thymus

incubation period: time between the reception of an antigen and initiation of clinical symptoms

infant mortality: number of infant deaths during the first year of life per 1,000 live births in any given year

infratentorial: below the plate that's under the cerebellum

interstitial compartments: spaces between tissues

intravascular compartments: spaces within blood vessels

left-to-right shunt: pressure from the left side of the heart pushing blood through a septal defect to the right side, thereby increasing blood flow to the lungs

medulloblastoma: highly malignant, fast-growing tumour in the cerebellum

metastasise: growing and spreading of malignant cells from the primary site to other tissues

morbidity: number of people in a population who are faced with a specific health problem at a particular point in time

mortality: number of deaths from a specific cause in a given year

national service framework for children, young people and maternity services: framework and standards for a range of multi-professional services mainly in the NHS

nephron: functional unit of the kidney responsible for the formation of urine

neurogenic bladder: dribbling of urine from the lack of spontaneous bladder emptying

nystagmus: involuntary, rapid, jerky movement of the eye

object permanence: awareness that objects exist while not in view

opisthotonos: spasmodic body posturing in which the back arches and the head and heels bend back

oligohydramnios: abnormally decreased amount of amniotic fluid in utero

oliguria: decreased urine formation manifested by low urine output

peer: individual who's the same as another in age, class or rank

polycythaemia: overproduction of red blood cells, resulting in increased blood viscosity and haematocrit

poverty: lack of money or resources necessary for survival

priapism: painful, prolonged and abnormal erection of the penis, usually unrelated to sexual desire

pruritus: itching

puberty: physical changes resulting in reproductive maturity

rumination: voluntary regurgitation and re-swallowing

scoliosis: lateral curvature of the spine

separation anxiety: manifested by crying and withdrawal; occurs when an infant or child recognises that their attachment figure isn't present

sinoatrial node: pacemaker of the heart; located within the right atrial wall near the opening of the superior vena cava

status asthmaticus: acute asthma exacerbation in which there's unrelenting, severe respiratory distress and bronchospasm

steatorrhoea: more than normal amounts of fat in the faeces resulting in foamy, light-coloured, bulky, foul-smelling, greasy stools

strabismus: condition in which the eyes are misaligned when fixating on the same object, from a muscle imbalance

stroke volume: amount of blood ejected by the heart with each heartbeat (or contraction)

subluxation: partial dislocation of any joint

sudden infant death syndrome: sudden death of a previously healthy infant in which a post-mortem examination fails to confirm the cause of death

supratentorial: within the cerebrum and above the tentorial plate

surfactant: phospholipid that lines the alveoli, preventing them from collapsing during exhalation

talipes: clubfoot; inability of the foot or ankle to attain correct alignment from twisting in any of multiple directions

toxoid: toxin that's rendered non-toxic

tracheostomy: surgically created opening in the anterior neck leading directly to the trachea; this opening is cannulated with a tracheostomy tube to serve as an airway

transitional object: object or comfort measure that represents parental security

umbilical arteries: two of the three blood vessels in the umbilical cord that carry deoxygenated blood from the foetus to the placenta; the other blood vessel is the umbilical vein

umbilical vein: one of the three blood vessels in the umbilical cord that carries oxygenated blood from the placenta to the foetus; the other two blood vessels are the umbilical arteries

veins: small, thin-walled blood vessels that carry deoxygenated blood from the capillaries to the heart

Selected references

Al-Gamal, E., and Long, T. Anticipatory grieving among parents living with a child with cancer. *Journal of Advanced Nursing* 66(9): 1980–1990, 2010.

Bowlby J. *Child Care and the Growth of Love*. Harmondsworth: Penguin, 1953.

Callery, P. Paying to participate: financial, social and personal costs to parents of involvement in their child's care in hospital. *Journal of Advanced Nursing* 25: 746–752, 1997.

Callery, P., and Smith L. A study of the role negotiation between nurses and parents of hospitalised children. *Journal of Advanced Nursing* 16: 772–781, 1991.

Chamley, C.A., Carson, P., Randall, D., and Sandwell, W.M. *Developmental Anatomy and Physiology of Children A Practical Approach*. Edinburgh: Elsevier, 2005.

Coles, I. Prevention of physical child abuse: concept, evidence and practice. *Community Practitioner* 81(6): 18–22, 2008.

Corlett, J., and Twycross, A. Negotiation of parental roles within family-centred care: a review of the research. *Journal of Clinical Nursing* 15: 1308–1316, 2006.

Darbyshire, P. *Living with a Sick Child in Hospital: The Experiences of Parents and Children*. London: Chapman & Hall, 1994.

Department of Health. *The National Service Framework for Children*. London: HMSO, 2004.

Fearnley R. Death of a parent and the children's experience: don't ignore the elephant in the room. *Journal of Inter-professional Care* 24(4): 450–459, 2010.

Foster, M., Whitehead, L., and Maybee, P. Parents' and health professionals' perceptions of family centred care for children in hospital, in developed and developing countries: a review of the literature. *International Journal of Nursing Studies* 47(9): 1184–1193, 2010.

Franck, L.S., and Callery, P. Re-thinking family-centred care across the continuum of children's healthcare. *Child: Care, Health and Development* 30(3): 265–277, 2004.

Gimbler-Berglund, I., Ljusegren, G., and Enskar, K. Factors influencing pain management in children. *Paediatric Nursing* 20(10): 21–24, 2008.

Glasper, A., Aylott, M., and Battrick, C., eds. *Developing Practical Skills for Nursing Children and Young People*. London: Hodder Arnold, 2010.

Jakubik, L.D., Cockerham, J., Altmann, A.R., and Grossman, M.B. The ABCs of pediatric laboratory interpretation: understanding the CBC with differential and LFTs. *Pediatric Nursing* 29(2): 97–103, 2003.

Livesley, J. Telling tales: a qualitative exploration of how children's nurses interpret work with unaccompanied hospitalised children. *Journal of Clinical Nursing* 12(5): 43–50, 2005.

MacKean, G.L., Thurston, W.E., and Scott C.M. Bridging the divide between families and health professionals' perspectives on family centred care. *Health Expectations* 8: 74–85, 2005.

Manworran, R.C.B. It's time to relieve children's pain. *Journal for Specialists in Pediatric Nursing* 12(3): 196–198, 2007.

Neill, S., and Knowles, H. *The Biology of Child Health*. Basingstoke: Palgrave, 2004.

Ranmal, R., Prictor, M., and Scott, J.T. Interventions for improving communication with children and adolescents about their cancer. *Cochrane Database of Systematic Reviews* Oct 8(4): CD002969, 2008.

Robertson, J. *Young Children in Hospital*, 2nd ed. London: Tavistock Publications, 1970.

Robertson, J. *Separation and the Very Young*. London: Free Association Books, 1989.

Royal College of Nursing. *The Recognition and Assessment of Acute Pain in Children: Update of Full Guideline*. London: RCN Institute, 2009.

Sheridan, M.D. *From Birth to Five Years*. Oxford: Routledge, 2007.

Shields, L., Pratt, J., Davis, L., and Hunter, L. Family-centred care for children in hospital. *Cochrane Database of Systematic Reviews* 1, Art no.: CD004811.DOI:10. 1002/14651858. CD004811.pub2, 2008.

Smith, L. and Coleman, V. *Child and Family-Centred Healthcare: Concept, Theory and Practice*. Basingstoke: Palgrave, 2010.

Unsworth, V., Franck,L., and Choonara, I. Parental assessment and management of children's postoperative pain: a randomised clinical trial. *Journal of Child Health Care* 11(3): 86–194, 2007.

Web resources

Action for Sick Children:
www.actionforsickchildren.org/

Allergy Academy:
www.allergyacademy.org

Alateen:
www.al-anonuk.org.uk/alateen

Association of British Paediatric Nurses:
www.abpn.org.uk/default.aspx

Association of Chief Children's Nurses:
www.accnuk.org/

Association for Spina Bifida and
Hydrocephalus:
www.asbah.org/

Asthma UK:
www.asthma.org.uk

Barnardo's:
www.barnardos.org.uk

Beat Eating Disorders:
www.b-eat.co.uk/Home

Baby Life Infant Support Systems:
www.bliss.org.uk

Brittle Bone Society:
www.brittlebone.org

Cardiac Risk in the Young:
www.c-r-y.org.uk/index.htm

Child and Adolescent Mental Health:
www.camh.org.uk/

Children's Cancer and Leukaemia Group:
www.cclg.org.uk

Child Health:
www.childhealth.co.uk

Children's Heart Federation:
www.childrens-heart-fed.org.uk/

Children's HIV Association:
www.chiva.org.uk

Children Living with Inherited Metabolic
Disease:
www.climb.org.uk

Contact a Family:
www.cafamily.org.uk

Cystic Fibrosis Trust:
www.cftrust.org.uk

Department of Health:
www.dh.gov.uk

Diabetes UK:
www.diabetes.org.uk/Guide-to-diabetes/
My-life/

Down's Syndrome Association:
www.downs-syndrome.org.uk/

Epilepsy Action:
www.epilepsy.org.uk/

European Academy of Allergy and
Clinical Immunology:
www.eaaci.net/index.php

Genetic Alliance UK:
www.geneticalliance.org.uk/index.html

GP Notebook:
www.gpnotebook.co.uk/homepage.cfm

Great Ormond Street Hospital for Children:
www.gosh.nhs.uk/

Healthtalkonline:
www.healthtalkonline.org

Hidden Hurt – Domestic Abuse Information
and Support:
www.hiddenhurt.co.uk/

Journal of Child Health Care:
http://chc.sagepub.com

Medical Conditions at School:
www.medicalconditionsatschool.org.uk

Muscular Dystrophy Campaign:
www.muscular-dystrophy.org/

National Children's Bureau:
www.ncb.org.uk

National Association for Children of
Alcoholics:
www.nacoa.org.uk

National Autistic Society:
www.autism.org.uk

National Society for Phenylketonuria:
www.nspku.org/

National Society for the Prevention of Cruelty
to Children:
www.nspcc.org.uk

NHS Evidence:
www.evidence.nhs.uk/default.aspx

Nursing and Midwifery Council:
www.nmc-uk.org

Paediatric Nursing Journal:
http://nursingchildrenandyoungpeople.
rcnpublishing.co.uk/

Patient UK:
www.patient.co.uk

Royal College of Midwives:
www.rcm.org.uk

Royal College of Nursing:
www.rcn.org.uk

Royal College of Paediatrics and Child health:
www.rcpch.ac.uk

Royal College of Psychiatrists:
www.rcpsych.ac.uk/
mentalhealthinfoforall/youngpeople.aspx

Self Help UK:
www.self-help.org.uk

Sickle Cell Society:
www.sicklecellsociety.org/

Scottish Intercollegiate Guidelines Network:
www.sign.ac.uk

The Anaphylaxis Campaign:
www.anaphylaxis.org.uk

Young Minds:
www.youngminds.org.uk/

Index

Note: Page numbers followed by c, i and t indicates chart, illustrations and table respectively.